"A broad and deep consensus exists, ever
ria, that alternative paradigms for diagnc
disorders must be developed if the field is to advance. But just w...... .,,
will be best? In this forward-looking volume, Hayes and Hofmann assemble the most sophisticated treatment models—all of which emphasize process, dimensionality, a functional analysis of behavior, and the ability to individualize and personalize diagnosis. Every mental health professional will benefit from these developments."

—**David H. Barlow, PhD, ABPP**, professor of psychology and psychiatry emeritus, and founder of the Center for Anxiety and Related Disorders (CARD) at Boston University

"Syndromal diagnosis provides a starting point for the classification of mental health disorders, but one that is inherently limited in terms of tracking underlying etiological pathways and principles of change. This volume describes a process-based approach that provides a far more compelling basis for organizing the causal processes underlying the etiology of mental health problems, be they diseases or disorders or the adaptations themselves that evolved to enhance reproductive fitness."

—**Steven D. Hollon, PhD**, Gertrude Conaway Vanderbilt professor of psychology at Vanderbilt University with a long-standing interest in the treatment and prevention of depression

"I LOVE this book. A surefire way to get a headache is to try to provide evidence-based care using empirically supported treatments for DSM syndromes while also attending to the evidence-based processes described in the basic science literature that appear to account for the struggles of the individual I'm caring for right now. This book addresses that dilemma, offering creative ideas for a unified science of psychopathology, its classification, and its treatment."

—**Jacqueline B. Persons, PhD**, director of the Oakland Cognitive Behavior Therapy Center; clinical professor in the department of psychology at the University of California, Berkeley; and author of *The Case Formulation Approach to Cognitive-Behavior Therapy*

"The DSM-based approach is unlikely to create a better understanding of, or more effective treatments for, mental health problems. Hayes and Hofmann offer a path forward. Open to various therapeutic traditions, based in science, and sensitive to client individuality, this book lays out multiple exemplars of understanding and treating mental health concerns based on the processes that create and maintain the problems—rather than the categories that describe them. This is a thought-provoking book that should be on the shelves of all clinicians and clinical researchers."

—**Douglas W. Woods, PhD**, dean of the Graduate School, and professor of psychology at Marquette University

"This impressive volume is a genuine advance in our efforts to understand psychological dysfunction. Hayes, Hofmann, and their contributing authors present exciting alternatives to traditional categorical diagnosis à la DSM and ICD—drawing from research that spans neuroscience, learning, coping, and culture. These new ideas can enrich the search for mechanisms that underlie psychopathology, guiding identification of treatment targets and the construction of principle-guided, individually tailored interventions."

—**John R. Weisz, PhD, ABPP**, is professor of psychology at Harvard University, and director of the Harvard Lab for Youth Mental Health, specializing in developing and testing transdiagnostic interventions for young people

"One would certainly expect Hayes and Hofmann to provide a thoughtful and integrative compendium on process-based approaches to assessing, diagnosing, and treating psychological problems. In this edited volume, they assemble cutting-edge thought leaders to effectively deliver on this expectation. Chapters provide a depth and breadth of focus that is detailed yet easy to consume, laying a solid foundation from which researchers and practitioners of various theoretical orientations can better understand and help shape a process-based future for psychotherapy."

—**Gordon J. G. Asmundson, PhD**, professor of psychology at the University of Regina, development editor for *Clinical Psychology Review*, and editor in chief of *Journal of Anxiety Disorders*

Beyond the DSM

Toward a Process-Based Alternative for Diagnosis *and* Mental Health Treatment

Edited by
STEVEN C. HAYES, PhD
STEFAN G. HOFMANN, PhD

CONTEXT PRESS
An Imprint of New Harbinger Publications, Inc.

Publisher's Note

This publication is designed to provide accurate and authoritative information in regard to the subject matter covered. It is sold with the understanding that the publisher is not engaged in rendering psychological, financial, legal, or other professional services. If expert assistance or counseling is needed, the services of a competent professional should be sought.

Distributed in Canada by Raincoast Books

Copyright © 2020 by Steven C. Hayes and Stefan G. Hofmann
                Context Press
                An imprint of New Harbinger Publications, Inc.
                5674 Shattuck Avenue
                Oakland, CA 94609
                www.newharbinger.com

The contributions to *Beyond the DSM* by authors who are employees of the National Institutes of Health (NIH), a part of the U.S. Department of Health and Human Services, were prepared as part of their official duties as employees of NIH and are works of the United States Government. The copyright status of these contributions is governed by 17 USC Section 105.

Cover design by Sara Christian; Acquired by Catharine Meyers;
Edited by Jenessa Jackson; Indexed by James Minkin

All Rights Reserved

Library of Congress Cataloging-in-Publication Data on file

Names: Hayes, Steven C, editor. | Hofmann, Stefan G, editor.
Title: Beyond the DSM : toward a process-based alternative for diagnosis and mental health treatment / [edited by] Steven C. Hayes, Stefan G. Hofmann.
Identifiers: LCCN 2020008075 (print) | LCCN 2020008076 (ebook) | ISBN 9781684036615 (trade paperback) | ISBN 9781684036622 (pdf) | ISBN 9781684036639 (epub)
Subjects: LCSH: Diagnostic and statistical manual of mental disorders. | Mental illness--Classification. | Mental illness--Diagnosis. | Mental illness--Treatment.
Classification: LCC RC455.2.C4 B494 2020 (print) | LCC RC455.2.C4 (ebook) | DDC 616.89/075--dc23
LC record available at https://lccn.loc.gov/2020008075
LC ebook record available at https://lccn.loc.gov/2020008076

Printed in the United States of America

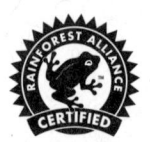

22   21   20

10   9   8   7   6   5   4   3   2   1   First Printing

Contents

1. Creating an Alternative to Syndromal Diagnosis: Needed Features of Processes of Change and the Models that Organize Them — 1
   Steven C. Hayes, PhD, *University of Nevada, Reno*;
   Stefan G. Hofmann, PhD, *Boston University*;
   Joseph Ciarrochi, PhD, *Australian Catholic University*

2. The NIMH Research Domain Criteria Project: A Decade of Behavior and Brain Integration for Translational Research — 23
   Uma Vaidyanathan, PhD; Sarah Morris, PhD;
   Ann Wagner, PhD; Joel Sherrill, PhD; David Sommers, PhD;
   Marjorie Garvey, MB BCh; Eric Murphy, PhD; Bruce Cuthbert, PhD, *National Institute of Mental Health*

3. Shifting Paradigms: From the DSM to the Process of Change — 47
   J. Scott Fraser, PhD, *Wright State University*

4. Psychological Vulnerabilities and Coping Responses: An Innovative Approach to Transdiagnostic Assessment and Treatment Planning in the Age Beyond DSM-5 — 73
   Rochelle I. Frank, PhD, *University of California, Berkeley & The Wright Institute*; Matthew McKay, PhD, *The Wright Institute*

5. Expectations and Related Cognitive Domains: Implications for Classification and Therapy — 97
   Winfried Rief, PhD, *The Philipps University of Marburg*

6. Learning, Language, and Derived Behaviors: Some Implications for a Process-Based Approach to Psychological Suffering — 115
   Dermot Barnes-Holmes, PhD; Yvonne Barnes-Holmes, PhD;
   Ciara McEnteggart, PhD, *Ghent University*

7   Cultural and Social Influences on Individual Variation in
    Emotion Processes   137
    Shruthi M. Venkatesh; Stacey N. Doan, PhD,
    Claremont McKenna College, Abigail L. Barthel;
    Stefan G. Hofmann, PhD, *Boston University*

8   What a Complex Systems Perspective Can Contribute to
    Process-Based Assessment and Psychotherapy   165
    Adele M. Hayes, PhD; Leigh A. Andrews, *University of Delaware*

9   Psychological Flexibility in Chronic Pain: Exploring the
    Relevance of a Process-Based Model for Treatment
    Development   199
    Lance M. McCracken, PhD, *Uppsala University*

10 A Multilevel, Multimethod Approach to Testing and
    Refining Intervention Targets   225
    Andrew T. Gloster, PhD, *University of Basel*;
    Maria Karekla, PhD, University of Cyprus

11 Building a Process-Based Diagnostic System:
    An Extended Evolutionary Approach   251
    Steven C. Hayes, PhD, *University of Nevada, Reno*;
    Stefan G. Hofmann, PhD, *Boston University*;
    Joseph Ciarrochi, PhD, *Australian Catholic University*

Index   281

CHAPTER 1

Creating an Alternative to Syndromal Diagnosis
Needed Features of Processes of Change and the Models that Organize Them

Steven C. Hayes, PhD
University of Nevada, Reno

Stefan G. Hofmann, PhD
Boston University

Joseph Ciarrochi, PhD
Australian Catholic University

For decades, intervention science has followed a primary analytic strategy—that of syndromal diagnosis—which has created a robust and progressive field but has now reached a dead end. Few now believe that an adequate field of evidence-based therapy will emerge from researchers continuing to evaluate psychosocial protocols and lists of approved medications focused on psychiatric syndromes. We must find a new strategy and way forward. The only question remaining is: "What will that strategy be?"

The *Diagnostic and Statistical Manual of Mental Disorders* (DSM; American Psychiatric Association, 2013) and the *International Classification of Diseases and Related Health Problems* (ICD; World Health Organization,

2018) have dominated the field for decades and left it with an intellectual hangover as it considers its future. Our discussion here will primarily focus on the DSM, but the same controversies also apply to the ICD.

Clinical programs have trained generations of students to take a topographical approach to human suffering based on the biomedical conviction that syndromes—collections of signs (things you see) and symptoms (things people complain of)—will lead to a deep, functional understanding of psychopathology. Students are trained to remember criteria, such as "five out of nine" or "four out of seven" signs and symptoms, and then pick the right set of organized techniques from approved lists of treatment protocols, all vetted by clinical randomized controlled trials (RCTs). In the minds of many, clinical skills mean the adherent delivery of techniques inside evidence-based protocols. Evidence-based therapy is synonymous with this "protocols-for-syndromes" strategy.

All of that is now changing—rapidly. After reviewing 30 years of effort on syndromal classification, the planning committee for the fifth version of the DSM (American Psychiatric Association, 2013) reached the conclusion that the entire enterprise is unlikely to ever lead researchers to the identification of functional entities: "All these limitations in the current diagnostic paradigm suggest that research exclusively focused on refining the DSM-defined syndromes may never succeed in uncovering their underlying etiologies. For that to happen, an as-yet unknown paradigm shift may need to occur" (Kupfer, First, & Regier, 2002, p. xix).

The Research Domain Criteria (RDoC) approach of the National Institute of Mental Health (NIMH) broke away from the hegemony of syndromal classification (Insel et al., 2010), perhaps in an attempt to create that "as yet unknown paradigm shift." We will review the history and current status of RDoC here. Whatever else eventually flows from RDoC, even a casual observer can see that the same agency that once lifted up the "protocols-for-syndromes" strategy has now turned away from it and toward a process-based direction. That opens the door to a new process-based look at evidence-based therapy and the diagnostic systems on which it stands. That is precisely the theme of the present volume.

In some ways, the current changes look like a return to the original agenda of behavior therapy (Davison, 2019). Evidence-based therapy was based on the extension of principles into ideographically useful functional analyses. These principles were high in precision (e.g., the definition of a "reinforcer" constrained when you could and could not use that term) and high in scope (e.g., a small number of principles were meant to be combined to explain a larger number of phenomena) and led to the generation of many applied methods.

However, this historical similarity is somewhat misleading because behavior therapy contained little guidance about how to develop *new* knowledge about processes of change. The greater emphasis was on applying principles already identified in the animal laboratory. Said another way, the steps needed to develop a more adequate set of processes of change were not originally a central concern to the field because, at first, the science of principles of psychological change appeared so advanced relative to the infant status of intervention science itself.

Instead, early behavior therapists put much of their attention on how to create replicable evidence-based methods of change that they could fit to the individual. You can see this clearly in the agenda laid out for evidence-based therapy by the late Gordon Paul: "What treatment, by whom, is most effective for this individual with that specific problem, under which set of circumstances, and how does it come about?" (Paul, 1969, p. 44). This "what" question was clearly meant technologically (what treatment), while the main focus was on how to deliver and fit that technology to the person (by whom, for what specific problem, and under which set of circumstances). The last six words about processes of change ("…and how does it come about") were almost an afterthought and were left out when this charge was first stated two years earlier (Paul, 1967). Paul did not mean "What new theory is needed to account for these effects?" He meant "How can we explain these results based on known principles?"

Indeed, behavior therapy was *defined* at the same time as experientially tested intervention methods, which were linked to and explained by "operationally defined learning theory" (Franks & Wilson, 1974, p. 7). Similarly, it was said that the defining feature of applied behavior analysis was its clarity of technique linked to the important social needs of people (Baer, Wolf, & Risley, 1968), while the only theory required was adherence to "behavioral principles."

The "protocols-for-syndromes" era of federal funding that soon followed fit comfortably into this technique-focused world of evidence-based psychosocial care. Cognitive behavioral therapy (CBT) researchers were particularly successful in establishing evidence-based therapy by testing protocols for syndromes in controlled, time-series designs and especially in RCTs

(Thompson-Hollands, Sauer-Zavala, & Barlow, 2014). These methods emerged as the dominant form of evidence-based psychosocial care (Hofmann, Asnaani, Vonk, Sawyer, & Fang, 2012). Concepts and theory were still important to the description of and rationale for various clinical methods, but they were not central. For example, meditational analyses were rare in CBT until only the last decade.

As this era of "protocol-for-syndromes" wanes, attention has returned to processes of change (Hayes & Hofmann, 2018; Hofmann & Hayes, 2019). Consensus-based processes inside the RDoC initiative and those inside CBT itself (Klepac et al., 2012) both agree that the future of intervention science is process-based. At this moment, we need greater clarity on how to search for processes of change and how to organize them into models and theories.

In this chapter, we will consider what researchers mean by "processes of change" and what properties these processes need to display so they can form the foundation for an alternative to syndromal diagnosis. We will examine what is needed by models or theories of such processes and will propose a way forward under the umbrella of evolutionary science.

Processes of Change

How can we best assemble a workable set of change processes, which are organized into simplified models, that enable the practitioner rapidly to answer this key question: "What core biopsychosocial processes should be targeted with this client given this goal in this situation, and how can they most efficiently and effectively be changed?" (Hofmann & Hayes, 2019, p. 47). We will begin with the key features of processes of change.

What Are Processes of Change?

Processes of therapeutic change are theory-based, dynamic, progressive, contextually bound, modifiable, and multilevel changes or mechanisms that occur in predictable, empirically established sequences oriented toward desirable outcomes (Hofmann & Hayes, 2019, p. 38). They are:

- *theory-based* because they are associated with a clear statement of relations among events and lead to testable predictions and method of influence;

- *dynamic* because processes may involve feedback loops and nonlinear changes;

- *progressive* because they may need to be arranged in an order to reach the treatment goal;

- *contextually bound and modifiable* to focus on their implications for practical changes and intervention kernels within reach of practitioners; and

- *multilevel* because some processes supersede or are nested within others.

There are several key features of importance in this definition, as we shall see. If we are to use processes to go beyond the DSM, they need to have particular characteristics.

High Precision, Scope, and Depth

A change process needs to have precision and scope, just as we discussed earlier regarding behavioral principles. It needs to be clear when a particular change process applies (*precision*), and the process needs to apply to a range of phenomena (*scope*). The requirement for precision eliminates general heuristics and loose metaphors as processes of change. The requirement for scope eliminates change processes that are merely restated versions of techniques and encourages processes of change that broadly apply. It would be neither scientifically nor practically useful to generate a myriad of change processes that apply only to narrow areas.

There is also a third requirement of adequate change processes: They must have *depth*. In a unified fabric of science, concepts at one level of analysis must not contradict well-established findings at other levels of analysis. Coherence across levels of analysis is an especially important criterion for a multidisciplinary area such as mental and behavioral health. Psychology is embedded in other levels of analysis, such as physiology, genetics, social process, and culture—to name only a few—and its concepts need to play well across that wide range of levels. For example, data from the neurobiology of emotion must not contradict an emotional change process that appears to be successful at the psychological level. If there is contradiction, then the scientific description of the change process is not adequate. We are not speaking of reductionism, as each level of analysis has its own work to do. Rather, the goal of a unified fabric of science needs to be ever in mind.

One implication of this perspective is that concepts in clinical science should link to viable basic science programs, since that is where the preparations exist that are needed to test concepts that have high levels of precision, scope, and depth. In that same vein, it is important not to stay entirely at the clinical level when researching change processes. We can find central change processes reflected in developmental studies, naturalistic longitudinal studies, experimental studies, and so on, and any process of change that we have not broadly vetted that way is likely not ready to be a cornerstone of process-based diagnostic systems.

Idiographic Processes

It is important to develop nomothetic knowledge about processes of change. There is no interest in the applied field in the "psychology of the one" because knowledge that does not apply to many people is not knowledge practitioners can afford to take the time to learn and use. That is part of what "scope" means. Processes of change need to apply across a reasonable range of people, problem areas, settings, and delivery methods for that knowledge to be useful. But there is a big difference between knowledge that can apply more generally and knowledge that is based on a collective level of analysis to begin with.

The behavioral and cognitive tradition has long dealt with arguments that cross-sectional group averages and longitudinal examinations of individuals are fundamentally different levels of analysis (e.g., Barlow, Hayes, & Nelson, 1984; Sidman, 1960; von Eye & Bergman, 2003), but the field in general has failed to appreciate how profoundly true that is. Western culture has embraced the empirically false idea of the "average person" for nearly 100 years (Rose, 2017), and Western science has followed suit. If all that matters is a single outcome, then it makes some sense. Yes, the pathways to get there might matter, but if 4 out of 10 people are no longer, say, avoiding work after this particular intervention (compared to 7 out of 10 in this other condition), then focusing on the collective may not create much harm.

At the level of processes of change, however, the picture is far less rosy. As we consider multiple variables, and their trajectories and interrelationships across time, our analysis at the level of the collective stops yielding information of known applicability to the individual. We might identify processes of change at the group level that not a single individual displays. It is also possible for these two levels of analysis to give different answers to the same question.

Consider the relationship between the speed of typing and the number of errors made while typing. If you gather virtually any large group of people, you will find that experts type faster (and with fewer errors) than hunt-and-peck typists. At the level of the collective, typing speed will be negatively related with errors. However, for every single individual, beginner and expert alike, trying to type faster will produce more errors. Therefore, typing speed and typing errors are negatively correlated in a group of people but positively correlated for every individual of the same group.

That is a commonsense example, so one could suppose that all you would need to do is add typing expertise as a covariate to clean up this mess. The problem is that in novel areas, you cannot say beforehand how to catch such errors and what covariates to add. Normally, when analyses at the level of the collective and at the level of the individual differ (e.g., Fisher, Medaglia, & Jeronimus, 2018; Turner & Hayes, 1996), we don't really know why, but we do know as a mathematical certainty that when we apply results from the analysis of change processes at the level of the group to a particular person, then we cannot assume the change process will benefit the individual (Fisher, 2015).

Why can we say that with mathematical certainty? Because that application of knowledge violates an accepted mathematical proof that has been established in the physical sciences for nearly 90 years: the ergodic theorem. In the early part of the last century, physicists wanted to know how individual gas molecules behaved, but they could only measure volumes of gas, not individual molecules. A mathematician worked out that the behavior of the two could be the same but only under rare and highly specific circumstances (Birkhoff, 1931). The resulting proof is called the ergodic theorem, and it has been considered settled in the physical sciences ever since, but it is little known in the behavioral sciences. The theorem did identify circumstances in which the collective reflects the subunits: When molecules are identical and do not change over time. A few ideal gases are actually like that (Volkovysskii & Sinai, 1971), but since psychologists and other behavioral health specialists do not treat frozen clones, these circumstances never apply in behavioral science.

The implications are stark. Statistical methods based on interindividual variation, such as the cross-product of the coefficients methods of classical meditational analysis (Preacher & Hayes, 2008), cannot properly model processes of change (Molenaar, 2008a, 2008b). Another way forward is needed.

This is a serious methodological and statistical issue that we can only fully solve over time, but taking the time to work on complex networks and dynamical systems opens the field up to a more progressive path forward (see chapter 8). We need to identify processes of change repeatedly at the level of the individual across time. We can then try to gather these patterns into nomothetic generalizations (either in the form of sub-populations or overall population parameters), provided that nomothetic statements do not distort what is found at the idiographic level. Processes of change identified or tested in time-series designs (Hayes, Barlow, & Nelson-Gray, 1999) are especially important examples for present purposes due to the breadth and depth of that research tradition in applied psychology. There is a lot we already know. In network analysis, there are also already available analytic tools that can make population estimates without ever treating idiographic data as "error," such as the Group Iterative Multiple Model Estimation method (GIMME; Gates & Molenaar, 2012).

Immediately and Repeatedly Measurable

The previous section helps explain why we need to assess processes of change using measurement methods capable of repeated longitudinal assessment, ideally at relatively high frequencies. For practical purposes, it is critical that these measurement methods are available at low cost and that they provide rapid feedback to the practitioner. In-session behavioral observations are a classic example of measures that can have those properties. There are good examples of transcript analysis and other in-session measures yielding evidence of functionally important processes of change (Hesser, Westin, Hayes, & Andersson, 2009). As natural language analysis software improves, practitioners' ability to receive feedback only minutes later regarding clients' in-session verbal patterns is on the close horizon. The growing base of smartphone-based ecological momentary assessment measures and automated assessment measures are another example. Measures that assess processes of change in this manner are preferable, in part because they can then provide immediate feedback to practitioners.

More troublesome is the state of evidence with self-report measures. Even well-known self-report measures have generally not been tested for high-frequency repeated use, and just a small collection of such measures would soon exhaust a client in any case. Certain solutions, such as taking the item with the highest loading and using it frequently, are mere rules of thumb and are not themselves based on well-established measurement logic. Part of the problem is that psychometrics and classical test theory also violate the ergodic theorem (Molenaar, 2008a), but a full solution to that problem has not yet been developed.

We should not view a self-report device as a successful measure of processes of change until we show it applies in high-density longitudinal analyses focused on the individual. Processes that we can measure in multiple modes—for example, via self-report and behavioral observation—are also much more likely to be robust and thus worthy of attention in building alternatives to the DSM.

Changeable and Contextual

Intervention science is a form of applied science—and, thus, processes of change (which are changeable and linked to contextual features that we can modify) are preferred over processes that are dependent variables alone without clear and known linkage to manipulable events. Using information about processes of change requires focusing on the interface between action and its changeable context: historical, situational, and internal.

Processes of change are functional sequences, not mere snapshots. Identifying correlates of outcome change is a fine first step, but it is far from adequate as a method of identifying change processes. If change processes are to serve as part of an alternative to the DSM, then these processes must directly and successfully lead to the selection and implementation of treatment kernels. For that reason, we should give preference to processes that are understood contextually and historically.

Functional Pathways of Change

A functionally important pathway of change is not a "cause" in any simple mechanistic sense because third variables are always possible, and change is not likely linear, unidirectional, or univariate. It is important, for example, to distinguish mere markers of treatment from mechanisms of treatment. Clients often learn to "talk the talk" of a given form of psychotherapy, and if the intervention is powerful, then any measure of that kind will yield analytic "vaporware" suggestive of processes of change. Researchers need to be cautious in such situations. If the process can be regularly detected in actual behavioral "walk-the-walk" measures, even without intervention, then it is more likely to be important. This is done in traditional meditational analysis by controlling for treatment in the "b path" (the mediator to the outcome path), which practically speaking means that the mediator-to-outcome relationship must exist in the control condition as well. In network analyses at an idiographic level, it is done more so by looking for similar patterns in untreated participants (Hayes et al., 2019).

With Coherent Moderators

If there was one finding that was revealed consistently in the syndromal era, it is that common-sense moderators are rarely powerful. For example, demographic factors, such as age, religion, and so on, generally do not predict replicable differential responses. The science of moderation, like the science of change processes, requires theoretical models that provide coherent leads and that make sense of the results. Processes of change linked to moderators of that kind are preferred.

Summary

A focus on processes of change has a clear chance to bring both researchers and practitioners together across theoretical divides. Many times, there are parallel concepts in different theoretical traditions. While agreement on overall models is often difficult, common interest in processes of change is far more established. If we know the features just described apply to a given process of change, then we are ready to consider the features as a building block in creating an alternative to the current psychiatric nosology.

Models of Change Processes

The list of proposed or identified broadly applicable or "transdiagnostic" change processes is lengthy. In one of the first book-length summaries, Harvey and colleagues (Harvey, Watkins, Mansell, & Shafran, 2004) identified over 100. That list has grown greatly in the last 15 years and appears now to number in the hundreds.

There is no practical way to use hundreds of processes of change to guide assessment and treatment. We must simplify the list by using theory and evidence. We will use the term "model" to describe an integrated set of change processes that are used as a guide to the selection and deployment of interventions.

Clear Philosophical Assumptions

Processes of change have meaning inside a network of concepts, data, and assumptions. Clarity of assumptions is key to preventing confusion with a model. For example, a developmental stage model may include concepts that are based on the idea that psychological events are similar to developing organic systems such as flowers or trees. In that organicist metaphor (Pepper, 1942), apparently disorganized or contradictory events come to be revealed as steps toward the final causes that are ultimately reflected in development. The rebellion of a teenager, for example, can later be understood to reflect healthy differentiation from parents and their behavioral control. Coherence is the implicit truth criterion in such analyses.

The philosophical assumptions that underlie a change process of that kind are quite different from those based on a formistic set of assumptions in which the goal is to characterize the particular event and name the classes of events it reveals. That same teenager might be diagnosed as having conduct disorder based on the type and frequency of their rebellious acts. Simple correspondence is the implicit truth criterion of that kind of nosological endeavor. Still another analyst might view the behavioral pattern contextually and suggest that the teenager deploys it to avoid, say, fear of rejection or failure. Workability is the truth criterion for such claims. Another might view it mechanistically as the result of an abnormal anatomical connectivity between the amygdala and the orbitofrontal cortex (Passamonti et al., 2012). Predictive verification is likely the underlying truth criterion.

If a model incoherently combines these sets of assumptions, then analytic confusion and wasted research energy will result. Concepts are vitalized by their connections to other concepts and by their accomplishment of underlying models of truth. For example, contextual theorists might show that with careful use of reinforcement, stages of development might be reordered, leading them to believe that they have revealed the inadequacy of a stage model or organicist position. That kind of research misses the whole point about normative stages in the vain attempt to turn a coherence model into an unwilling workability model. An acorn is "meant to be" an oak tree if the normal organic process is allowed to occur *and not* if the acorn can end up as part of an autumn stew.

This example points to the futility of turning philosophical differences into empirical battles, but when we mix assumptions incoherently within a single model, useless conflicts occur *within* that research program. That possibility helps explain why consensus processes among intervention science educators have led to calls for routine training in philosophy of science in graduate education (Klepac et al., 2012).

Philosophy of science is little more than owning one's own assumptions. There is a degree of philosophical incommensurability between distinct models, but if we allow the data to be interpreted from different vantage points, then scientific cooperation is still viable across assumptions once people know what they are assuming.

Comprehensive, Coherent, and Functional

Models of change processes need to cover enough key processes over a sufficient range of problems and sub-issues with a client to serve as a reasonable guide to care. The processes identified in the model need to address key dimensions of the human experience, such as motivation to change, sense of self, or affect. Ideally, the process selected will focus not only on ameliorating problems but also on establishing prosperity. The reasons for these statements are pragmatic. If models of change processes are to form the basis of an alternative to the DSM, then they must be simple and few. Scores and scores of models are just as practically problematic as scores and scores of diagnoses, or scores and scores of individual change processes.

The processes of change included in any given model must fit together in a coherent fashion, and there needs to be evidence that the set is complete or at least not clearly limited. The nomothetic knowledge displayed in a model needs to tell researchers and practitioners what is likely going on at the level of the individual. At its highest level, that means models of change processes should lead to new forms of functional analysis that allow practitioners to select treatment elements that produce better outcomes. Research on the impact of suggested components and kernels should itself be extensive and theoretically coherent, and there should be an encouragement to go beyond brand-name techniques in the testing program if these methods fit the underlying model. We must show clear links between the process model and the treatment element choice, and the practitioner should find these links to be useful.

Another way to say this is that the treatment utility of individual functional analysis emerging from the model is the key outcome for models of change processes (Hayes, Jarrett, & Nelson, 1987). However, conceptual utility is also important, such as the ability of the models to account for data in related areas, including the role of the therapeutic relationship, the impact across means of delivery, the role of cultural background, and so on.

Broadly Applicable and Potent

Finally, the model must be applicable and potent across a broad range of clients. The field of intervention science needs the initial 20 percent of process focus to do 80 percent of the work in terms of outcome. The 80 percent of additional process focus, which accounts for the last 20 percent of outcomes, can wait for later.

Summary

Models of change processes that hope to vie for status as alternatives to syndromal diagnosis have a heavy burden to carry. They need to be broadly applicable across clients, reasonably comprehensive as applied to the individual client's issues, and still philosophically and theoretically coherent. Most of all, they need to be potent in leading to individual treatment choices that increase client outcomes.

Creating a Model of Models

In recent writings, we have argued that model developers need a way of organizing their work that avoids local theoretical disputes, empowers effective communication, and leads toward the needed features of proposed change processes and models of those processes (Hayes et al., 2019). Having a common communication system is one benefit of the DSM, and it is worth trying to develop such a system within process-based approaches. Of all the alternatives available, only one overarching approach seems to have the heft and breadth needed to accomplish all those goals. It is our position that we should structure our efforts around the queen of all theories in the life sciences: a multidimensional, multilevel extended evolutionary account (Hayes, Monestès, & Wilson, 2018; Wilson & Hayes, 2018).

There was recently a time when evolution could be straightforwardly defined as a "change in gene frequencies in a species due to selective survival" (Bridgeman, 2003, p. 325), and to this day, the word "evolution" is generally heard to mean "genes." It is an irrelevant echo from the past. Today, the progress of evolutionary science has fundamentally changed that view.

Mapping of the human genome has conclusively shown that genes do not code for specific phenotypic attributes (Jablonka & Lamb, 2014), in psychopathology or anywhere else. As an example, a recent study with genomic mapping of nearly half a million participants examined the 18 most-studied candidate genes for depression and compared them to randomly selected genes (Border et al., 2019). They concluded "no clear evidence was found for any candidate gene polymorphism associations with depression phenotypes or any polymorphism-by-environment moderator effects. As a set, depression candidate genes were no more associated with depression phenotypes than noncandidate genes" (p. 376). Other studies have reached similar conclusions with mental health syndromes (e.g., Cross-Disorder Group of the Psychiatric Genomics Consortium, 2013), putting a dagger through the heart of the behavioral genetics dreams of yesteryear in which it was thought small sets of genes would prove critical in the development of specific forms of psychopathology. That hypothesis has been conclusively disproven.

This does not mean genes do not matter. They do—but as part of entire networks of evolving dimensions, including gene systems, epigenetic regulation of gene systems, neurobiological processes, environment, behavior, learning, symbolic events, culture, the gut biome, and so on (Jablonka & Lamb, 2014). As evolutionary science becomes that broad, we can use a multidimensional, multilevel extended evolutionary account to organize behavioral interventions (Wilson, Hayes, Biglan, & Embry, 2014) and to provide a structure for models of processes of change (Hayes et al., 2019).

Learning to Be VRSCDL: Six Key Concepts from Evolutionary Science

There are six key concepts and four key questions needed in an evolutionary approach. The six concepts can be expressed in the acronym VRSCDL (pronounced as if it is the word "versatile"), which stands for **V**ariation and **R**etention of what is **S**elected in **C**ontext at the right **D**imension and **L**evel (Hayes, Stanton, Sanford, Law, & Ta, in press). In a well-rounded evolutionary account, these concepts are applied to any phenomenon using Niko Tinbergen's (1963) four central questions: function, history, development, and mechanism.

Variation is the seed corn of evolution. Initially, variation is blind, but because variation is so central to the successful development of complex systems, variation itself evolves. For example, when facing stressful environments, various life-forms—ranging from bacteria to mammals—increase mutation rates and decrease DNA repair (Galhardo, Hastings, & Rosenberg, 2007). "The collection of species we have with us today is not only the product of the survival of the fittest, but also that of the survival of the most evolvable" (Wagner & Draghi, 2010, p. 381).

Selection and *retention* are the processes of noting the impact of environment-behavior interactions and keeping variants that have beneficial impact. In natural selection, success is a matter of life and death, and retention occurs through genetic and other forms of heritability being passed on from the living. In behavior, contingencies of reinforcement may help establish habits, and in cognition, coherence and problem solving may lead to schemas and core beliefs.

Variation and selective retention occur within a *context*. It is context that determines selection pressures, but it becomes a focus of conscious attention only when the goal is intentional evolutionary change. For example, some new forms of emotional expression may only take hold if an individual deploys this expression in the context of a loving relationship. Concerns over natural contingencies, cultural fit, social support, and so on are all typical ways that practitioners speak of context in an evolutionary sense.

All species capable of contingency learning can select environments by their behavior ("niche selection"), but many can also create physical and social contexts that alter production and reproduction, what is called "niche construction." Humans are especially adept at niche construction. For example, they may deliberately create the kinds of relationships in which emotional growth is possible. That impact is one reason learning is the ladder of evolution (Bateson, 2013).

Variation, selection, retention, and context apply across different streams of inheritance or *dimensions*: genes, epigenes, and so on. Within the psychological domain, several dimensions can be readily discerned, including affect, cognition, attention, motivation, self, and overt behavior.

Finally, selection operates simultaneously at different *levels* of organization. For instance, the normal human adult is composed of over 37 trillion cells (Bianconi et al., 2013). Millions of them die each second, but overall, they do better as part of an organism than they would on their own. If even one "decides" to just make more of itself, the body will try to detect and kill it; and if the body fails to do so, the person develops cancer. This shows how multilevel selection works. Cooperation at the level of a group can be selected (such as the major evolutionary transition that led to multicell organisms), provided the selfishness of lower levels of organization can be restrained.

We can apply VRSCDL features in a robust evolutionary account to any or all Tinbergen's questions (1963): how the *function* of variants alters adaptation (a topic central to "functional analysis"); how these variants emerge and are retained over time in their evolutionary *history*; how these variants *develop* within the lifetime of the organism; and how specific external and internal *mechanisms* combine to produce particular phenotypes, physical or behavioral.

The Extended Evolutionary Meta-Model

We can now combine these ideas into an extended evolutionary meta-model (Hayes et al., 2019). We are using the phase "meta-model" to refer to the idea that we are proposing a model that can incorporate a number of specific models, that is, a model of models. While not comprehensive, we can classify processes of change in intervention science into six key psychological dimensions (affect, cognition, attention, self, motivation, and overt behavior), nested into two additional levels of selection (sociocultural and physiological). In each of these dimensions and levels, variation, selection, retention, and context are key, or to use terms that are more familiar to practitioners, each of these involve processes and procedures related to change, function, habits or patterns, and fit and support. Finally, these can be adaptive or maladaptive.

Figure 1.1 presents the meta-model. We claim that a process-based model will be relatively adequate to the extent that it has most of these rows and columns specified in their targeted processes of change and intervention kernels or kernel selection criteria. All other things being equal, models that cover more of this matrix will be more useful; those that cover less of it will be less useful.

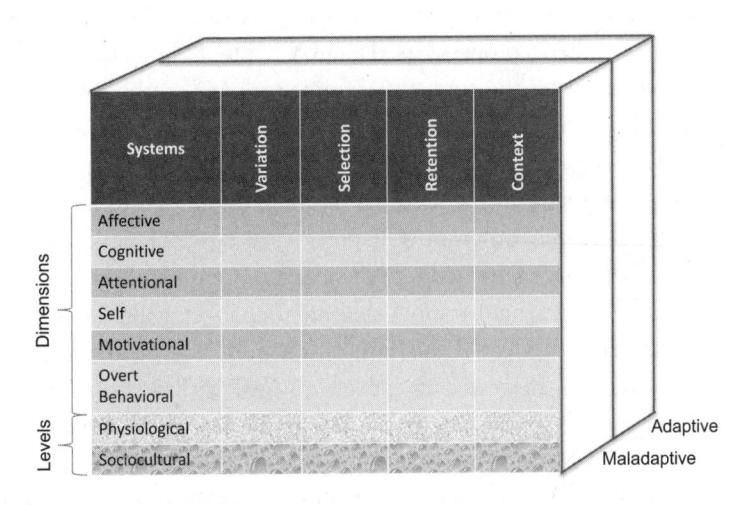

Figure 1.1. The Extended Evolutionary Meta-Model of Processes of Change

We present the criteria and this model as a kind of organizational structure within which to consider the arguments and data presented in this volume.

In the first section of this book, we explore the movement toward process-based models and theories. In particular, chapter 2 discusses the RDoC initiative by NIMH, describes the motivation and approach of RDoC, and provides an update on its current status and future directions. Chapter 3 describes the shifting paradigms from the DSM to processes of change by exploring a social constructionist and systems perspective on a process-based approach. Chapter 4 identifies and discusses various psychological vulnerabilities and coping strategies that can inform a transdiagnostic, process-oriented, and treatment-relevant classification system.

In the second section of the book, we examine domains critical to our understanding of processes of change. One powerful patient variable that influences treatment response to virtually any approach is the role of expectancy, and chapter 5 examines the implications of this patient variable on classification and treatment. Chapter 6 explore some implications of learning, language, and derived symbolic relations for a process-based approach. Chapter 7 discusses the cultural and social influences on individual variation in emotional responses, suggesting that psychopathology is also a sociocultural construct.

In the third and final section of the book, we examine various methodological and level-of-analysis issues, and we explore examples of research programs that have taken a process-based focus. Chapter 8 shows that a complex systems approach offers the conceptual framework and methodological tools to create a process-based system. Chapter 9 discusses the importance of psychological flexibility as a key change process and shows how exploration of psychological flexibility in the area of chronic pain has led to a progressive process-based research program. Chapter 10 discusses how a multilevel, multi-method approach can facilitate the identification of functionally based mechanisms of action that promote treatment change, again using psychological flexibility as a focal point. Finally, chapter 11 evaluates this metamodel and discusses how well it appears to deal with a diverse range of findings and concepts as researchers and practitioners alike begin to take a process-based approach to the elements that need to be considered to create an alternative to the DSM. This final chapter also explores some of the practical issues the field will face and provides a glimpse into a future in which process-based assessment and process-based therapy are the recognized core of evidence-based treatment.

We are at an exciting choice point as a field. The visionary dreams of the founders of evidence-based care are being revisited and viewed now through the decades of effort that led both to successes and dead ends. If the future of evidence-based treatment is process-based, then we need to create an alternative to the DSM. It is time to begin.

References

American Psychiatric Association. (2013). *Diagnostic and statistical manual of mental disorders*. (5th ed). Arlington, VA: Author.

Baer, D. M., Wolf, M. M., & Risley, T. R. (1968). Some current dimensions of applied behavior analysis. *Journal of Applied Behavior Analysis, 1,* 91–97.

Barlow, D. H., Hayes, S. C., & Nelson, R. O. (1984). *The scientist practitioner: Research and accountability in clinical and educational settings.* New York: Pergamon.

Bateson, P. (2013). Evolution, epigenetics and cooperation. *Journal of Biosciences, 38,* 1–10.

Bianconi, E., Piovesan, A., Facchin, F., Beraudi, A., Casadei, R., ... Canaider, S. (2013). An estimation of the number of cells in the human body. *Annals of Human Biology, 40,* 463–471.

Birkhoff, G. D. (1931). Proof of the ergodic theorem. *Proceedings of the National Academy of Sciences of the United States of America, 17,* 656–660.

Border, R., Johnson, E. C., Evans, L. M., Smolen, A., Berley, N., Sullivan, P. F., & Keller, M. C. (2019). No support for historical candidate gene or candidate gene-by-interaction hypotheses for major depression across multiple large samples. *American Journal of Psychiatry, 176*(5), 376–387. doi: 10.1176/appi.ajp.2018.18070881

Bridgeman, B. (2003). *Psychology and evolution: The origins of mind.* Thousand Oaks, CA: Sage.

Cross-Disorder Group of the Psychiatric Genomics Consortium. (2013). Identification of risk loci with shared effects on five major psychiatric disorders: A genome-wide analysis. *Lancet, 381,* 1371–1379.

Davison, G. C. (2019). A return to functional analysis, the search for mechanisms of change, and the nomothetic-idiographic issue in psychosocial interventions. *Clinical Psychological Science, 7*(1), 51–53.

Fisher, A. J. (2015). Toward a dynamic model of psychological assessment: Implications for personalized care. *Journal of Consulting and Clinical Psychology, 83,* 825–836. doi: 10.1037/ccp0000026

Fisher, A. J., Medaglia, J. D., & Jeronimus, B. F. (2018). Lack of group-to-individual generalizability is a threat to human subjects research. *Proceedings of the National Academy of Sciences, 115*(27), E6106–E6115.

Franks, C. M., & Wilson, G. T. (1974). *Annual review of behavior therapy: Theory and practice.* New York: Brunner/Mazel.

Galhardo, R. S., Hastings, P. J., & Rosenberg, S. M. (2007). Mutation as a stress response and the regulation of evolvability. *Critical Reviews in Biochemistry and Molecular Biology, 42,* 399–435.

Gates, K. M., & Molenaar, P. C. M. (2012). Group search algorithm recovers effective connectivity maps for individuals in homogeneous and heterogeneous samples. *NeuroImage, 63,* 310–319.

Harvey, A., Watkins, E., Mansell, W., & Shafran, R. (2004). *Cognitive behavioral processes across psychological disorders: A transdiagnostic approach to research and treatment.* New York: Oxford University Press.

Hayes, S. C., Barlow, D. H., & Nelson-Gray, R. O. (1999). *The scientist-practitioner: Research and accountability in the age of managed care* (2nd ed.). New York: Allyn & Bacon.

Hayes, S. C., & Hofmann, S. G. (Eds.). (2018). *Process-based CBT: The science and core clinical competencies of cognitive behavioral therapy.* Oakland, CA: Context Press/New Harbinger Publications.

Hayes, S. C., Hofmann, S. G., Stanton, C. E., Carpenter, J. K., Sanford, B. T., Curtiss, J. E., & Ciarrochi, J. (2019). The role of the individual in the coming era of process-based therapy. *Behaviour Research and Therapy, 117*, 40–53. doi: 10.1016/j.brat.2018.10.005

Hayes, S. C., Monestès, J-L, & Wilson, D. S. (2018). Evolutionary principles for applied psychology. In S. C. Hayes & S. G. Hofmann (Eds.), *Process-based CBT: The science and core clinical competencies of cognitive behavioral therapy* (pp. 155–171). Oakland, CA: Context Press/New Harbinger Publications.

Hayes, S. C., Nelson, R. O., & Jarrett, R. (1987). Treatment utility of assessment: A functional approach to evaluating the quality of assessment. *American Psychologist, 42*, 963–974. doi: 10.1037//0003-066X.42.11.963

Hayes, S. C., Stanton, C. E., Sanford, B. T., Law, S., & Ta, J. (in press). Becoming more versatile: Using evolutionary science to suggest innovations in ACT. Chapter to appear in M. E. Levin, M. P. Twohig, & J. Krafft (Eds.), *Recent innovations in ACT.* Oakland, CA: New Harbinger Publications.

Hesser, H., Westin, V., Hayes, S. C., & Andersson, G. (2009). Clients' in-session acceptance and cognitive defusion behaviors in acceptance-based treatment of tinnitus distress. *Behaviour Research and Therapy, 47*, 523–528. doi: 10.1016/j.brat.2009.02.002

Hofmann, S. G., Asnaani, A., Vonk, J. J., Sawyer, A. T., & Fang, A. (2012). The efficacy of cognitive behavioral therapy: A review of meta-analyses. *Cognitive Therapy and Research, 36*, 427–440. doi: 10.1007/s10608-012-9476-1

Hofmann, S. G., & Hayes, S. C. (2019). The future of intervention science: Process-based therapy. *Clinical Psychological Science, 7*(1), 37–50. doi: 10.1177/2167702618772296

Insel, T., Cuthbert, B., Carvey, M., Heinssen, R., Pine, D. S., Quinn, K., ... Wang, P. (2010). Research Domain Criteria (RDoC): Toward a new classification framework for research on mental disorders. *American Journal of Psychiatry, 167*, 748–751. doi: 10.1176/appi.ajp.2010.09091379

Jablonka, E., & Lamb, M. J. (2014). *Evolution in four dimensions* (2nd ed.). Cambridge, MA: MIT Press.

Klepac, R. K., Ronan, G. F., Andrasik, F., Arnold, K. D., Belar, C. D., Berry, S. L., ... Strauman, T. J. (2012). Guidelines for cognitive behavioral training within doctoral psychology programs in the United States: Report of the inter-organizational task force on cognitive and behavioral psychology doctoral education. *Behavior Therapy, 43*, 687–697. doi: 10.1016/j.beth.2012.05.002

Kupfer, D. J., First, M. B., & Regier, D. A. (2002). Introduction. In D. J. Kupfer, M. B. First, & D. A. Regier (Eds.), *A research agenda for DSM-V* (pp. xv–xxiii). Washington DC: American Psychiatric Association.

Molenaar, P. C. M. (2008a). Consequences of the ergodic theorems for classical test theory, factor analysis, and the analysis of developmental processes. In S. M. Hofer & D. F. Alwin (Eds.), *Handbook of cognitive aging: Interdisciplinary perspectives* (pp. 90–104). Thousand Oaks, CA: Sage. doi: 10.4135/9781412976589.n5

Molenaar, P. C. M. (2008b). On the implications of the classical ergodic theorems: Analysis of developmental processes has to focus on intra-individual variation. *Developmental Psychobiology, 50*, 60–69. doi: 10.1002/dev.20262

Passamonti, L., Fairchild, G., Fornito, A., Goodyer, I. M., Nimmo-Smith, I., Hagan, C. C., & Calder A. J. (2012). Abnormal anatomical connectivity between the amygdala and orbitofrontal cortex in conduct disorder. *PLoS ONE, 7*(11), e48789. doi: 10.1371/journal.pone.0048789

Paul, G. L. (1967). Strategy of outcome research in psychotherapy. *Journal of Consulting Psychology, 31*(2), 109–118.

Paul, G. L. (1969). Behavior modification research: Design and tactics. In C. M. Franks (Ed.), *Behavior therapy: Appraisal and status* (pp. 29–62). New York: McGraw-Hill.

Pepper, S. C. (1942). *World hypotheses: A study in evidence.* Berkeley: University of California Press.

Preacher, K. J., & Hayes, A. F. (2008). Asymptotic and resampling strategies for assessing and comparing indirect effects in multiple mediator models. *Behavior Research Methods, 40,* 879–891. doi: 10.3758/BRM.40.3.879

Rose, T. (2017). *The end of average.* San Francisco: Harper One.

Sidman, M. (1960). *Tactics of scientific research.* Oxford, UK: Basic Books. doi: 10.1126/science.1225244

Thompson-Hollands, J., Sauer-Zavala, S., & Balrow, D. H. (2014). CBT and the future of personalized treatment: A proposal. *Depression and Anxiety, 31;* 909–911. doi: 10.1002/da.22301

Tinbergen, N. (1963). On aims and methods of ethology. *Journal of Animal Psychology (Zeitschrift für Tierpsychologie), 20*(4), 410–433.

Turner, A. E., & Hayes, S. C. (1996). A comparison of response covariation viewed idiothetically and nomothetically. *Psicologia Conductual, 4,* 231–250.

Volkovysskii, R. L., & Sinai, Y. G. (1971). Ergodic properties of an ideal gas with an infinite number of degrees of freedom. *Functional Analysis and Its Applications (Funktsional'nyi Analiz i Ego Prilozheniya), 5*(3), 185–187.

von Eye, A., & Bergman, L. (2003). Research strategies in developmental psychopathology: Dimensional identity and the person-oriented approach. *Development and Psychopathology, 15*(3), 553–580. doi: 10.1017/S0954579403000294

Wagner, G. P., & Draghi, J. (2010). Evolution of evolvability. In M. Pigliucci & G. B. Müller (Eds.), *Evolution: The extended synthesis* (pp. 379–399). Cambridge, MA: MIT Press.

Wilson, D. S., & Hayes, S. C. (Eds.). (2018). *Evolution and contextual behavioral science: An integrated framework for understanding, predicting, and influencing human behavior.* Oakland, CA: Context Press/New Harbinger Publications.

Wilson, D. S., Hayes, S. C., Biglan, T., & Embry, D. (2014). Evolving the future: Toward a science of intentional change. *Behavioural and Brain Sciences, 34,* 395–416. doi: 10.1017/S0140525X13001593

World Health Organization. (2018). *International classification of diseases and related health problems* (11th rev.). Geneva, Switzerland: Author.

CHAPTER 2

The NIMH Research Domain Criteria Project
A *Decade of Behavior and Brain Integration for Translational Research*

Uma Vaidyanathan, PhD; Sarah Morris, PhD;
Ann Wagner, PhD; Joel Sherrill, PhD;
David Sommers, PhD; Marjorie Garvey, MB BCh;
Eric Murphy, PhD; and Bruce Cuthbert, PhD

National Institute of Mental Health

It has been approximately 10 years since the inception of the Research Domain Criteria (RDoC) initiative by the National Institute of Mental Health (NIMH). The principles it espouses, such as the focus on transdiagnostic mechanisms and a dimensional conceptualization of mental disorders, have become more widespread and commonly accepted frameworks among the United States and European research communities. The goal of this chapter is to provide an introduction to RDoC, provide an update on its current status, describe its relevance to treatment, and offer insight into its potential future directions.

The Motivation for RDoC

NIMH's motivation for initiating RDoC was two-fold: First and foremost, scientific progress in understanding and treating mental disorders in recent decades has been disappointing, despite considerable advances in genetics, behavior, and molecular, cellular, and circuit-based neuroscience. With some exceptions, new insights provided by basic science have not translated into new discoveries about disease etiology, novel treatment targets, or more effective treatments. Disability due to mental illness is high and projected to increase (Prince et al., 2007), suicide mortality in the United States remains stubbornly elevated (and has increased for middle-aged men; Fond et al., 2016), and pharmaceutical companies are finding the return on investment for the development of new central nervous system medications to be unacceptably low (Hyman, 2012; Kaitin & Milne, 2011). Some of these difficulties result from unavoidable and inherent challenges of understanding illnesses that arise from complex combinations of psychological, environmental, genetic, and neural factors, but self-imposed constraints—specifically, the de facto mandate confining psychiatric research to traditional diagnostic categories—could be addressed.

Contemporary research has identified a variety of problems with current diagnostic systems, which contain nearly identical categories for both the *Diagnostic and Statistical Manual of Mental Disorders* (DSM; American Psychiatric Association, 2013) and the *International Classification of Diseases and Related Health Problems* (ICD; World Health Organization, 2018) (e.g., Clark, Cuthbert, Lewis-Fernández, Narrow, & Reed, 2017; Jablensky, 2016; Markon & Krueger, 2005; Widiger & Samuel, 2005). The current dominant model of mental disorders conceptualizes these phenomena as categorical conditions reflecting a simple binary distinction between "well" and "sick," even though it is widely accepted that this is more a matter of convention rather than positing or implying that such distinctions exist in nature. Indeed, most research to date indicates that mental disorders are likely best modeled as a set of underlying dimensions (Hettema, Prescott, Myers, Neale, & Kendler, 2005; Krueger, 1999; Slade & Watson, 2006). Further, it is increasingly recognized that current disorder categories represent broad and heterogeneous syndromes rather than specific disease entities (Hyman, 2010). A related and additional issue is the proliferation of the number of such categorical mental disorder conditions in official diagnostic manuals—resulting in a diagnostic manual whose categories are simultaneously too broad (i.e., heterogenous) and too narrow (i.e., resulting in excess comorbidity) (Casey et al., 2013).

Another problem concerns the lack of strong correlates or knowledge about mechanisms that reliably characterize disorders and distinguish one disorder from another. As it is well-known, the current diagnostic format—

which requires numerous self-report and behavioral measures of symptoms—was devised in the DSM-III era to aid in standardizing diagnoses of mental disorders to allow for precise communications between various stakeholders. It was acknowledged around this time that such symptoms formed a part of the "clinical description" of a disorder that would presumably, in conjunction with other types of research, such as laboratory and family studies, eventuate in valid characterizations of mental disorders (Feighner et al., 1972; Robins & Guze, 1970; Spitzer, Endicott, & Robins, 1978).

However, this approach has been largely unsuccessful in validating diagnostic categories that can be identified by biomarkers or predict optimal treatment approaches (Kapur, Phillips, & Insel, 2012). Deeper philosophical matters underlie the issues raised in seminal papers and books—such as the question of whether mental disorders have biological correlates (Fodor, 1968; Miller, 2010)—to which we cannot do justice here. Regardless of the reader's perspective on such debates, however, it is apparent that beyond the self-report or behavioral domain, and despite the plethora of studies to date, much remains to be discovered about the etiology and pathophysiology of mental disorders (Kupfer & Regier, 2011).

While perhaps unintended, the current diagnostic nosology has had far-reaching consequences. Whether this nosology is being taught to students in training, adopted by researchers or clinicians, or employed for clinical trials or insurance purposes, this model tends to be utilized by the entire mental health system. As one example, grant applications submitted to NIMH for funding have overwhelmingly focused on specific diagnostic categories for research proposals—an enterprise that has yielded limited results in reducing the overall burden of mental disorders (Insel, 2009). Despite investigators' awareness that using arbitrary diagnostic cutoffs and group comparisons may not yield generative results, this system has continued, given that it has been the only consensus nosology available.

RDoC resulted from this set of concerns as a broad strategy for opening up clinical and translational research that could be more directly informed by the considerable advances in contemporary basic behavioral neuroscience research. Rather than continuing to focus psychiatric research endeavors on existing diagnostic classifications, which do not appear to align with patterns of dysfunction in neural circuits, behavior, or genetics, RDoC encourages researchers to instead anchor their hypotheses in the understanding of behavioral, cognitive, and affective neuroscience and to consider how psychiatric symptoms might arise from abnormalities in these systems. The intent was to remain agnostic with regard to existing diagnostic criteria (Sanislow et al., 2010).

A more tactical aim was related to this change in scientific perspective and approach, and it addressed a pragmatic concern. As we mentioned earlier, before the introduction of RDoC, the use of DSM or ICD categories had become a de facto standard requirement in research designs for clinical grant applications to NIMH. This constraint blocked efforts to study psychopathology from other viewpoints, particularly in light of emerging data that the current diagnoses were inadequate mirrors of nature. However, prior experience at NIMH suggested that efforts to move the field to explore new ways of conceptualizing and classifying mental disorders would likely fail unless some additional guidance were provided as a starting point. In other words, if the field adopted a stance of agnosticism toward longstanding diagnostic categories, then it would likely flounder without a framework to constrain the innumerable potential alternative approaches. The RDoC initiative provided investigators, reviewers, and journal editors with a starting point of shared vocabulary, nominated constructs and suggested research principles and implicit hypotheses to support a paradigm change.

The RDoC Framework

RDoC comprises a multifaceted framework that is intended to accommodate and integrate major perspectives on current psychopathology research. Many viewpoints advocated by RDoC are not novel. Various aspects, such as the focus on dimensionality rather than categorical conditions and a move to understanding mechanisms rather than focusing on overt symptoms alone, have been promulgated by various researchers and clinicians (Krueger & Markon, 2011; Wilson & Sponheim, 2014). Rather, RDoC attempts to gather all these principles in a way that allows for a more unrestricted conceptualization of mental disorders and the mechanisms that may contribute to them and that molds them into a larger, usable framework that researchers can implement in their studies.

The core of RDoC is centered on the notion of functional constructs that connect biology and behavior. What differentiates an RDoC construct from a more conventional one is that it must satisfy the following criteria: (a) it must be linked to actions, behavior, or cognition; (b) it must also be associated with an implementing neural circuit; and (c) it must be related to psychopathology. Put simply, such constructs reflect the biological implementations of behaviors that are relevant to psychopathology (Yee, Javitt, & Miller, 2015).

An additional, and important, consideration is that the constructs are defined as dimensional in nature and span a spectrum of human functioning from normal to abnormal, which is intended to encourage studies of the range where dysfunction gradually emerges with respect to psychopathology. Current RDoC constructs are grouped into six broader domains of human behavior that span the range from wellness to increasingly severe degrees of dysfunction—namely, Positive Valence Systems, Negative Valence systems, Cognitive Systems, Social Processes, Arousal/Regulatory Systems, and Sensorimotor Systems. These domains are intended as heuristic divisions in the overall framework, but it is clear that systems interact in producing adaptive behavior. For example, emotional stimuli likely affect not only Negative or Positive Valence Systems, but Cognitive Systems as well. RDoC is based upon the premise that current conceptualizations of mental disorders and their symptoms involve gradations of abnormal functioning in one or more of these domains and constructs, as well as the interactions among them.

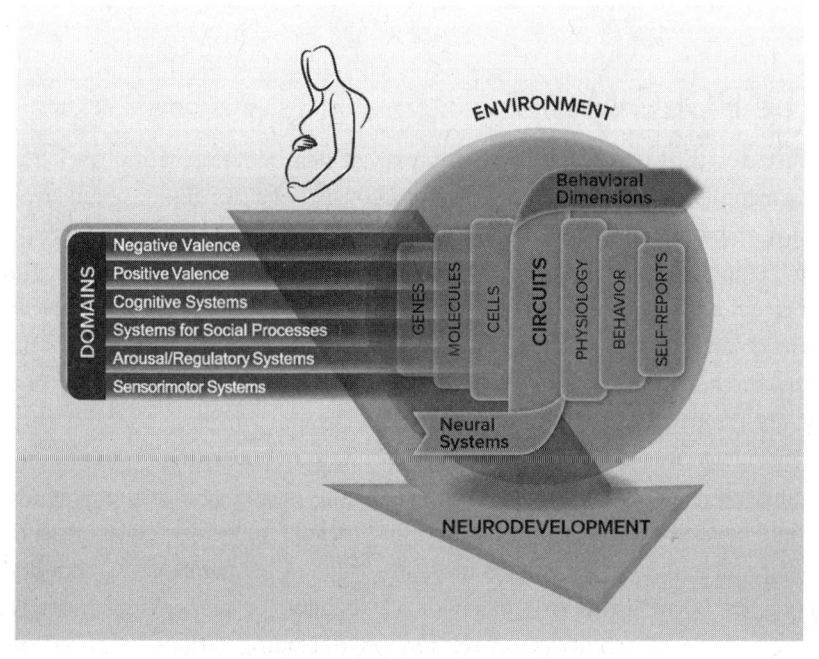

Figure 2.1. The RDoC Framework

As a research framework attempting to integrate knowledge about the etiology of psychopathology, RDoC incorporates two essential aspects that are generally underrepresented in the "presenting-problem" orientation of current diagnostic frameworks. First, mental disorders are increasingly recognized to involve disruptions in developmental processes, from both biological and psychological perspectives (Casey et al., 2013). The importance of this factor is reflected in the fact that approximately half of the RDoC-oriented grants funded by NIMH over the past decade have focused on developmental issues. Second, the effects of environmental circumstances are well-recognized as significant risk or protective factors for mental disorders (and have complex interactions with the points in development at which various events occur). However, a mechanistic approach to environmental effects has been hampered by the narrow focus on studying individual diagnostic categories. For instance, the consequences of trauma may be seen in various diagnostic categories, such as post-traumatic stress disorder (PTSD), depression, anxiety disorders, personality disorders, and substance abuse. The emphasis on studying one specific disorder at a time blurs a more comprehensive examination of transdiagnostic mechanisms and obscures appropriate consideration of the heterogeneity within disorders.

The RDoC Matrix

Nested within the overarching contexts of neurodevelopmental and environmental influences, the RDoC matrix consists of a two-dimensional layout with domains (and nested constructs) in the rows, and units of analysis as the columns (see Figure 2.1). Constructs represent functions identified through an extensive workshop process (Cuthbert & Kozak, 2013) that are particularly well-established—and thus exemplify promising areas for study and further development—and domains are face-valid groupings of constructs. For instance, the Positive Valence domain currently contains three constructs of Reward Responsiveness, Reward Learning, and Reward Valuation. The units of analysis depict various classes of measurement that could be used to study the constructs and include molecules, cells, measures of circuit activity, physiological measures (such as heart rate or adrenocorticotropin hormone levels), behavior (in behavioral tasks or quantitative observations of activity), and self-reports (including ratings by clinicians, family, and others). An additional column lists various paradigms that have been used to study each construct. Given that a central goal of RDoC is to study brain-behavior relationships, investigators are strongly encouraged to include measures from multiple units of analysis in order to conduct multivariate analyses that can lead to a more integrative understanding.

Both the rows and columns of the matrix are intended as heuristic exemplars, not as fixed sets that must be followed. The constructs are viewed as model examples that demonstrate the idea of dimensions that can be jointly defined by evidence for a particular function and by evidence for an implementing circuit. But a central goal within RDoC involves both revising constructs on the basis of new data and studying potentially brand-new constructs that could be added. Units of analysis are meant to suggest the classes of measures that could be included in study designs but are not meant to be an exhaustive list. For instance, the self-report column could be broken down into questionnaires that participants complete and instruments that the interviewer fills out. Similarly, the behavior column could include responses to behavioral tasks or observer measurements of behavior, such as a toddler approach-avoidance test. The notion is to give investigators a general illustration of thinking about multi-measurement designs, not to spell out in rigid detail the measurement classes that are allowed.

Various features of the RDoC matrix instantiate the principles of RDoC research. In order to encourage research that uses behavioral neuroscience as its starting point (rather than starting with clinical signs and symptoms), the sets of domains and associated constructs in the matrix are organized around normative processes. The constructs were selected and defined in workshops (one per domain) attended by experts with relevant expertise who evaluated pertinent literatures. To constrain the selection among the many possible constructs, attendees were asked to develop a set of constructs that have a documented behavioral or psychological function, that have evidence of an implementing neural circuit, and that have an empirically demonstrated relationship to some aspect of psychopathology. The goal of the workshop process was to develop a set of constructs that had an appropriate degree of granularity so they could be studied across the various units of analysis. Ongoing and future research will help to clarify the extent to which narrower or broader constructs are optimal and whether other constructs are useful for the ultimate goal of improving psychiatric classification. The matrix is not definitive or comprehensive, so the current domains and constructs should be thought of as exemplars. Further, it is anticipated that the matrix will evolve as new discoveries are made.

In addition, RDoC constructs are not operationally defined in the sense of having a one-to-one correspondence with any specific task or measure. Rather, the elements in the cells of the matrix for each construct are considered to be convergent measures of the construct, and the tasks and measures listed in the paradigms column are suggestions for studying constructs. There are also a few symptoms, such as hallucinations in the Perception and Understanding of Self construct, included among the elements of the matrix. Most behavioral and self-report elements are normative and may be present among individuals along a dimension or continuum, such as response inhibition or risk assessment. The hypothesis inherent to the RDoC framework is that psychopathology—whether it manifests as self-report symptoms, observable signs, impaired functioning, or a combination of these—arises at one or both extremes of the dimension.

Research that includes non-help-seeking individuals and psychiatric patients will reveal the nature of the dimensions, including the degree to which they are skewed or multimodal and whether there are naturally occurring discontinuities that may provide empirical definitions of disorders. These types of analyses, which are based on an assumption of dimensionality between health and illness and are agnostic regarding diagnostic criteria, require some clinical researchers to move away from the between-groups, "patients-versus-controls" models that may be most familiar to them. Instead, the desideratum focuses on evaluating the validity of novel cut-points or clusters for the purpose of predicting treatment response or illness course or for isolating illness mechanisms. The RDoC approach also encourages analyses that span units of analysis and that avoid assumptions about the primacy of any particular type of data. For example, although psychiatry relies heavily upon self-report of internal experiences, there may be signals detectable in other systems, such as circuit-based measures of cognitive performance, that are more informative for understanding and treating psychopathology or that can be detected earlier in the course of development than self-report symptoms.

Another important point to note is that RDoC constructs are considered to be attributes of individuals rather than of the environment, and environmental features are thus not represented in the matrix. As mentioned earlier, though, neurobehavioral constructs are affected by various aspects of the physical, social, and psychological environment. Determining the role of environmental influences on constructs, and their contribution to symptoms and impairment in functioning, is an important part of the RDoC project.

The framework eschews a listing of specific types of environmental factors in order to avoid any implied priorities in this regard, instead encouraging investigators to pursue those aspects that they view most salient.

Designing an RDoC Study

We hope that our comments thus far will give the reader information and context about how the overall framework has been conceived and a broad notion of how it is intended to encourage translational research. How does one go about distilling these various principles into a research design to examine psychopathology from an RDoC perspective? In brief, designing a study consistent with RDoC postulates involves the following steps:

1. Start with what is known about normal neurobehavioral processes rather than with DSM- or ICD-disorder categories.

2. Focus on specific clinical problems that span diagnoses or on identifying meaningful, valid subgroups of patients that can be related to one or more RDoC constructs.

3. Assume that that there are neurobehavioral continuities from normal to abnormal across various aspects of psychopathology and that neurobehavioral processes can and do cut across disorders. However, this does not mean a linear gradient throughout, and marked inflection points along dimensions may contribute to useful cut-off points for defining a disorder or its severity.

4. Do not necessarily assume self-reports of symptoms are the "gold standard." As an example, the original behavior therapies, such as those for phobias, relied upon behavior tests, as well as symptom reports, for the initial assessments.

5. Assume interactions among constructs. For example, emotion affects cognition and vice versa.

It bears reiterating that the RDoC matrix provides exemplars of the instantiation of such constructs. The matrix is not meant to be exhaustive or comprehensive; rather, it serves as a starting point for research on constructs relevant to psychopathology. It is hoped that as research using RDoC principles accumulates, the matrix can and will evolve in multiple ways. If investigators wish to use their own constructs when designing studies for an RDoC funding opportunity, then they may do so to the extent that the constructs they propose fit the notion of an RDoC construct. Again, the intent of RDoC is to encourage a multidisciplinary and integrative perspective on mental health and illness rather than to emphasize specific diagnostic categories or constructs in a prescriptive manner.

RDoC and Treatment

While the primary goal of this chapter is to describe RDoC as a framework for understanding and studying psychopathology, RDoC also has the potential to advance the conceptualization of interventions, to facilitate intervention development and testing, and to ultimately guide the delivery of interventions. RDoC domains, and the constructs and mechanistic substrates they subsume, represent potential intervention targets both within and across traditional diagnostic classes of mental disorders. In this sense, considering treatment targets in terms of RDoC constructs is redolent of the formal behavioral assessment approaches of several decades ago (Hersen & Bellack, 1981).

The RDoC framework also has implications for conceptualizing the timing of intervention delivery—in terms of both illness trajectories (from early signs and symptoms to fully syndromal) and lifespan development. Its emphasis on understanding pathology on a continuum, including a focus on inflection points that might represent transitions from healthy/functional to pathological/impaired, incorporates developmental considerations as a parallel continuum and allows for the identification of potential targets for preventive, as well as curative, interventions. Similarly, RDoC's emphasis on lifespan development as a cross-cutting consideration underscores its potential to inform targets and identify critical periods for intervening, not only early in the illness trajectory, but also early in the life course. While moving away from a categorical conceptualization adds layers of complexity, RDoC offers the potential to represent a more valid understanding of how psychopathology develops and persists compared to other extant models.

As a field, psychology has always been interested in individual differences (cf. Anastasi, 1958), and it is clear that the field has asked the question of "which intervention for whom" for decades (e.g., Fonagy, 2010; Paul, 1969).

Although the typical clinician is aware of the need to consider this question in the context of case formulation, the field has been limited by a standard set of intervention options that are fit to a relatively broad and heterogeneous group of patients seen over time. This might be roughly analogous to the use of a broad-spectrum antibiotic for a lingering upper respiratory infection (URI). It might work, or might not, but in either case, the URI was likely not bacterial, intervention with an antibiotic is administered without a sound rationale, and we gain no understanding (from the onset of the pathology to the cure) as to what really happened. What if the patient doesn't improve? Would a more carefully constructed diagnosis of the underlying pathology have made sense? Certainly, these diagnostic procedures would come later if the patient were not to improve, and indeed, URIs can be caused by a wide variety of pathogens.

Similarly, most psychopathologies labeled under the common nomenclature of the DSM and the ICD can be caused by multiple pathologies in underlying systems (e.g., Galatzer-Levy & Bryant, 2013). This is where RDoC has the potential to be useful, as it is applied to intervention development. Rather than starting broadly and drilling down when a patient exhibits no response or a partial response, it would be preferable to start at a point of precision in pursuit of an optimal intervention response. The domains and subsumed constructs in the RDoC matrix represent these potential precision points (Kozak & Cuthbert, 2016). While still "under construction," RDoC aims to better understand the causation of overt psychopathology to allow for the development of more efficacious and efficient interventions. The cost of getting closer to a more precise understanding of etiology is that the data become several orders of magnitude more complex, perhaps unmanageably so. However, "big data" approaches and machine-learning algorithms have already proven capable in allowing for the extraction of meaningfulness and in identifying ideas for interventions.

RDoC's approach to understanding and studying psychopathology is consistent with rational, mechanism-based intervention development and testing programs such as the NIMH experimental therapeutics approach (Insel, 2015). In this manner, RDoC-consistent constructs and associated assessment strategies might guide the selection of individuals who could benefit from a specific intervention, the selection of targets for the intervention, and the approach to assessing whether the intervention, if it works, achieves its benefit via the putative targets (i.e., the mechanism of action, which could be psychological, biological, or both). This is precision medicine.

In terms of identifying relevant patients or candidates for the intervention (i.e., caseness or inclusion criteria for a trial), RDoC represents a framework for identifying individuals with deficits in the specific domains associated with symptoms and impairment in functioning or with a common underlying structural or functional pathology—and, in turn, for enrolling those potential trial participants for whom the candidate targets and strategies might be most relevant (e.g., Krystal et al., 2019).

In addition, RDoC's multilevel approach to assessment offers options for identifying valid and feasible alternatives for assessing whether a candidate intervention strategy can be administered in a sufficient dose (e.g., the number, frequency, or duration of sessions) to engage RDoC-consistent targets. In turn, the RDoC approach also allows for an examination of whether intervention-induced changes in these proximal targets drive clinical benefits (i.e., for selecting assessment strategies that span levels of analyses for purposes of assessing target engagement and target validation).

RDoC-consistent mechanism-driven approaches to conceptualizing and designing interventions also have implications that ultimately guide the delivery of these interventions. A focus on developing interventions that target the causative foundation of pathology might facilitate the deployment of simpler, more focal, or modularized interventions that could be delivered in a more prescriptive, personalized, and precise manner. Moreover, such focal, modular approaches might be more inherently scalable. First, training clinicians in a set of specific strategies that can be flexibly but broadly implemented might be more feasible and sustainable than promulgating multicomponent intervention manuals for the various mental health conditions encountered in clinical practice (Barlow, Allen, & Choate, 2016; Hayes et al., 2019; Hofmann & Hayes, 2019). In addition, a suite of more focal interventions that could be more flexibly deployed might be better suited to clinical realities, where patients commonly present with multiple comorbidities and the problem focus often varies over time (Chorpita, Daleiden, & Weisz, 2005). For example, in process-based therapies, the emphasis on procedures and techniques is secondary to the attention paid to the therapeutic change processes impacting the individual. RDoC allows for the advancement of specific hypotheses about such processes that can be tested and verified or falsified. This, in turn, allows for modifications of the therapies that are more precisely suited to the individual (Hayes et al., 2019; Hofmann & Hayes, 2019).

An important question to ask here is whether our intervention on an RDoC variable generates an effect on a person's overall health or illness. While RDoC will encourage improved targeting of interventions to underlying mechanisms, it is not yet clear how an intervention specific to a particular construct or mechanism (e.g., diminished reward valuation), while successful, would relate to overall response or remission regarding traditional concepts of caseness (e.g., depression). It might work fully, to some extent, or not at all. On the other hand, the fact that current interventions seldom exceed 50 percent in effectiveness suggests that treatment development aimed at heterogeneous (and frequently comorbid) syndromes is not a viable strategy for long-term improvements in therapeutic success. These are questions that remain to be addressed in future research regarding precision treatments for mental disorders.

Exemplary Findings from RDoC-Themed Studies

Data from studies funded explicitly under RDoC funding announcements are just beginning to emerge, but there are already promising findings that illustrate the potential of the approach. In addition, some research projects initiated before the start of the RDoC program have also reported results that are equally illustrative and significant. A few of the most salient findings are summarized here, and literature searches will reveal new findings that are being published with increasing frequency.

Some of the most generative RDoC-themed results have been reported by the Bipolar and Schizophrenia Network for Intermediate Phenotypes (BSNIP) program (Clementz et al., 2016). The initial study in this effort obtained a wide variety of symptomatic, behavioral, electrophysiological, magnetic resonance imaging (MRI), and other measures in patients with psychotic disorders (schizophrenia, schizoaffective disorder, and psychotic bipolar disorder), their first-degree relatives, and healthy controls (total N of nearly 2,000). The investigators factor-analyzed their multiple measures and found two major factors—one comprising cognitive measures plus a stop-signal task ("cognitive control") and another involving EEG and event-related potential responses to tone and light stimuli ("sensorimotor reactivity")—which are compatible with the RDoC "cognitive control" and "perception" constructs, respectively. A cluster analysis of the factor scores revealed three "biotypes" in the patient group comprising different combinations of the two factors that cut across diagnostic categories and were validated by other measures varying systematically across the groups (such as cortical gray-matter loss) and by similar patterns in first-degree relatives (Clementz et al., 2016; Tamminga et al., 2017). This study has contributed significantly to revised views of psychosis phenotypes (Vinogradov, 2019).

Another example of RDoC-themed research comes from a program of translational anxiety disorders studies, which stemmed from basic psychophysiological research into fear and threat (Lang & Bradley, 2010). In an initial transdiagnostic analysis, patients with anxiety disorders were grouped into quintiles based upon a composite reactivity measure of heart rate and emotion-modulated startle response to imagery of clinically relevant material. Perhaps counterintuitively, lowered reactivity was associated with greater degrees of negative affectivity and functional impairment independent of formal diagnosis (Lang, McTeague, & Bradley, 2016). In a more recent study of emotional picture processing, functional magnetic resonance imaging (fMRI) data were collected to analyze relationships between symptom scores (such as trauma history and negative affect) and amygdala and ventral visual cortex activity (Sambuco, Bradley, Herring, Hillbrandt, & Lang, 2019). Consistent with prior results, patients showing the smallest fMRI reactivity reported the highest trauma scores, independent of PTSD diagnosis, indicating that greater exposure to trauma is associated with disruptions in threat reactivity. This type of transdiagnostic "reactivity phenotype" has obvious implications when it comes to etiology, prevention, and precision treatment.

In a third example, children with attention deficit/hyperactivity disorder were divided into three phenotypes related to RDoC constructs using an advanced clustering method based on graph theory to analyze parental ratings of child temperament. The groups, termed "mild," "surgent," and "irritable," were validated using several behavioral and autonomic methods as well as clinical outcomes (Karalunas et al., 2014). As in the two prior examples, more precise phenotypes could be pinpointed by analyses of functional dimensions using behavioral and biological measures in the analysis, suggesting new ideas for nosology and treatment.

Evolution and Future of RDoC

As an experimental research framework, there has always been an intention that the RDoC framework would change considerably over time, both in response to advances in the scientific literature and in various procedural and administrative aspects. One notable improvement was the instantiation of a process for evaluating proposed changes to the RDoC framework, which had been envisioned from the outset but took some time to develop. The process is coordinated by the Changes to the RDoC Matrix (CMAT) workgroup, which is a small steering committee formed of current and former members of NIMH's National Advisory Mental Health Council (NAMHC) along with other experts from the field. The group considers potential changes to the matrix and determines the scope of the evaluation for each, ranging from minor revisions with a few consultants to extensive modifications that may involve a large number of experts and that require attending in-person workshops. Recommendations are drafted in a report submitted to the full NAMHC for approval. The CMAT workgroup has already overseen revisions to the positive valence domain and the addition of a new sensorimotor processes domain, with other proposed changes under consideration.

Other activities have involved efforts to enhance outreach and training regarding the overall framework. To this end, several webinars have been held on various RDoC-related topics (including a series of three events organized in collaboration with the Delaware Project on clinical science training in psychology). Further, RDoC staff have held virtual office hours for over a year in order to discuss RDoC principles and research designs with interested investigators and students. RDoC staff have also organized an in-person workshop specifically devoted to issues regarding the training of MD and PhD students in learning about RDoC-related concepts and conducting research from an RDoC perspective; more recently, another workshop was conducted to discuss ways to highlight the importance of developmental processes and environmental influences in studies of RDoC constructs.

More significantly, there have been substantial changes in the scientific approaches associated with RDoC. In its current state, RDoC is clear that the matrix essentially constitutes a set of hypotheses. The expectation is that over time, research will lead not only to enhanced validation or modification of the RDoC domains and constructs, but also to the ways in which the overall framework is conceived and evaluated. At present, the RDoC domains and constructs are essentially the product of an expert consensus process, albeit based upon careful consideration of basic and clinical literatures. Better measures of RDoC concepts are needed, which will allow for further validation of the domains.

Fortunately, innovations in research designs, mathematical models, and data storage and analysis have burgeoned in the decade since RDoC began. One of the most promising innovations has been the rapid development of a broad effort termed "computational psychiatry." This new field comprises several different aspects, including biophysical modeling of neuronal and synaptic processes, computational modeling of behavior or brain-behavior relationships, and computational phenotyping that utilizes a variety of analytic techniques to uncover new phenotypes that may cut across current diagnostic categories (Clementz et al., 2016). In fact, development of this latter aspect was partly prompted by the RDoC framework, which offered examples of how mechanistic approaches to functioning could be used to study alternative phenotypes to traditional disorder categories (Adams, Huys, & Roiser, 2016).

There are detailed descriptions available that provide thorough summaries of computational psychiatry and its methods (Ferrante et al., 2018; Paulus, Huys, & Maia, 2016). In brief, the study of brain-behavior relationships with computational models relies upon two classes of analysis. Theory-driven models involve the development of a very specific mathematical model of behavior-brain relationships (or, in some cases, behavior only) that include a variety of parameters, thus permitting a detailed test of the model that can lead to further refinements and, ultimately, a precise delineation of how particular functions operate. Data-driven approaches typically apply one or more of the many machine-learning techniques that have recently emerged and are useful for initial exploratory analyses that can suggest new models for study.

It is notable that, at the current time, NIMH supports funding that focuses exclusively on parametrically oriented behavioral tests, such as a recent call for R21 applications on computationally-defined behaviors in psychiatry. Computational phenotyping is a related effort that uses a variety of machine learning, clustering techniques, and latent class or latent dimensional models to suggest new clinical phenotypes. One approach to computational phenotypes that is particularly relevant to RDoC involves normative models (Marquand, Wolfers, Mennes, Buitelaar, & Beckmann, 2016), which specifically address the heterogeneity and dimensionality of disorder categories by expressing scores for patients in terms of distributions for healthy subjects (analogous to height and weight charts for children's growth). This analytic approach has already shown a strong potential for transcending standard clinical diagnoses in order to provide more fine-grained information about biomarkers and clinical phenotypes (Wolfers et al., 2018). Such analyses can lead to precision-medicine approaches for new treatments across all therapeutic modalities (Paulus et al., 2016)—a strong theme of several chapters in this book.

A related trend has been the accelerating use of "big data" methods for data processing. Clearly, very large data sets are required for analyses of highly dimensional data that can provide more precise insights into the unique, multivariate nature of individuals or precisely defined homogeneous groupings. Recent advances have included two different aspects of large-N analyses. One development has been an increased number of large, multisite studies that recruit several hundred subjects to accommodate more powerful computational approaches. The BSNIP study provides an excellent example, as the initial cohort has been followed by two replication and extension studies that bring the total database to several thousand subjects.

As the RDoC approach has gained visibility, more investigators are employing the framework to conceive and explore large-scale, critical hypotheses regarding mechanisms of similar clinical phenotypes across disorders. An example of such an effort is the Psychiatric Ratings using Intermediate Stratified Markers (PRISM) project, which is a large, multisite project funded by the European Union's Innovative Medicines Initiative that is exploring similarities and differences in social withdrawal across patients with schizophrenia, Alzheimer's Disease, and depression from an explicitly RDoC perspective (Bilderbeck et al., 2019). This project will recruit several hundred subjects and employ computational modeling methods in the analysis, with an ultimate aim of providing a pathway toward regulatory approvals (potentially transdiagnostic) for treatments of social withdrawal.

The other trend in "big data" has been the creation of very large databases that house data from multiple studies. This practice obviously can achieve even larger data sets for analyses, facilitating machine-learning approaches to find hidden trends and subgroups in the data. A good example of this effort is the National Institute of Mental Health Data Archive (NDA).

However, one of the barriers to successful implementation of these approaches is the fact that different measures are used in different studies, and even when the same putative measure is used, various task parameters vary across studies. These factors hamper the ability of these resources to achieve their full potential. Nevertheless, an increasing number of studies have been published from NDA data, and the advent of common data elements that are included in all studies, along with newly implemented requirements for data sharing with virtually all clinical grants at NIMH, highlight the potential of such databases for more powerful computational analyses.

Conclusion

RDoC has frequently been viewed as the instantiation of a specific type of approach to psychopathology, which includes processes that refine the structure over time. Actually, the converse is closer to the actual goal: RDoC was established as a conceptual strategy for conducting research on psychopathology that is informed by contemporary behavioral and brain research, and the framework was established in the spirit of providing guidelines that could evolve over time in order to facilitate the progress. As noted in a recent commentary, "A common misunderstanding is that the published matrix *is* RDoC. On the contrary, RDoC is more a strategic proposal than it is a content proposal" (Yee et al., 2015, p. 1159). The specific intent was to free investigators to pursue research into psychopathology that is independent of traditional disorder categories rather than constraining them with a new set of strictures.

The inclusion of biological units of analysis in the framework, as well as some funding announcements that require both behavioral and biological measures, has understandably prompted the assumption that RDoC is a reductionistic enterprise in which behavior has a diminished role. On the contrary, RDoC is an attempt to focus attention on the understudied interstices between primarily behavioral and primarily biological views of psychopathology. One working assumption is that progress can be made most efficiently when each aspect informs the other. Behavioral scientists emphasize the fact that nervous system activity can best be understood in terms of the behavior that it implements. Similarly, psychological constructs are more scientifically compelling when grounded in a consideration of nervous system operations. Given the extensive adaptability of human behavior that is supported by the evolution of nervous system plasticity, interventions that target behavior will remain a staple of treatment development efforts and can be enhanced when informed by biology, as in a recent observation: "Given the limitations of systemic medications for treating specific neural pathways, the treatments that RDoC fosters will likely be behavioral, honed for neuromodulatory impact" (Yee et al., 2015, p. 1160).

From this perspective, the RDoC process aligns strongly with behavioral and cognitive approaches. The key element for any treatment is to think mechanistically about functional deficits and to develop interventions that target these mechanisms in therapy. Psychological mechanisms are core elements in behavioral therapies and can be enhanced through increased knowledge of the implementing neural systems (Bechtel, 2007). One marked advantage of behavioral treatments in the current clinical environment is the potential of such interventions to be developed and fielded more rapidly than drug or device therapies with their complex regulatory pathways. In the spirit of Hersen and Bellack (1981), behavioral and cognitive therapies are able to target specific mechanisms for individual patients as informed by contemporary research and thus have the potential to play a pioneering role in precision medicine for mental disorders. Similarly, behavioral treatments have long been salient contributors to prevention research and are well-placed to increase this role in a framework that emphasizes dimensional measurements of validated functions and mechanisms (Foa et al., 2005; Weisz, Sandler, Durlak, & Anton, 2005).

In conclusion, behavioral and cognitive therapies will have a major role in developing treatments of the future. Clearly, we are not there yet, and much work remains to be done. It is hoped that the perspectives generated by the RDoC framework can, in the words of Steve Jobs, provide an "enabling technology" that will enhance efforts within and across disciplines to hasten urgently needed interventions for psychopathology.

References

Adams, R. A., Huys, Q. J. M., & Roiser, J. P. (2016). Computational psychiatry: Towards a mathematically informed understanding of mental illness. *Journal of Neurology, Neurosurgery, and Psychiatry, 87*(1), 53–63. doi: 10.1136/jnnp-2015-310737

American Psychiatric Association. (2013). *Diagnostic and statistical manual of mental disorders.* (5th ed). Arlington, VA: Author.

Anastasi, A. (1958). *Differential psychology: Individual and group differences in behavior* (3rd ed.). Oxford, UK: Macmillan.

Barlow, D. H., Allen, L. B., & Choate, M. L. (2016). Toward a unified treatment for emotional disorders—republished article. *Behavior Therapy, 47*(6), 838–853. doi: 10.1016/j.beth.2016.11.005

Bechtel, W. (2007). Reducing psychology while maintaining its autonomy via mechanistic explanation. In N. Shouten & H. Looren de Jong (Eds.), *The matter of the mind: Philosophical essays on psychology, neuroscience and reduction* (pp. 172–198). Oxford, UK: Blackwell Publishers.

Bilderbeck, A. C., Penninx, B. W. J. H., Arango, C., van der Wee, N., Kahn, R., Wintervan Rossum, I., … Dawson, G. R. (2019). Overview of the clinical implementation of a study exploring social withdrawal in patients with schizophrenia and Alzheimer's disease. *Neuroscience & Biobehavioral Reviews, 97,* 87–93. doi: 10.1016/j.neubiorev.2018.06.019

Casey, B. J., Craddock, N., Cuthbert, B. N., Hyman, S. E., Lee, F. S., & Ressler, K. J. (2013). DSM-5 and RDoC: Progress in psychiatry research? *Nature Reviews Neuroscience, 14*(11), 810–814.

Chorpita, B. F., Daleiden, E. L., & Weisz, J. R. (2005). Identifying and selecting the common elements of evidence based interventions: A distillation and matching model. *Mental Health Services Research, 7*(1), 5–20.

Clark, L. A., Cuthbert, B., Lewis-Fernández, R., Narrow, W. E., & Reed, G. M. (2017). Three approaches to understanding and classifying mental disorder: ICD-11, DSM-5, and the National Institute of Mental Health's Research Domain Criteria (RDoC). *Psychological Science in the Public Interest, 18*(2), 72–145. doi: 10.1177/1529100617727266

Clementz, B. A., Sweeney, J. A., Hamm, J. P., Ivleva, E. I., Ethridge, L. E., Pearlson, G. D., … Tamminga, C. A. (2016). Identification of distinct psychosis biotypes using brain-based biomarkers. *The American Journal of Psychiatry, 173*(4), 373–384. doi: 10.1176/appi.ajp.2015.14091200

Cuthbert, B. N., & Kozak, M. J. (2013). Constructing constructs for psychopathology: The NIMH research domain criteria. *Journal of Abnormal Psychology, 122*(3), 928–937. doi: 10.1037/a0034028

Feighner, J. P., Robins, E., Guze, S. B., Woodruff, R. A., Winokur, G., & Munoz, R. (1972). Diagnostic criteria for use in psychiatric research. *Archives of General Psychiatry, 26*(1), 57–63.

Ferrante, M., Redish, A. D., Oquendo, M. A., Averbeck, B. B., Kinnane, M. E., & Gordon, J. A. (2018). Computational psychiatry: A report from the 2017 NIMH workshop on opportunities and challenges. *Molecular Psychiatry, 24*(4), 479–483.

Foa, E. B., Cahill, S. P., Boscarino, J. A., Hobfoll, S. E., Lahad, M., McNally, R. J., & Solomon, Z. (2005). Social, psychological, and psychiatric interventions following terrorist attacks: Recommendations for practice and research. *Neuropsychopharmacology, 30*(10), 1806–1817. doi: 10.1038/sj.npp.1300815

Fodor, J. A. (1968). *Psychological explanation: An introduction to the philosophy of psychology.* New York: Crown Publishing Group/Random House.

Fonagy, P. (2010). Psychotherapy research: Do we know what works for whom? *The British Journal of Psychiatry, 197*(2), 83–85. doi: 10.1192/bjp.bp.110.079657

Fond, G., Llorca, P. M., Boucekine, M., Zendjidjian, X., Brunel, L., Lancon, C., ... & Boyer, L. (2016). Disparities in suicide mortality trends between United States of America and 25 European countries: retrospective analysis of WHO mortality database. *Scientific Reports, 6*, 20256.

Galatzer-Levy, I. R., & Bryant, R. A. (2013). 636,120 ways to have posttraumatic stress disorder. *Perspectives on Psychological Science, 8*(6), 651–662.

Hayes, S. C., Hofmann, S. G., Stanton, C. E., Carpenter, J. K., Sanford, B. T., Curtiss, J. E., & Ciarrochi, J. (2019). The role of the individual in the coming era of process-based therapy. *Behaviour Research and Therapy, 117*, 40–53. doi: 10.1016/j.brat.2018.10.005

Hersen, M., & Bellack, A. S. (1981). *Behavioral assessment: A practical handbook* (2nd ed., Vol. 22). Oxford, UK: Pergamon Press.

Hettema, J. M., Prescott, C. A., Myers, J. M., Neale, M. C., & Kendler, K. S. (2005). The structure of genetic and environmental risk factors for anxiety disorders in men and women. *Archives of General Psychiatry, 62*(2), 182–189.

Hofmann, S. G., & Hayes, S. C. (2019). The future of intervention science: Process-based therapy. *Clinical Psychological Science, 7*(1), 37–50. doi: 10.1177/2167702618772296

Hyman, S. E. (2010). The diagnosis of mental disorders: The problem of reification. *Annual Review of Clinical Psychology, 6*, 155–179.

Hyman, S. (2012). Revolution stalled. *Science Translational Medicine, 4*(155).

Insel, T. R. (2009). Translating scientific opportunity into public health impact: A strategic plan for research on mental illness. *Archives of General Psychiatry, 66*(2), 128–133. doi: 10.1001/archgenpsychiatry.2008.540

Insel, T. R. (2015). The NIMH experimental medicine initiative. *World Psychiatry: Official Journal of the World Psychiatric Association (WPA), 14*(2), 151–153. doi: 10.1002/wps.20227

Jablensky, A. (2016). Psychiatric classifications: Validity and utility. *World Psychiatry, 15*(1), 26–31. doi: 10.1002/wps.20284

Kaitlin, K. I., & Milne, C. P. (2011). A dearth of new meds: Drugs to treat neuropsychiatric disorders have become too risky for Big Pharma. *Scientific American. 305*(2). doi: 10.1038/scientificamerican0811-16

Kapur, S., Phillips, A. G., & Insel, T. R. (2012). Why has it taken so long for biological psychiatry to develop clinical tests and what to do about it? *Molecular Psychiatry, 17*(12), 1174–1179.

Karalunas, S. L., Fair, D., Musser, E. D., Aykes, K., Iyer, S. P., & Nigg, J. T. (2014). Subtyping attention-deficit/hyperactivity disorder using temperament dimensions: Toward biologically based nosologic criteria. *JAMA Psychiatry, 71*(9), 1015–1024. doi: 10.1001/jamapsychiatry.2014.763

Kozak, M. J., & Cuthbert, B. N. (2016). The NIMH research domain criteria initiative: Background, issues, and pragmatics. *Psychophysiology, 53*(3), 286–297.

Krueger, R. F. (1999). The structure of common mental disorders. *Archives of General Psychiatry, 56*(10), 921–926.

Krueger, R. F., & Markon, K. E. (2011). A dimensional-spectrum model of psychopathology: Progress and opportunities. *Archives of General Psychiatry, 68*(1), 10–11.

Krystal, A. D., Pizzagalli, D. A., Mathew, S. J., Sanacora, G., Keefe, R., Song, A., … Potter, W. (2019). The first implementation of the NIMH FAST-FAIL approach to psychiatric drug development. *Nature Reviews Drug Discovery, 18*(1), 82–84. doi: 10.1038/nrd.2018.222

Kupfer, D. J., & Regier, D. A. (2011). Neuroscience, clinical evidence, and the future of psychiatric classification in DSM-5. *American Journal of Psychiatry, 168*(7), 672–674.

Lang, P. J., & Bradley, M. M. (2010). Emotion and the motivational brain. *Biological Psychology, 84*(3), 437–450. doi: 10.1016/j.biopsycho.2009.10.007

Lang, P. J., McTeague, L. M., & Bradley, M. M. (2016). RDoC, DSM, and the reflex physiology of fear: A biodimensional analysis of the anxiety disorders spectrum. *Psychophysiology, 53*(3), 336–347. doi: 10.1111/psyp.12462

Markon, K. E., & Krueger, R. F. (2005). Categorical and continuous models of liability to externalizing disorders: A direct comparison in NESARC. *Archives of General Psychiatry, 62*(12), 1352–1359. doi: 10.1001/archpsyc.62.12.1352

Marquand, A. F., Wolfers, T., Mennes, M., Buitelaar, J., & Beckmann, C. F. (2016). Beyond lumping and splitting: A review of computational approaches for stratifying psychiatric disorders. *Biological Psychiatry: Cognitive Neuroscience and Neuroimaging, 1*(5), 433–447.

Miller, G. A. (2010). Mistreating psychology in the decades of the brain. *Perspectives on Psychological Science: A Journal of the Association for Psychological Science, 5*(6), 716–743. doi: 10.1177/1745691610388774

Paul, G. L. (1969). *Behavior modification research: Design and tactics.* New York: McGraw-Hill.

Paulus, M. P., Huys, Q. J. M., & Maia, T. V. (2016). A roadmap for the development of applied computational psychiatry. *Biological Psychiatry: Cognitive Neuroscience and Neuroimaging, 1*(5), 386–392. doi: 10.1016/j.bpsc.2016.05.001

Prince, M., Patel, V., Saxena, S., Maj, M., Maselko, J., Phillips, M. R., & Rahman, A. (2007). No health without mental health. *The Lancet, 370*(9590), 859–877.

Robins, E., & Guze, S. B. (1970). Establishment of diagnostic validity in psychiatric illness: Its application to schizophrenia. *American Journal of Psychiatry, 126*(7), 983–987.

Sambuco, N., Bradley, M., Herring, D., Hillbrandt, K., & Lang, P. J. (2019). Transdiagnostic trauma severity in anxiety and mood disorders: Functional brain activity during emotional scene processing. *Psychophysiology*, e13349. Advanced online publication. doi: 10.1111/psyp.13349

Sanislow, C. A., Pine, D. S., Quinn, K. J., Kozak, M. J., Garvey, M. A., Heinssen, R. K., … & Cuthbert, B. N. (2010). Developing constructs for psychopathology research: research domain criteria. *Journal of Abnormal Psychology, 119*(4), 631.

Slade, T. I. M., & Watson, D. (2006). The structure of common DSM-IV and ICD-10 mental disorders in the Australian general population. *Psychological Medicine, 36*(11), 1593–1600.

Spitzer, R. L., Endicott, J., & Robins, E. (1978). Research diagnostic criteria: Rationale and reliability. *Archives of General Psychiatry, 35*(6), 773–782.

Tamminga, C. A., Pearlson, G. D., Stan, A. D., Gibbons, R. D., Padmanabhan, J., Keshavan, M., & Clementz, B. A. (2017). Strategies for advancing disease definition using biomarkers and genetics: The Bipolar and Schizophrenia Network for Intermediate Phenotypes. *Biological Psychiatry: Cognitive Neuroscience and Neuroimaging, 2*(1), 20–27. doi: 10.1016/j.bpsc.2016.07.005

Vinogradov, S. (2019, March 29). Cognitive training for neural system dysfunction in psychotic disorders. *Psychiatric Times*. Retrieved from https://www.psychiatrictimes.com/article/cognitive-training-neural-system-dysfunction-psychotic-disorders

Weisz, J. R., Sandler, I. N., Durlak, J. A., & Anton, B. S. (2005). Promoting and protecting youth mental health through evidence-based prevention and treatment. *American Psychologist, 60*(6), 628–648. doi: 10.1037/0003-066X.60.6.628

Widiger, T. A., & Samuel, D. B. (2005). Diagnostic categories or dimensions? A question for the Diagnostic and Statistical Manual of Mental Disorders—fifth edition. *Journal of Abnormal Psychology, 114*(4), 494–504. doi: 10.1037/0021-843X.114.4.494

Wilson, S., & Sponheim, S. R. (2014). Dimensions underlying psychotic and manic symptomatology: Extending normal-range personality traits to schizophrenia and bipolar spectra. *Comprehensive Psychiatry, 55*(8), 1809–1819.

Wolfers, T., Doan, N. T., Kaufmann, T., Alnæs, D., Moberget, T., Agartz, I., … Marquand, A. F. (2018). Mapping the heterogeneous phenotype of schizophrenia and bipolar disorder using normative models. *JAMA Psychiatry, 75*(11), 1146–1155. doi: 10.1001/jamapsychiatry.2018.2467

World Health Organization. (2018). *International classification of diseases and related health problems* (11th rev.). Geneva, Switzerland: Author.

Yee, C. M., Javitt, D. C., & Miller, G. A. (2015). Replacing DSM categorical analyses with dimensional analyses in psychiatry research: The Research Domain Criteria Initiative. *JAMA Psychiatry, 72*(12), 1159–1160.

CHAPTER 3

Shifting Paradigms
From the DSM to the Process of Change[1]

J. Scott Fraser, PhD
Wright State University

In 1962, American physicist Thomas Kuhn published a book that became so influential that it outsold copies of the Bible the subsequent year. His book, *The Structure of Scientific Revolutions* (Kuhn, 1962), introduced the concept of paradigms and paradigm shifts as an explanation of how all mature domains of scientific inquiry evolve and advance. Kuhn used the term in two ways. First, he pointed to what members of the scientific community have in common in terms of viewpoints, approaches, assumptions, and values. Second, he used it to orient toward a particular set of assumptions, premises, and rules of investigation defining a coherent tradition of investigation.

Kuhn placed unique emphasis on how groups of scientists decided to follow a particular paradigm, believing that the process of choosing a paradigm is as important as the nature of the paradigm itself. By his reckoning, the community of practitioners and investigators within a domain of science hold particular sway over what paradigm is adopted and sustained at any given time. Thus, the investigators and the paradigm are, in some ways, inseparable.

While there are gray areas over what is and is not a paradigm, in the realm of psychological problems and their resolution, few would disagree that the predominant paradigm over the past fifty years has been the medical model. In accord with Kuhn, the medical model not only established a set of premises and related practices, but it also became the predominant vehicle

---

[1] Adapted from Fraser, J. S. (2018). *Unifying effective psychotherapies: Tracing the process of change.* Washington, DC: APA Books.

shaping the search for what works in psychotherapy and the research findings that resulted. Shifting this paradigm is a momentous task, yet the time has come for such a shift (Fraser, 2018; Hayes & Hofmann, 2017, 2018; Hayes et al., 2019; Hofmann & Hayes, 2018).

In this chapter, I will note the nature of the medical model in psychological intervention and the tension it caused between the search for specific and common factors of change. I will explore this tension from a social constructionist and systems perspective on process-oriented therapy and attempt to link this approach to the more cognitive behavioral perspective to process-based therapy represented by the editors of this volume. While these two visions are not identical, I will try to show that the overlap suggests that a paradigm shift may be underway that crosses traditional boundaries defined by a school or therapeutic approach.

The Nature of the Problem in Psychotherapy

Thanks to sixty-five years of intensive research, we now know that psychotherapy is clearly effective. Despite being one of the best-validated interventions in health care, psychotherapy still lacks a scientifically grounded theory of psychological *change*.

Part of that asymmetry is due to the medical model, which cast psychological intervention as a specific set of techniques that could address the mental health manifestations of latent diseases that were reflected by specific psychiatric syndromes. This general approach was much in keeping with the history of medical science and practice. In the early 1900s, following a philosophy of science that emphasized *objectivism*, medicine began to emphasize observable results (mainly in the organismic, biological, or materialistic sphere of observations). In this approach, researchers looked for *specific effects* that proved that a specific treatment or medication was more effective than placebos for a specific disorder or medical diagnosis. If so, the search could eventually continue for a *specified cause or explanation* that altered a specifiable *mechanism of change*.

In many areas of medicine, this approach worked quite well. For example, over the past century, the medical model has been relatively effective for determining, through research, what specific medication or practice components work for specific physical health diagnoses. In the case of psychotherapy, however, the identification of successful mechanisms of action has been delayed almost indefinitely as specific protocols have targeted specific syndromes and sub-syndromes. Over the last thirty years, the list of "evidence-based" psychotherapies has grown so large that it is hard for a therapy practitioner to even know what they are, and learning and practicing all these techniques in a satisfactory manner is simply not possible. A visit to the website for the American Psychological Association's Society of Clinical Psychology finds a list of eighty (and counting) current evidence-supported treatments (ESTs) for a variety of disorders, many of which claim to require many months or even years of training in order to apply them properly (see http://www.div12.org/PsychologicalTreatments/faq.html).

Psychotherapy Wars
THE SEARCH FOR SPECIFIC FACTORS

As can be seen, once psychotherapy was generally found to be effective, the field turned to determine which approach to psychotherapy was most effective and what specific techniques or other factors contributed to that effectiveness. Such approaches were termed ESTs, and there is a very strong literature backing up these ESTs. An all-time classic text reviewing research on psychotherapy, *Bergin and Garfield's Handbook of Psychotherapy and Behavior Change* (Lambert, 2013), is in its fifth edition. Nathan and Gorman's book on ESTs, *A Guide to Treatments That Work* (Nathan & Gorman, 2015), is now in its fourth edition and covers a wide range of ESTs, and it is one of Oxford Press's best sellers. Building on this trend, Oxford Press is now publishing an extensive set of treatment manuals and workbooks on specific ESTs for specific disorders in their *Treatments That Work* series. David Barlow has now published the fifth edition of the best seller, *Clinical Handbook of Psychological Disorders: A Step-by-Step Treatment Manual* (Barlow, 2014), which offers both research and clinical examples of applications of EST approaches to a similarly wide range of specific disorders.

This growing literature has made ESTs more accessible to practitioners and fueled the movement toward disseminating ESTs into everyday clinical practice. While eminently reasonable, the focus on technique over processes of change has provided no restraint on an ever-growing list of specific approaches for specific problems. The frequent finding that different ESTs produce similar effects has weakened interest in finding the one "best" approach, but the absence of evidence regarding process of change means that practitioners face a confusing collection of often rather unrelated approaches.

THE COMMON FACTORS REJOINDER

Building upon the growing research evidence emphasizing the influence of so-called common factors, as indicated by Lambert (Lambert, 1992) and Wampold (Wampold, 2001; Wampold & Imel, 2015), there has emerged an equally strong and competing voice calling attention to the influence of common factors across the entire spectrum of psychotherapy. Based on meta-analyses of extensive psychotherapy research studies, a competing set of researchers have concluded that such common factors account for the lion's share of the variance related to change as opposed to only minor contributions from factors specific to any given approach and rationale. This competing voice might be termed ESRs, or evidence-supported relationships. Based upon the collected efforts of the American Psychological Association's Division of Psychotherapy, an overview of the research evidence supporting common factors in psychotherapy was published. Now in its second edition, *Psychotherapy Relationships That Work: Evidence-Based Responsiveness, Second Edition* (Norcross, 2011) offers an accessible overview of research supporting the influence of the *therapeutic alliance, empathy, goal consensus and collaboration, client state of change,* and a range of other factors found to be quite powerful in accounting for client success in psychotherapy. Another influential edited book emphasizing the power of common factors in psychotherapy is *The Heart and Soul of Change: What Works in Therapy*, now also in its second edition (Duncan, Miller, Wampold, & Hubble, 2010; Hubble, Duncan, & Miller, 1999). It is worth noting that these identified common factors are less technological and specific and more focused on the processes within the relationship between the practitioner and client. As might be expected, these two warring camps have battled over the better part of a decade in what might be termed therapy wars, and the war still rages.

A MOVEMENT TOWARD FLEXIBILITY AND FIT

However, there is a growing agreement that common factors cannot stand alone, nor can specific factors. They are always embedded within and facilitated by a given agreed-upon *therapeutic rationale*. Therapy without an explanation is not sufficient. Laska and Wampold (2014) reiterate this point as they say, "One of the aspects of all treatments is that the patients are provided an explanation for their disorder and that there are treatment actions consistent with that explanation" (p. 520). The particular theoretical explanation or rationale used is most likely to emerge from a *best fit between the perspectives of the client and therapist*. Agreement on tasks and goals of therapy is highly correlated with successful treatment and is facilitated further by agreement on a therapeutic rationale to explain the nature of the client problem and to imply a direction to move toward resolution. This is an evolution from the recent polarities of the specific factors versus common factors debate that alters the definition of "what works" in psychotherapy.

Thus, with all of the positions on the debate about what works in psychotherapy in mind, what conclusions may we draw? There is now no doubt that psychotherapy can and does work, but exactly how the *process* comes together is still evolving. Evidence supports a growing number of approaches to treatment, such as cognitive behavioral therapy (CBT), acceptance and commitment therapy (ACT), interpersonal therapy (IPT), emotion-focused therapy (EFT), behavioral activation, prolonged exposure, and mindfulness-based therapy, to name but a few. Yet the field is moving toward agreement that effective treatment is not all about techniques or one theoretical rationale. It must include considerations such as the *qualities and expertise of the therapist;* the *qualities, values, cultures, and preferences of clients;* and consideration of the *best evidence we have on what has been found to work with different problems*. To this end, the field is moving toward addressing *context*, toward clarifying *the nature of change and the theories of change*, and toward identifying *principles of change*. While the future is hopeful for identifying these unifying concepts and practices, the outcome remains to be seen.

Shifting Paradigms

Currently, there are unanimous calls for practitioners to use only evidence-based approaches, yet for the most common psychological problems seen in clinicians' offices—anxiety and depression—there are several ESTs for each. Most of them have different premises for how the problems developed and how they are to be effectively treated. Yet they are all equally effective. How can this be? The positivist premises underlying the rational empirical and clinical trial approaches assume that there will be one correct and most effective approach tracing the cause of these problems and their effective treatment. Currently, there is no unifying perspective to account for such widespread yet diverse effectiveness. This cries out for a more transdiagnostic and transtheoretical meta-theory or point of view. As the field has begun to move beyond terms like "transdiagnostic," which still implies traditional use of medical model notions of diagnoses, it is adopting a more process-based way of conceptualizing and describing personal and interpersonal distress. In answer to this need, a process of change perspective, linked with dynamical systems theory, is emerging as an alternative paradigm to fill this void, as is reflected in this volume (Fraser, 2018; Hayes & Hofmann, 2017, 2018; Hayes et al., 2019; Hofmann & Hayes, 2018). This change is now allowing a more integrative conversation between the different wings of the field, such as traditional CBT and relationship-oriented approaches.

SHIFTING PHASES

Kuhn (1962) suggests that while shifts in paradigms typically make watershed differences in the way a given discipline views its subject and interacts with it, those shifts are usually long and fraught with conflict. Based on a historical examination of many such shifts, Kuhn describes a characteristic set of phases that are likely to occur, each of which carries implications for the field in focus. First, the predominant paradigm begins accumulating a growing set of anomalies not well explained or predicted within that paradigm. This may sound familiar in the domain of psychotherapy, where the underlying cause of problems remains elusive, numerous effective therapies exist, and their mechanisms of action are unknown or unsupportive of their putative model. Once the set of anomalies nears a critical number of unaccounted-for problems, the discipline is thrown into a crisis where alternate ideas or perspectives are tried, some of which may have existed all along. A process view of systemic change has long existed in parallel to a medical view. Eventually, camps of followers of new perspectives form and begin to clash with those holding to the old paradigm, and often vicious attacks and debates follow for years (sometimes ending only as the old guard dies out). This long battle stands in contrast with some popular ideas of "paradigm shifts" happening in the blink of an eye. The intense arguments between the so-called specific factor advocates versus the common factor camp in explaining the effects of psychotherapy could be an example of such a debate. Different forms of a process perspective appear to be emerging out of both camps, suggesting that a paradigm shift may indeed be underway (Fraser, 2018; Hayes & Hofmann, 2017, 2018; Hayes et al., 2019; Hofmann & Hayes, 2018).

Shifting to a Process View: A Constructionist and Systems-Oriented Perspective

From the social constructionist (cf. Gergen, 2015) and systems-oriented process view I represent, there is a unity that connects all effective psychotherapies (Fraser, 2018). This unity transcends both diagnosis and theoretical perspectives—it is transdiagnostic and transtheoretical—or, better said, beyond traditional diagnoses. It represents an alternative paradigm to the current medical model, which is guided by positivism, reductionism, and linear research designs. From the view of the philosophy of science, this unity follows from the process view of Alfred North Whitehead (Whitehead, 1978). Whitehead's process system view suggests that everything is a process. The appearance of enduring substance or structures is only a product of our limited point of view or ideas on what we are observing. The universe is a set of relationships between relationships between relationships—all of which change over time. This is a nonlinear process view. What we view as a system is merely an observation of events in the process of change at a given segment of time. A patient's panic attacks, a couple's struggles, or a nation's changes are all a product of our focus and definitions of those interactions. This alternate perspective has watershed effects in resolving current muddles and conflicts in the domain of effective psychotherapies.

With regard to the process perspective, Nicholas Rescher (1996) has said, "The guiding idea of this approach is that natural existence consists in and is best understood in terms of *processes* rather than *things*—of modes of change rather than fixed stabilities" (p. 7, emphasis added). This idea is not new. In ancient Greece, Heraclitus launched this approach in his dictum "everything flows." Later, Leibniz (1646-1717) became a proponent of process theory in modern philosophy, suggesting that all things are mere phenomena and not unified substances at all. Moreover, Hegel (1770-1831), through his dialectic view of the interaction of opposites, argued that whatever exists in the world of things or ideas is never stable but always in the process of evolving and changing. Nonetheless, while there are other key figures along this recent history, the work of Alfred North Whitehead (1861-1947) in his seminal work, *Process and Reality* (Whitehead, 1978), has become synonymous with the constructivist and systems-oriented process view in recent times and has clear links to pragmatic perspectives that underlie other process-based accounts.

Summarizing the process view, Rescher (1996) suggests the following:

- Process philosophy "is really less of a theory than a point of view taking the line that one must prioritize processes over things and activities over substances... Process philosophy thus prioritizes change and development in all of its aspects over fixity and persistence" (p. 35).

- Process in this view represents "a coordinated group of changes in the complexion of reality, an organized family of occurrences that are systematically linked to one another either causally or functionally... Processes are correlated with occurrences or events: Processes always involve various events, and events exist only in and through processes" (p. 39).

- Processes may also evolve over time and can encompass changes without themselves changing. In this sense, "things" should always be viewed as processes. Therefore, a "thing" such as a river becomes an enduring entity while still flowing and changing.

- Referring to Heraclitus's famous dictum "You can never step into the same river twice," Rescher (1996) suggests, "Heraclitus was only half right: We indeed do not step twice into the same *waters*, but we can certainly step twice into the same *river*" (p. 52–53). Practically speaking, a client may experience panic attacks in different situations and with different intensity, yet that person remains the same client with the same repeating panic attack process. Thus, the emphasis in a process view is upon constant change within *systems*, and these systems are dependent in their definition upon the *observer*.

What we view as observers and describers within our worlds depends upon the nature of our language, constructs, culture, and the focus of our interests and attention. Furthermore, our concepts and related actions develop through an ongoing process of interaction with our world. This is a co-creative process. From this process view, the universe is a set of relationships between relationships between relationships, all of which change over time, and none of these relationships are ever static. In the process view, process is primary, and what we call substance is merely a temporary pattern produced by that process. Thus, our description of a given problem as "anxiety" or "depression" may reflect a description of what we view as a common process within our cultural context at a given time and from a given set of concepts on the nature of such problems. The appearance of enduring substances is thus merely a product of our limited point of view. The description of static reality as simply the product of our limited perspective of an ongoing pattern at a given time has also led us to the postmodern views of socially constructed realities and cultural and cross-cultural diversity in perspectives. This represents a social constructionist view (Gergen, 2015). Thus, the frames we use to construct our world constrain the process of interactions, and those interactions further refine and evolve our frames.

The same is true for the therapeutic rationales we use to guide different approaches to psychotherapy. They each become both enlightening and self-confirming. In open social systems, a given problem may have a range of different causes or starting points, and from the same starting point, a wide range of eventual states may evolve. What is viewed as a problem and is expressed one way within one culture may not be expressed the same way or even be seen as a problem within another culture. Something that may seem to be an outrageous, paradoxical, or counterintuitive solution to a given problem may be just the right resolution. Understandably, this process view may seem vague and abstract at this time. However, when winnowed down, it offers a way of thinking that solves some of the current challenges, muddles, and controversies facing the idea of psychological problems and effective treatments in psychotherapy. This is very different from the underlying assumptions of the medical model, which focuses on which treatments are best for which problems.

Strange Attractors and Common Human Problems

Culture, language, history, and norms define what we perceive as problems and what we are to do about them. They define what are termed first-order solutions or "first-order change," which target problem resolution (Fraser & Solovey, 2007; Fraser, 2018). They represent simple rules like "pull back from potential pain" or "try again if at first we don't succeed."

Such first-order solutions persist because they usually work. However, when they fail, solution patterns often redouble in characteristic escalating *vicious cycles,* which only exacerbate the problem they aim to resolve. This becomes a self-organizing pattern around a targeted domain and a goal or a "strange attractor" in dynamical systems terms. It becomes a *solution-generated problem.* It is self-perpetuating, escalating, and tends to be constrained by characteristic ideas and roles of behavior within a given context of culture, language, norms, and rules of behavior that usually work. Thus, the repeatedly failed solutions nevertheless "make sense" to the problem solvers. Furthermore, each iteration of such solution patterns is self-similar to others in classic repeated patterns within the system.

COMMON PROBLEMS

Some common examples of such self-organizing, strange attractors with self-similar patterns are anxiety, grief, and post-traumatic stress disorder (PTSD), to name but a few. These classic problems usually pattern around the rule of "mastery by avoidance." They include solutions whose goal is to move away from or to control potential anxiety-provoking, grief-inducing, or traumatic stimuli or memories. As noted, such solutions "make sense" within the history, culture, language, norms, and traditions of the people involved. Therefore, they typically redouble with variations of intensity, frequency, location, and so forth—yet each represents the same self-similar pattern with classic escalating results.

RESOLUTIONS

Solutions different from these dominant, repeated patterns usually seem "counterintuitive" or "paradoxical" from within the constraints of the problematic system. This is similar to the classic children's finger trap toy, where logical attempts to free one's fingers by pulling them out is only solved by the counterintuitive solution of pushing them in. Such counterintuitive yet effective solutions most often resolve, redirect, or dissolve their classic problem cycles. This class of solutions is termed "second-order change." It originates from outside the typical first-order constraints, ideas, and patterned rules of the problematic system pattern (Fraser & Solovey, 2007).

Regarding the common problems of anxiety, grief, and PTSD, all effective psychotherapies converge on the same class of pattern disruption involving pattern reversal. They target second-order change. To do so, however, they must link with the patterned constraints, ideas, and solutions of the self-organizing system. They must offer frames for the problem and associated rationales for new solutions that "make sense" to all involved, both clients and therapists. From this view, such frames and related rationales represent the theories and related practices of the various effective psychotherapies available. Some approaches will *fit* with the client and therapist alike, and some will not. Therapists must therefore be *flexible* so they can fit the theory and related rationales to both themselves and the client-systems in question to enable the pattern reversals and to allow significant differences to be initiated and subsequently supported toward resolution. Once new concepts or solution patterns begin, they are then reinforced to initiate new *virtuous cycles* from the former vicious cycles of the problematic, classic patterns of anxiety, grief, or PTSD. From the process view and dynamical systems perspective, all effective therapies do this. Problems often evolve from small yet meaningful differences or triggers, and similarly, therapeutic solutions often evolve from small yet significant differences that make a difference (Fraser, 2018).

Depression as a Case in Point

Turning to the example of depression, let us examine three very different yet strongly evidence-supported psychological treatments summarized in Table 1. Such a diverse array of effective approaches presents a challenge for the medical model. The medical model would assume a specific cause or origin of the latent disease that underlies depression and would assume that it is best treated or cured by a specific treatment. The medical model struggles with the existence of multiple different effective approaches, each of which assumes a different set of causes and applies different treatment procedures.

Table 1. Evidence-Supported Psychological Treatments for Depression
(from http://www.div12.org/psychological-treatments/disorders/depression/)

Therapy	Basic Premise	Essence of Therapy
Cognitive Therapy	Aaron T. Beck's cognitive theory of depression proposes that people susceptible to depression develop inaccurate and unhelpful core beliefs about themselves, others, and the world as a result of their learning histories. These beliefs can be dormant for extended periods of time and are activated by life events that carry specific meaning for that person. Core beliefs that render someone susceptible to depression are broadly categorized into beliefs about being unlovable, worthless, helpless, and incompetent. Cognitive theory also focuses on information-processing deficits, selective attention, and memory biases toward the negative.	In cognitive therapy, clients are taught cognitive and behavioral skills so they can develop more accurate and helpful beliefs and so they can eventually become their own therapists.
Interpersonal Therapy	Depression often follows changes in one's interpersonal environment (e.g., struggles with a significant other, loss of a loved one). Once depressed, symptoms can lead to compromised interpersonal functioning, which can precipitate continued stressful events. The goal in therapy is to address both the stressful life events and improve social support.	Interpersonal therapy focuses on improving problematic interpersonal relationships or circumstances that are directly related to the current depressive episode.
Behavioral Activation	When people get depressed, they may increasingly disengage from their routines and withdraw from their environment. Over time, this avoidance exacerbates depressed mood as individuals lose opportunities to be positively reinforced through pleasant experiences, social activity, or experiences of mastery.	Behavioral activation seeks to increase the patient's contact with sources of reward by helping them get more active and, in so doing, improves their life context. One version of behavioral activation (BATD) is briefer, focusing specifically on identifying values that will guide the selection of activities. In addition to a focus on increasing activities, the second version of behavioral activation also works on identifying processes that inhibit activation and encourage avoidance as well as on teaching problem-solving skills.

However, what if the root cause of depression is not what creates the problem? Instead, what if *the current pattern of interaction of the system* (or in this case, the way a person is struggling to rid themself of depression) is what creates the problem? Given that the manner in which each person is struggling to recover "makes sense" to them, altering the pattern of their current solutions for being depressed is hard for them to conceive. Such alternatives may not make sense or may even feel somehow uncomfortable. They need someone who understands their plight and who is supportive of their goal to feel better. They need an explanation for their situation that makes sense or that fits in some way with the way they view themself and their world. Yet they also need a rationale that makes sense of how and why they should take action on their depression in a new way that may actually help them recover. Finally, they need a compassionate, supportive, and skilled guide to help them through that journey to change. Each of these evidence-supported approaches in question (as well as other equally effective treatments for depression) represents a different yet equally plausible description of the reasons why a person may have become depressed, and each approach offers a reasonable path toward change. The extent to which each approach makes sense or fits with the client and the therapist as they negotiate an alliance is the extent to which each approach is likely to be effective in shifting the vicious cycle patterns of the client's conceived problem.

Process and Change in Depression

It is worth recalling that a systems-oriented process perspective views all problems as vicious cycles of clients' often well-meaning solutions (or first-order changes) within the context of the way they explain their circumstances and what "makes sense" to resolve their dilemma. Group theory (cf. Fraser, 2018) suggests that such problems cannot be resolved from within the premises, rules, and patterns of the group. Clients must step out of their problem-generated system to a meta-level (or make a second-order change) in order to reflect on their assumptions and solution patterns and consider alternative courses. Each of the effective approaches listed in Table 1 does just this. Most often, the new solution patterns will appear counterintuitive or paradoxical from the original group level and will rarely be considered. Each of these effective approaches offers a new frame for the client's problem and a related rationale to make sense of formerly counterintuitive solutions.

In many ways, all treatments seek to initiate some form of problem pattern disruption or difference, but that difference must be a difference that *makes* a difference. First-order changes within the current rules and patterns of a client's problem simply reaffirm the problem and are more of the same patterns. Second-order change *changes the system itself.* Clients must effectively join a meta-level group with therapists to form a working alliance to resolve their problems. Joining in this working alliance is the first step in the second-order change process. Each of these effective approaches first allies with clients and then offers frames and rationales to make sense of formerly paradoxical pathways toward resolution. Therapists' empathy, warmth, genuineness, and validation of the client's struggle and pain open this alliance. Each of the approaches in Table 1 emphasizes such empathic joining as at least a precondition for change and sometimes as a major change itself for the client who feels flawed and unlovable.

The next step involves agreeing on a frame that helps "make sense" of the problem and its patterns for the client in new ways. This new frame enables the client and therapist to agree on a related rationale for treatment. This rationale will help formerly unconsidered or counterintuitive options make sense for the client. Most therapeutic interventions make sense within a given frame for a problem and its related treatment rationale—yet they are inherently paradoxical from the level of the client's initial understanding and related solution patterns. For example, CBT offers a cognitive frame to explain depressive self-fulfilling prophesies and encourages new actions to check out a client's negative assumptions about themselves, their situation, and their future. IPT offers an interpersonal frame to validate the client's depression and make sense of taking action on new solutions to those interpersonal issues. Behavioral activation explains the downward cycle of withdrawal from anticipated negative situations and feelings and helps clients make sense of taking opposite actions from their current avoidant solutions.

There are other equally effective approaches, and in each case, the same comments apply. For example, EFT offers an emotion-based frame for the recurrent avoidant patterns of clients' depressive cycles and explains that re-experiencing these intense emotions is the pathway toward resolving them. Acceptance and mindfulness-based approaches explain the vicious cycles of clients' depressive patterns and then teach clients to go toward depressive thoughts and triggering situations while not judging them or becoming caught into their former vicious cycles. Each effective treatment offers clients a compelling new frame to reconceptualize their cycles of depression that makes new sense of interdicting former downward cycles by taking opposite action to resolve them. Finally, the treatment alliance with the therapist supports, amplifies, and generalizes the new pattern shifts once they begin to evolve a new, virtuous cycle. Each of these effective approaches echoes the premises of a process paradigm and nonlinear dynamical theory.

While the frames and foci of these approaches may differ, if the process view I am presenting here holds true, then the process of problem pattern reversal should hold constant. As we can see, all of these different approaches converge on the same goal of pattern disruption and reversal in the vicious cycle patterns common to depression in the dominant culture. If there is general agreement that clients with depression tend to react to distressing perceived losses and life changes by withdrawing, avoiding, and ruminating in a downward spiral, then effective interventions will reverse these patterns in some way. This is process-based unification.

The Process of Unifying Effective Therapies

In human social systems, norms, social conventions, concepts, and expectations reflect the constraints of a given social system. The context of our clients' lives, including their culture, language, personal histories, and identities, channel the flow of their lives. The same applies to therapists. Shifting frames and metaphors through therapy rationales and interventions may rechannel that flow. Similarly, rechanneling their behavior or interactions may alter their frames, metaphors, and context.

The relevance of this approach can be seen by revisiting how therapy works from the perspective of the medical model. Given the constraints of the medical model, clinicians can explain how therapy works from their given theoretical perspective. At the same time, perspectives cannot go outside of themselves to explain how other therapies work. Clinicians trained in CBT can explain what they think they are doing from a CBT perspective, but they cannot explain how IPT works. The reverse is also the case for the IPT perspective. If both therapies are equally effective and operate on different premises, then the credibility of the premises that underlie each therapy is suspect. The best we can say is that both work for unknown reasons.

A unity emerges as we understand psychotherapy from a systems-oriented process view. From this unity, practitioners of all theoretical persuasions note, interrupt, and redirect vicious cycles. At this meta-level, the goals of effective interventions are to note, create, and then support virtuous cycles. This may sound easier said than done, and it often is. However, this process is at the heart of all effective psychotherapies. The case of depression is simply one example.

Unifying Effective Psychotherapies Through a Process Paradigm

So what does all of this have to do with integrating psychotherapies that work? The answer is that, from a process view, all problems are vicious cycle patterns rooted in context. The goal of all treatments that work from this process perspective is therefore a *pattern shift* in those vicious cycles. From the process view, context and process combine to shape change. A shift in context, process, or both around vicious cycles *defines success across all treatments that work.* Thus, when psychotherapies work, from the process view, they all achieve a pattern shift in one way or another. This focus on pattern shift or change is lacking in all current approaches to integrating psychotherapies that work. The process perspective offers a platform that unifies all psychotherapies that work around these principles of context, process, and change. All of this emerges from the process paradigm.

Principles of a Process Paradigm

Given the twists and turns we have taken through our discussion of systems and process theories, a summary of key points might be helpful. These may be viewed as more explicit and testable hypotheses of this version of a process-based approach to therapy. Therefore, to be more explicit on the general assumptions of this process of change view, the following principles characterize relatively open, complex systems like social relationships:

- *Observers define systems.* There are no systems out there that exist separately from the concepts, focus, and interests of observers. Whitehead's process system view suggests that everything is a process. The appearance of enduring substance or structures is only a product of our limited point of view or ideas on what we are observing. The universe is a set of relationships between relationships between relationships—all of which change over time. What we view as a system is merely an observation of events in the process of change at a given segment of time. A patient's panic attacks, a couple's struggles, or a nation's changes are all a product of our focus and definitions of those interactions.

- *Change is constant and can be rapid.* Stability and structure are a product of an observer's description of ongoing process at a specific time and space in the life of a system. Yet, as in the succeeding phases of Heraclitus's river—as it moves from wide ponds to steeper narrows with boulders to cascading waterfalls—change can also be rapid as the system often rapidly shifts in intensity, direction, or both over time. This applies equally to the lives of our clients and to the life of the process of therapy.

- *Process is primary.* Because in open systems, you can get to any arbitrary end from a wide variety of beginnings—and conversely, because the same beginning point may result in widely different arbitrary ends—*contingencies and interacting processes are critical. Current process is the best definition and access point into any given system.* History is always relevant but does not always predict the same end, such as a panic attack, a dissolved relationship, or the fall of the Berlin wall.

- *The goal of psychotherapy is shifting patterns.* Patterns are a sample of a chosen process of interaction at a given point in time and space in the ongoing system. The interacting patterns of a couple leading to their eventual breakup is just one example. One might choose different samples and punctuate them in different ways, yet they would all reflect the couple's distress. Furthermore, patterns repeat in self-similar cycles across time and scope. This is especially true around the vicious cycles of clients' problems.

- *A small sample of current patterns may reflect much larger system patterns.* As in the fractal principle of self-similar patterns occurring at successively larger scales in dynamical systems, such as human interaction (cf. Briggs & Pete, 1989), a smaller sample of patterned process may suffice to surmise an overriding similar process over time. From this view, just a few examples or iterations of a college student's attempts to control his panic become emblematic of variations on the same patterned and escalating cycles over time. John Gottman (1999) has shown that a five-minute sample of a couple disagreeing can predict eventual divorce with a high degree of accuracy.

- *Small changes can have cascading large results.* The overriding effects of positive feedback loops within the regularities of an open social system will tend to amplify change over time. As reported, a misinterpreted message delivered on one night in Berlin led to the cascading and dramatic opening of the monolithic Berlin wall. A slight difference while plotting weather patterns led a researcher to the idea of the "butterfly effect" (Briggs & Peat, 1989). Similarly, a key reframe in psychotherapy, or a random difference in a client's life outside of treatment, may quickly lead to problem resolution for clients.

- *Not all small changes will initiate cascading change.* Each system has certain sensitive points of information that are more likely to create a reaction. The system may react to the same difference by viewing it as a potential threat to the system or by viewing it as a potential opportunity, and so on. The point is that each system has parameters that will identify *a difference that may make a difference.* Some call these "vulnerabilities" (Barlow & Kennedy, 2016; Moses & Barlow, 2006). This is the influence of context. The college student's panic attacks might have been initiated by perceived situations that threatened to make him lose control. A husband's jealous rages may have been triggered by his history of a prior partner's deceit and lost relationships. The fall of the Berlin wall was likely triggered by a critical misperceived message (cf. Fraser, 2018).

- *Positive and negative feedback loops are complementary.* In response to a perceived difference, attempts at balance through negative feedback at one level may have the successive results of creating a positive escalating feedback over time. Our college student's attempt to calm down in the face of potential panic may have only fed back into cycles of anxiety and growing panic. His solutions would have become the problem, just as a husband's jealous attempts to prevent his wife's potential attraction to another man may have only driven a wedge between them.

- *Constancy/stability and change are interrelated.* As we see in Heraclitus's river, the water in the river might change in multiple ways while the identity of the river remains the same. The banks of the river may erode more slowly while the turbulence of the stream may increase and create sudden shifts; but the identity of the stream remains constant. Constancy and change exist at different levels while both are in the process of change. Clients who attempt the same solutions with more intensity and variations on the same theme perpetuate and escalate their problem. Their solutions become the problem and perpetuate its identity.

- *Rules, regularities, and constraints within open systems channel their ongoing interaction patterns.* In Heraclitus's river, the constraints of the riverbank, the steepness (or angle) of the river bottom, and the placement of boulders constrain and channel the flow of water in the stream. In human social systems, norms, social conventions, concepts, and expectations reflect the constraints of a given social system. The context of our clients' lives, including their culture, language, personal histories, and identities channel the flow of their lives. Shifting frames and metaphors through therapy rationales and interventions may rechannel that flow. Similarly, rechanneling their behavior or interactions may alter their frames, metaphors, and context.

Cycling Back

The above principles of a systems-oriented process view help unify effective psychotherapies transdiagnostically and transtheoretically—and in many ways beyond diagnoses and theories as we use them now. Some practical, more explicit, and testable applications for therapists and researchers thus emerge as follows:

- How problem patterns begin is less important than the current patterns or solutions clients are using as they wrestle with it here and now. There is no single invariant cause for any general psychological problem as postulated by the medical model.

- A small sample of clients' current solutions should generalize to repeating patterns across time and situations, as they represent self-similar patterns. As noted above, this has been clearly shown, for example, with distressed couples where very limited interaction samples have shown high predictive power for divorce.

- The dominant culture's research literature on typical or general problem patterns for the most common problems offers guidance on what a clinician might expect to see for any given client within that cultural context. Culture and context are thus seen as moderators of common problem patterns. Traditional research should not be discarded, in that it tends to show regularities in problem patterns within a given dominant culture. However, clinicians and researchers must always be open to unique or idiographic variations based upon clients' unique histories, culture, language, norms, and so on. Further, as we will discuss in the final section of this chapter, alternate research methods, often using more idiographic approaches, will be needed to empirical study generic and specific variations of problem patterns and to fit effective treatment approaches to those variations.

- The cultural and personal contexts of clients will then combine to form the unique constraints that shape the specific vicious cycles for each client. There are generic and idiographic variations of depression, based on context and history, across different clients.

- The dominant culture's research literature on effective treatments for various problems offers valuable frames, rationales, and tools that work to create successful vicious cycle pattern shifts for each general problem. These contribute to *flexibility* and *fit*.

- *Fitting* these various treatment approaches to what "makes sense" for the client and therapist is the task of treatment planning. This implies that therapists have knowledge of multiple effective approaches for a given problem and remain *flexible* to fit them to each client, as well as to deliver them authentically themselves.

- The result of a good fit is the working alliance, with positive bonds, goal consensus, and related treatment procedures targeting the ultimate goal of pattern shifts or change in the vicious cycle at hand.

- As clients gain trust and join in a meta-level alliance with their therapist or helpful other, they can gain perspective as they now reflect on the failed cyclical patterns of their problem-generating vicious cycles.

- Because all pattern reversals in vicious cycles are *counterintuitive* or *paradoxical* from the level of clients' problems, new explanations or *frames* for their problems and their related *treatment rationales* help clients "make sense" of formerly counterintuitive solutions.

- Ongoing feedback within and between sessions allows continuous adjustments maintaining the trajectory toward the ultimate outcome of pattern shift.

- As clients achieve the targeted pattern shifts, therapists support those changes and applaud clients' achievements as *personal, positive,* and *pervasive*.

- As clients resume the process of their lives, practitioners enhance resilience and instill relapse prevention by supporting flexibility, encouraging practice, predicting future challenges, and remaining open to future contact.

Finally, all of these premises, propositions, and predictions of the process view and this version of process-based therapy are open to future research. Such investigation should verify, modify, and completely revise the assumptions and propositions of the process view—and such research will require equally alternative research methods compared with those used for study within the prior medical model paradigm.

Research from a Process-Based View

I have been discussing a systems-oriented process-based perspective and showing how it can be used to move from a very broad set of concepts and assumptions to some very specific propositions and predictions about behavioral problems and their resolution. My intent in being so specific in these extrapolations is to foster their ability to be subjected to future research and to reinforce the commonalities evident in all of the approaches represented in this volume. However, the kind of research needed in this domain shows how profoundly a process-perspective impacts our field, or stated another way, why a process-based view may represent a true paradigm shift.

A process-based view calls for a set of alternative research approaches to fit its assumptions. This final section will highlight some potential alternative methods and analyses that may best fit the assumptions of the process approach underlying many chapters of this book. I will consider these issues in the context of the work on process-based therapy developed by the editors of this volume (cf. Hayes & Hofmann, 2017, 2018; Hayes et al., 2019; Hofmann & Hayes, 2018).

THERAPEUTIC PROCESS DEFINED

Hofmann and Hayes (2018) suggest "a process-based approach is the key for the future of evidence-based care" (p. 2). They go on to distinguish between *therapeutic processes* and *therapeutic procedures*. Whereas therapeutic *procedures* describe the methods or techniques used by a therapist to achieve a client's goals, therapeutic *processes* involve the following:

> *Therapeutic processes* are the underlying change mechanisms that lead to the attainment of a desirable treatment goal. We define therapeutic processes as a set of theory-based, dynamic, progressive, and multilevel changes that occur in predictable empirically established sequences oriented toward the desirable outcomes. These processes are *theory-based* and associated with falsifiable and testable predictions, they are *dynamic* because processes may involve feedback loops and nonlinear changes, they are *progressive* in the long term in order to be able to reach the treatment goal, and they form a *multilevel system* because some processes supersede others (p. 38).

PATTERNS

As noted earlier in this chapter, a process view turns our attention to interactional *patterns* around defined areas of interest—no matter whether those patterns revolve around what is described as a problem or if they address the patterns surrounding interventions that effectively interdict, redirect, or change those defined problem patterns. Advocating for more individually based models of change processes, Hofmann and Hayes (2018) suggest that a "complex network approach can offer an analytic alternative to the latent disease model. The approach holds that psychological problems are not expressions of underlying disease entities but rather are interrelated elements of a complex network" (p. 8). In our discussions earlier in this chapter, such interaction networks might be the repeated escalating vicious cycle patterns around clients' perceived problems or the evolving patterns of problem resolution through effective interventions.

BOTTOM-UP RATHER THAN TOP-DOWN ANALYSES

As opposed to the common top-down group designs of the typical randomized clinical trial approaches of the medical model, a process-based view lends itself best to a bottom-up design using more idiographic, single-subject approaches. Whereas group clinical trial research models strive for within-group homogeneity, treating individual differences as nuisance factors to be controlled for, individual designs seek to study such variations. A bottom-up approach implies that repeated observations of similar interaction patterns around a problem of interest or successful intervention may imply a broader, generalizable conclusion. Hayes, Hofmann, and colleagues (2019) suggest that "by identifying the processes responsible for promoting psychological well-being at the level of the individual and then summarizing them into nomothetic generalizations, process-based therapies can be implemented to apply specific procedures to individualized problems that are designed to modify biopsychosocial change processes in specific contexts" (p. 5). Furthermore, more idiographic approaches allow for the study of patterns over time, as well as the relation of these pattern shifts or evolution to problem development or problem resolution criteria—the heart of a process-based model's focus and predictions. Turning to idiographic research models brings several options to light.

PROMISING RESEARCH MODELS FOR A PROCESS-BASED VIEW

Without going too deeply into each approach, there are ranges of alternate research models that may fit quite well with a process-based view. Experience sampling methods (ESM) and ecological momentary assessment (EMA) collect self-reported behaviors, cognitions, and emotions from individuals in real time or at predetermined intervals in real-world settings. They collect multiple assessments over time to study how events and responses to everyday events relate to one another. Such analyses can detect shifts following interventions or events and detect moderating factors that may alter typical patterns expected in a problem in focus or an intervention studied. Measures of process in session have also been greatly aided through mechanized transcript analyses.

Time series analyses can bring light to intraindividual change processes throughout treatment, allowing statistical models of the relationship between changes in relevant variables to be determined. This hones in on the idea of tracking patterns and pattern shifts predicted in either the evolution of problems or the successful intervention in those problem patterns. Such approaches might allow us to test the proposition that vicious cycle pattern reversal accompanies subsequent symptom relief.

Complex network approaches hold even more potential for tracking the evolution of problem patterns and subsequent pattern shifts. Hayes, Hofmann, and associates (2019) note that several statistical frameworks have recently been adopted to study dynamic processes, such as the evolution of problems and successful intervention. They state, "In dynamic networks, nodes reflect features of psychopathology (e.g., anhedonia, insomnia, etc.), and directed edges can be specified to represent partial regression coefficients connecting different nodes. Because directed edges specify the direction of a relationship, such networks can provide potential information about causality using intensive time-series data" (p. 7). These sorts of analyses can show how certain processes unfold for individuals, and they can potentially be used to track predicted pattern shifts in psychotherapy. Another strength of such dynamical system analyses is that it can both plot and track potential sudden shifts predicted in psychotherapy, such as "flashes of insight" or all-or-nothing shifts from significant reframes or behavioral tasks. These sorts of analyses hold promise in conducting tipping point analyses and the like, which are reflected in chaos and catastrophe theories applied to problem development and resolution. The explicit assumptions and predictions of the process-based model presented in the previous sections of this chapter represent just one example of a process-based therapy model that is open to such research.

The deep resonance between my approach to a process-based perspective from a social constructionist and system-perspective and the work on process-based therapy by Hayes and Hofmann from a behavioral and cognitive perspective underlines how profoundly a process-view reorganizes our field.

Shifting Paradigms to the Process of Change

Psychological problems and psychotherapy are all about change. Change is what our clients want from therapy. Desire to change unwanted difficulties is what triggers their struggles to return to what they view as normal. *Their struggle to change their identified problems is the real problem.* The problem is not the trigger. The client's response to that trigger shapes their problems and their vicious cycles of first-order solutions. Therefore, from a process of change view, *change is the problem, change is the goal, and change is the solution.* According to the process-based approach described in this chapter, knowingly or not, second-order change is the target of all effective psychotherapies. This is a change in how clients are attempting to change their problem. To make this shift, clients need a fitting frame or rationale that steps them out of their current level of logical views and solutions and that enables new and, quite often, opposite solutions. All clients and therapists seek this second-order change. All effective treatments target and achieve this change. And as I've argued, it unifies them (Fraser, 2018).

All of this naturally flows from a process perspective. The coherence of such a profound set of changes suggests that a paradigm shift is implied by the movement toward a process-based view. Shifting paradigms is likely to be fraught with conflicts and dilemmas, as Thomas Kuhn warned us long ago. However, the time has come. The dominant medical model underlying the *Diagnostic and Statistical Manual of Mental Disorders* (DSM) has failed us. A process-based approach simply fits the data better.

References

Barlow, D. H. (Ed.). (2014). *Clinical handbook of psychological disorders: A step-by-step treatment manual* (5th ed.). New York: Guilford Press.

Barlow, D. H., & Kennedy, K. A. (2016). New approaches to diagnosis and treatment in anxiety and related emotional disorders: A focus on temperament. *Canadian Psychology/Psychologie Canadienne, 57*(1), 8–20.

Briggs, J., & Peat, F. D. (1989). *Turbulent mirror: An illustrated guide to chaos theory and the science of wholeness.* New York: HarperCollins Publishers.

Duncan, B. L., Miller, S. D., Wampold, B. E., & Hubble, M. A. (Eds.). (2010). *The heart and soul of change: Delivering what works in therapy.* Washington, DC: American Psychological Association.

Fraser, J. S. (2018). *Unifying effective psychotherapies: Tracing the process of change.* Washington, DC: American Psychological Association.

Fraser, J. S., & Solovey, A. D. (2007). *Second-order change in psychotherapy: The golden thread that unifies effective treatments.* Washington, DC: American Psychological Association.

Gergen, K. J. (2015). *An invitation to social construction* (3rd ed.). Los Angeles, CA: Sage.

Gottman, J. M. (1999). *The marriage clinic: A scientifically based marital therapy*. New York: W. W. Norton & Company.

Hayes, S. C., & Hofmann, S. G. (2017). The third wave of CBT and the rise of process-based care. *World Psychiatry, 16*, 245–246.

Hayes, S. C., & Hofmann, S. G. (Eds.). (2018). *Process-based CBT: The science and core clinical competencies of cognitive behavioral therapy*. Oakland, CA: Context Press/New Harbinger Publications.

Hayes, S. C., Hofmann, S. G., Stanton, C. E., Carpenter, J. K., Sanford, B. T., Curtiss, J. E., & Ciarrochi, J. (2019). The role of the individual in the coming era of process-based therapy. *Behaviour Research and Therapy, 117*, 40–53. doi: 10.1016/j.brat.2018.10.005

Hofmann, S. G., & Hayes, S. C. (2019). The future of intervention science: Process-based therapy. *Clinical Psychological Science, 7*(1), 37–50. doi: 10.1177/2167702618772296

Hubble, M. A., Duncan, B. L., & Miller, S. D. (Eds.). (1999). *The heart and soul of change: What works in therapy*. Washington, DC: American Psychological Association.

Kuhn, T. S. (1962). *The structure of scientific revolutions*. Chicago, IL: University of Chicago Press.

Lambert, M. J. (1992). Psychotherapy outcome research: Implications for integrative and eclectical therapists. In J. C. Norcross & S. L. Garfield (Eds.), *Handbook of psychotherapy integration* (pp. 94–129). New York: Basic Books.

Lambert, M. J. (2013). *Bergin and Garfield's handbook of psychotherapy and behavior change* (5th ed.). New York: John Wiley & Sons.

Laska, K. M., & Wampold, B. E. (2014). Ten things to remember about common factor theory. *Psychotherapy, 51*(4), 519–524.

Moses, E. B., & Barlow, D. H. (2006). A new unified treatment approach for emotional disorders based on emotion science. *Current Directions in Psychological Science, 15*(3), 146–150.

Nathan, P. E., & Gorman, J. M. (Eds.). (2015). *A guide to treatments that work*. New York: Oxford University Press.

Norcross, J. C. (Ed.). (2011). *Psychotherapy relationships that work: Evidence-based responsiveness*. New York: Oxford University Press.

Rescher, N. (1996). *Process metaphysics: An introduction to process philosophy*. Albany, NY: SUNY Press.

Wampold, B. E. (2001). *The great psychotherapy debate: Models, methods, and findings*. Mahwah, NJ: Lawrence Erlbaum Associates.

Wampold, B. E., & Imel, Z. E. (2015). *The great psychotherapy debate: The evidence for what makes psychotherapy work* (2nd ed.). New York: Routledge/Taylor & Francis Group.

Whitehead, A. N. (1978). *Process and reality: An essay in cosmology*. New York: The Free Press.

CHAPTER 4

Psychological Vulnerabilities and Coping Responses

An Innovative Approach to Transdiagnostic Assessment and Treatment Planning in the Age Beyond DSM-5

Rochelle I. Frank, PhD
University of California, Berkeley & The Wright Institute

Matthew McKay, PhD
The Wright Institute

For many decades, the gold standard of care in psychology and other helping disciplines has been manualized treatments that have been successfully evaluated in randomized controlled trials (RCTs) targeting symptoms of singular psychiatric diagnoses, such as obsessive-compulsive disorder, major depressive disorder, and generalized anxiety disorder. This approach has been subjected to a number of critiques. First, experimental and naturalistic practice settings rarely compare, which renders dissemination difficult—at best—for manuals crafted for research purposes (e.g., Barlow, 1981; Barlow, Levitt, & Bufka, 1999; Dattilio, Piercy, & Davis, 2014; Silverman, 2001). Moreover, the diagnosis-specific, manualized approach to treatment provides very limited information on mechanisms of change within psychotherapy because it does not consider the countless variables, and their complex interplay over time, specific to each patient and therapeutic dyad (Dattilio, Edwards, & Fishman, 2010; Kazantzis, Dattilio, & Dobson, 2017).

This might include moderator variables (such as personality characteristics, motivational factors, available resources, or internal and external stressors) and a myriad of possible mediator variables (such as automatic thoughts, dysfunctional attitudes, and other cognitive distortions) in psychotherapy that influence outcomes in clinical practice. Citing Barlow and Knock's (2009) call to action to integrate and emphasize idiographic approaches alongside nomothetic ones, Dattilio and colleagues (2010) argue for a "mixed methods" design that blends close examination of single cases with clinical trials as the new gold standard of evidence-based treatments (Fishman, Messer, Edwards, & Dattilio, 2017).

Defining the Problem

Consistent with these concerns, behavioral health care is increasingly advancing toward transdiagnostic approaches aimed at treating the underlying mechanisms hypothesized to drive and maintain patients' presenting problems. This trend is due, in part, to the growing recognition that traditional psychiatric diagnoses—and thus, the treatments that focus on them—are flawed because of the inherent limitations of our current diagnostic system, the *Diagnostic and Statistical Manual of Mental Disorders, Fifth Edition* (DSM-5; American Psychiatric Association, 2013). Meidlinger and Hope (2017) identify three main problems with the DSM: (a) categorical overlap, (b) high comorbidity rates, and (c) loss of relevant clinical information. These problems have contributed toward a burgeoning interest in new process-based models of psychotherapy.

Toward a Transdiagnostic Approach

The National Institute of Mental Health (NIMH) created an alternative to the use of the DSM as a way of improving and prioritizing clinical and empirical psychiatric research in the form of the Research Domain Criteria (RDoC; Insel et al., 2010). Rather than focusing on clinical observation and clustering of symptoms, RDoC emphasizes observable behavior, cognitive constructs, inheritable traits, and underlying neural structures as hypothesized mechanisms of action that can modify emotional and behavior problems and their associated functional impairments. The desired benefits of systematically targeting putative mechanisms of change, versus relying on categorical symptom clusters, include a broadened understanding of the etiological and maintaining factors driving mental illness, which could ultimately lead to more efficacious treatments and preventative measures (Sanislow et al., 2010).

Over the past twenty years, several transdiagnostic classification systems emphasizing common psychological processes have been introduced by researchers. For example, Hayes and colleagues (1996) identified experiential avoidance (i.e., one's unwillingness to remain in contact with internal experiences, such as thoughts, feelings, behavioral urges, and physical sensations) and the related process of psychological inflexibility as principal factors maintaining psychological distress and functional impairments across multiple disorders. In addition, Leahy (2002) identified fourteen emotional schemas (i.e., beliefs about the acceptability of one's emotional responses) hypothesized to cause emotional disorders. Similarly, Harvey, Watkins, Mansell, and Shafran (2004) isolated twelve processes (e.g., attentional avoidance, emotional reasoning, recurrent negative thinking) within the domains of attention, memory, reasoning, thought, and behavior that are shared across disorders and account for the etiology, maintenance, and comorbidity of psychological problems. Finally, based on their research on rumination, Nolen-Hoeksema and Watkins (2011) proposed a tripartite model to explain convergent and divergent trajectories of transdiagnostic risk factors across disorders and individuals.

Treatments Focused on Transdiagnostic Mechanisms

The growing database on shared psychological processes is giving rise to the development of transdiagnostic treatment protocols that target one or more of these mechanisms. For example, cognitive behavioral therapy for intolerance of uncertainty (CBT-IU; Robichaud, 2013) is an evidence-based protocol that was developed for generalized anxiety disorders. In addition to intolerance of uncertainty, CBT-IU targets the related constructs of cognitive avoidance (Borkovec, Alcaine, & Behar, 2004), metacognitive beliefs about the usefulness of worry (Wells, 2009), and negative problem orientation (Nezu, Nezu, & D'Zurilla, 2013). Other forms of CBT have been similarly developed. For example, cognitive behavioral treatment of perfectionism (Egan, Wade, Shafran, & Antony, 2014) targets perfectionism as a known process that is involved in the onset and maintenance of anxiety, depression, and eating disorders (Egan, Wade, & Shafran, 2012; Lloyd, Schmidt, Khondoker, & Tchanturia, 2014; Riley, Lee, Cooper, Fairburn, & Shafran, 2007). Rumination-focused CBT for depression (Watkins, 2016) utilizes mindfulness, cognitive behavioral interventions, and compassion to reduce depressive rumination and avoidance and to help patients build healthier coping responses.

Barlow's Unified Protocol (Barlow et al., 2018) is yet another transdiagnostic treatment that was developed to target multiple mechanisms (cognitive misappraisals, experiential avoidance, and emotion-driven behaviors) across emotional disorders—specifically, comorbid anxiety and unipolar depressive disorders. Even though the Unified Protocol targets a range of conditions, it does at least as well as more diagnosis-specific treatments that would be more difficult to disseminate (Steele et al., 2018). Likewise, McKay, Fanning, and Zurita Ona (2011) developed a protocol for improving emotion regulation and overall coping by integrating skills from acceptance and commitment therapy, CBT, and dialectical behavior therapy. Norton's (2012) group CBT for anxiety disorders is another example of transdiagnostic treatment, as this approach targets perfectionism, negative schemas, cognitive misappraisals, and other mechanisms. Moreover, this protocol yields at least equivalent efficacy for anxiety disorders as diagnosis-specific treatments (Norton, 2017) and perhaps even superior efficacy when it comes to comorbid anxiety and negative emotional disorders (Norton & Paulus, 2017).

Propelling the transdiagnostic movement even further, Hayes and Hofmann (2018) compiled a volume integrating acceptance-based, behavioral, cognitive, and mindfulness strategies to help clinicians target core psychological change processes rather than diagnostic entities. By focusing on functional analyses of presenting problems, therapists can select evidence-based interventions—such as exposure, problem solving, cognitive defusion, arousal reduction, and many other proven strategies—to help clients gain objectivity in viewing and accepting their difficulties while building skills to navigate them and mitigate problematic coping behaviors. Whereas this compilation of strategies is rooted in decades of empirical research on standardized protocols, it underscores an idiographic, non-pathologizing, and efficacious approach to helping clients improve functioning and engage in values-based living.

The Transdiagnostic Road Map: Searching for a Practical Solution

While transdiagnostic protocols may be useful in targeting multiple problems, they are limited by their RCT genesis—and thus do not address the complex array and interplay of variables unique to each patient and therapist (Kazantzis et al., 2017). Based on Persons's (2008) case formulation model, Frank and Davidson's (2014) "transdiagnostic road map" offers an innovative and practical step toward (a) identifying specific transdiagnostic mechanisms (TDMs) to explain the etiology and maintenance of patients' presenting problems, and (b) targeting them in treatment with evidence-based interventions that clinicians select based on their functional utility in modifying mechanisms and achieving treatment goals at varying points in therapy.

Based on a comprehensive review of the empirical literature, the authors define TDMs as "underlying vulnerabilities and patterns of responses that are hypothesized to trigger and maintain cognitive, behavioral, emotional, and physiological symptoms and functional impairments across diagnostic categories" (Frank & Davidson, 2014, p. 10). TDMs are organized as either vulnerability mechanisms or response mechanisms, and all may be directly targeted in treatment with functionally-based clinical interventions (see Table 1). Frank and Davidson's compilation of the empirical database on psychological mechanisms and transdiagnostic processes provides a systematic way of identifying specific mechanisms for patients' presenting problems.

78 Beyond the DSM

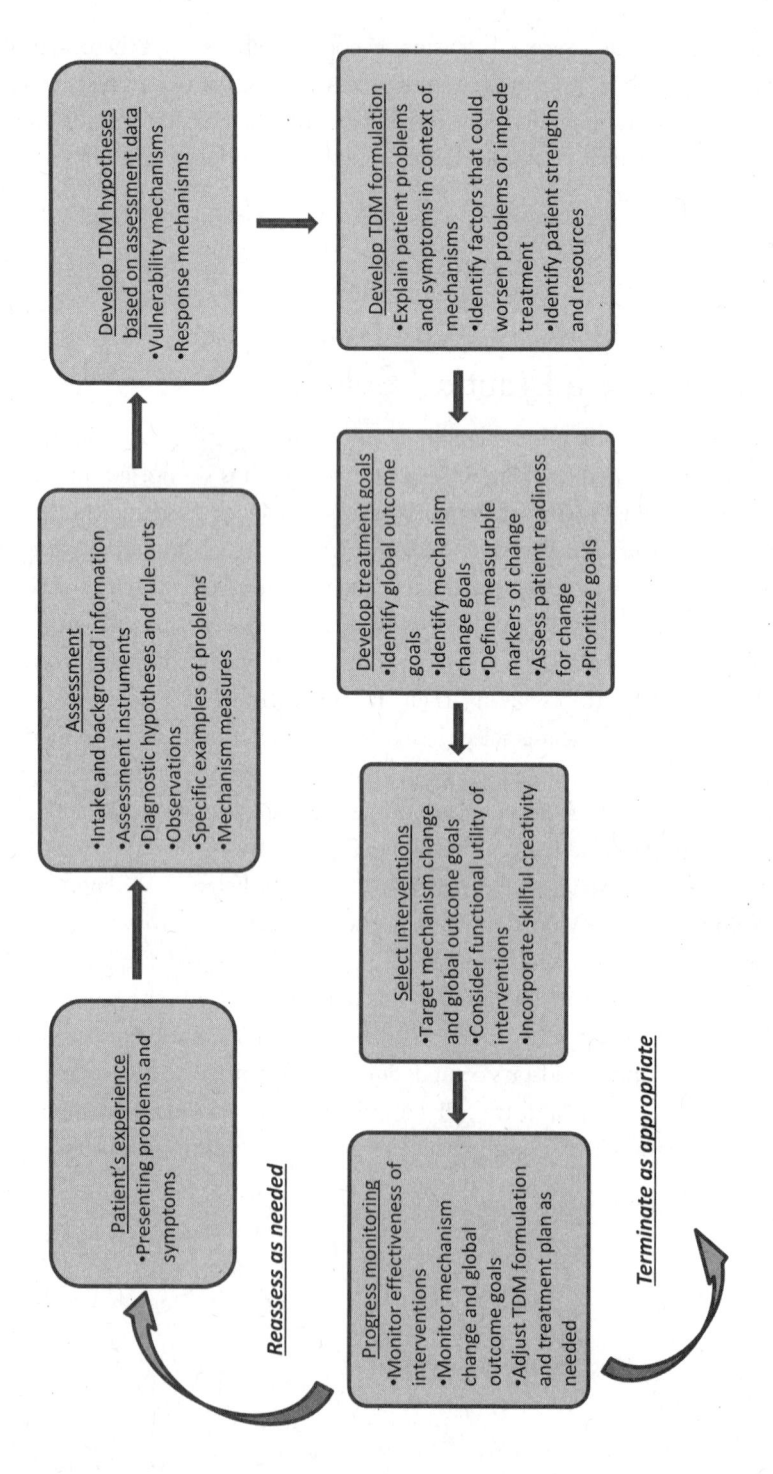

Figure 4.1 TDM-Based Case Formulation

Table 1. Transdiagnostic Mechanisms

Vulnerability Mechanisms	Response Mechanisms

Neurophysiological Predispositions
• Deficits in:
  • Arousal regulation/inhibitory control
  • Respiratory and cardiac control
  • Executive functioning
  • Information processing
  • Information storage and retrieval
  • Emotion regulation
  • Sleep regulation
 	
Learned Responses
• Conditioned responses to stimuli
• Reinforced responses
• Modeling
 	
Pervasive Beliefs
• Negative schemas
• Metacognitive beliefs
 	
Specific Cognitive Constructs
• Anxiety sensitivity
• Perceived control
• Intolerance of uncertainty
• Perfectionism
• Fear of evaluation
• Negative problem orientation
• Inflated responsibility and threat estimation
• Illness/injury sensitivity
 	
Multidimensional Construct
• Distress tolerance
	Experiential Avoidance
	• Avoidance and escape strategies
	  • Safety seeking
	  • Reassurance seeking
	  • Compulsions
	• Behavioral (situational) avoidance
	• Cognitive avoidance
	  • Thought control
	  • Thought suppression
	  • Worry
	• Interoceptive (somatic) avoidance
	• Emotional avoidance
	• Emotion-driven behaviors
	
	Cognitive Misappraisals
	
	Attentional Focus
	
	Attributional Bias
	• Internalizing
	• Externalizing
	
	Repetitive Negative Thinking
	• Worry
	• Rumination
	• Post-event processing

© 2014 Frank & Davidson

Psychological Vulnerabilities and Coping Responses

Vulnerability mechanisms are trait-like constructs that predispose individuals to psychological problems as a result of genetic risk factors, physiological predispositions, regulatory deficits, and early learned experiences (Frank & Davidson, 2014). They may be cognitive, emotional, perceptual, behavioral, or multidimensional, and they typically co-occur. Whereas the majority of vulnerability mechanisms may be measured in the present, early learning provides a context for the expression of TDMs and is identified through history gathering and functional behavioral analysis of specific examples of presenting problems (Frank and Davidson, 2014). Vulnerability mechanisms are susceptible to internal and external stressors, triggering maladaptive behavioral responses—that is, response mechanisms—that serve to mitigate and cope with the psychological vulnerabilities. For example, experiential avoidance, cognitive misappraisals, and repetitive negative thinking (such as worry and rumination) are posited to arise within this system when psychological vulnerabilities (such as intolerance of uncertainty, executive functioning deficits, and negative schemas) are activated by stress. While both types of TDMs may act as mediators and moderators of presenting symptoms and functional impairments, the response mechanisms often reflect attempts to cope with or avoid unpleasant emotional states, compensate for actual and perceived deficits, or control outcomes (Frank & Davidson, 2014). In sum, the vulnerability and response mechanisms represent different components of patients' problems, and transactions among these mechanisms contribute to continuous feedback loops that exacerbate existing problems and often perpetuate additional ones (Frank & Davidson, 2014).

The transdiagnostic road map offers a possible way to turn the large and growing literature on TDMs into a practical and flexible guide for clinicians, providing an ideographic, empirical approach to assessment and treatment. Because the primary categories apply broadly, new TDMs can be added as they arise in the empirical literature. As an alternative to psychiatric diagnosis, the road map encourages therapists to treat a broad range of simple, complex, singular, and comorbid problems by selecting interventions that will fit their patients' needs and that best target the mechanisms driving and maintaining those problems. Moreover, by framing problems in the context of (a) vulnerabilities that everyone is susceptible to and has some combination thereof, and (b) responses that represent natural attempts to manage psychological pain, clinicians can bypass the aforementioned limitations of the existing psychiatric nosology. Also, by coming to understand their presenting problems in this framework, patients may arrive at a less stigmatizing view of themselves—potentially mitigating shame and distress and facilitating engagement in treatment.

Transdiagnostic Classification

A transdiagnostic classification system, unlike the DSM, can lead directly to case conceptualization and thus identify both the causal and maintaining factors of a patient's symptoms. The central assumption of the transdiagnostic road map approach is that the resulting case formulation should distinguish and identify:

1. *Vulnerability mechanisms:* an individual's hardwired and "hard-baked" susceptibilities to stress.

2. *Stressors:* specific and relevant triggers (or adverse situations or events) that activate TDMs.

3. *Response mechanisms:* an individual's maladaptive coping strategies to control stress and mitigate unpleasant emotional experiences.

To the degree that client problems are driven by the activation of vulnerability and response mechanisms, treatment procedures and interventions aimed at TDMs rather than DSM classifications should have broader applicability. Rigid, multicomponent protocols, with interventions that are unnecessary or inappropriate for a particular patient and components that may be both untested and untargeted, can ultimately be replaced by discrete intervention kernels aimed at patient vulnerability and response mechanisms.

To effectively replace the DSM, a transdiagnostic classification system of this kind will require assessment instruments to measure each of the vulnerability mechanisms (exclusive of learned responses, which are identified through comprehensive history gathering) and each of the response mechanisms (Frank & Davidson, 2014). In principle, this may significantly improve our current psychiatric nosology because:

1. TDM-based measures target *causes* of symptoms rather than the symptoms themselves;
2. TDM-based measures lead directly to case formulation;
3. TDM-based measures assess improvement in the mechanisms that cause (and potentially mediate) patient distress and functional impairments; and
4. TDM-based measures of vulnerability and response mechanisms can be tied directly to treatment because each can be targeted by one or more specific treatment processes or interventions.

A major problem in developing such a set of measures is that TDMs need to apply to individuals over time, since trajectories of these processes and their combination will vary between people. However, psychometrics and RCTs both require ergodic assumptions in order for results to apply to individuals, and these assumptions are that individuals do *not* differ in the change processes that apply nor in their trajectories (Molenaar, 2013). Said another way, the very reason to focus on TDMs suggests that new methods of evaluating assessment quality and treatment impact need to be developed.

While we recognize this need, it is one that is difficult to satisfy and is shared by the entire field. In the following section, we will examine our attempt to use traditional psychometric methods to provide measures that fit the transdiagnostic road map approach.

The General Vulnerabilities Questionnaire (GVQ)

The GVQ (Choudri, 2018) is a 90-item instrument developed to measure the 16 vulnerability mechanisms (exclusive of learned responses) within the remaining categories identified by Frank & Davidson (2014): neurophysiological deficits, pervasive beliefs, specific cognitive constructs, and distress tolerance. The GVQ remains in development, and some of its subscales may be modified pending the outcome of validation and reliability studies.

The Comprehensive Coping Inventory-Revised (CCI-R)

The CCI was originally developed as a measure of 49 positive and negative coping strategies to deal with stress (Zurita Ona, 2007). After a period of testing, the CCI was modified to measure 7 transdiagnostic response mechanisms targeted by the Mind and Emotions Protocol (McKay et al., 2011). These maladaptive coping responses included experiential avoidance, rumination, emotional masking, short-term focus, response persistence, hostility/aggression, and negative appraisal. The protocol was tailored so components could be dropped or included depending on whether a patient had elevated scores on a particular TDM. The CCI was modified a second time (Birnbaum, 2015) and expanded to measure the 16 transdiagnostic response mechanisms identified by Frank and Davidson (2014).

Preliminary Validation Study

A preliminary validation study by Birnbaum (2015) examined the performance of the CCI-R. There were 191 participants in the study, with 92 in the clinical group (patients receiving services at a low-fee community-based CBT clinic) and 99 in the non-clinical group (respondents to a broadly distributed online survey). Participants' mean age was 42, and 80 percent were Caucasion. Seventy-nine percent of the sample completed college, and 66 percent endorsed being in the middle class. Internal consistency of the subscales was examined using Cronbach's alpha with the expectation of a minimum alpha of .75. Of the 16 subscales of the CCI-R, only Safety Seeking (.73) and Emotion-Driven Behavior (.67) failed to meet that criterion. With these exceptions, questions were appropriately clustered within their corresponding subscales. Across all 16 subscales, Cronbach's alpha averaged .82, with a median value of .82 and a range from .67 to .92. The data that follow derive from this study.

The sensitivity of the CCI-R in distinguishing between clinical versus non-clinical populations was analyzed for the 16 subscales using a MANOVA. For 11 of the 16 subscales, there were statistically significant differences between clinical and non-clinical means (see Table 2).

Table 2. MANOVA Results for the CCI-R Subscales

	Clinical Mean	Clinical SD	Non-Clinical Mean	Non-Clinical SD	F	p
Safety Seeking	13.043	4.317	11.919	4.149	3.551	0.004
Reassurance Seeking	15.533	4.449	13.465	4.104	3.445	0.005
Compulsions	13.413	4.433	11.040	4.660	6.302	0.000
Situational Avoidance	15.870	4.786	12.859	4.658	6.785	0.000
Thought Control	2.500	4.155	12.939	4.763	1.781	0.119
Thought Suppression	12.989	3.675	12.414	4.302	4.605	0.001
Worry	16.033	5.134	12.162	4.903	5.878	0.000
Interoceptive Avoidance	12.152	5.626	11.061	4.973	0.885	0.492
Emotional Avoidance	13.424	4.292	10.778	4.308	6.776	0.000
Emotion-Driven Behavior	14.696	4.878	11.687	3.521	5.807	0.000
Misappraisals	16.967	4.285	13.798	4.274	7.077	0.000
Threat Focus	14.533	5.377	11.687	4.469	5.220	0.000
Externalizing	11.196	4.160	10.566	3.637	0.359	0.876
Internalizing	17.957	4.946	16.354	5.306	1.884	0.099
Rumination	17.033	5.057	14.141	5.307	4.339	0.001
Post-Event Processing	16.761	4.993	15.131	5.130	1.332	0.252

Subscales bolded in Table 2 are capable of differentiating clinical from non-clinical populations at a statistically significant level. The five subscales that did not significantly differentiate clinical from non-clinical populations were Thought Control, Interoceptive Avoidance, Externalizing Attributional Bias, Internalizing Attributional Bias, and Post-Event Processing. These subscales appear to represent coping mechanisms that are readily found in both clinical and non-clinical groups. This could indicate that these constructs are not true transdiagnostic response mechanisms that should be targeted by treatment processes, or it could be that these processes are harmful only in the context of various vulnerabilities or clinical moderators. More research will be needed to untangle these possibilities.

The next step in a traditional psychometric approach would be to examine the distinguishability of the targeted processes using exploratory factor analysis. Unfortunately, in the very development of factor analysis, a decision was made to focus on consistency in a collective of people at a given point in time versus consistency of patterns within people across time—what

Cattell (1988) has called "p methods." Thus, it is not clear that traditional factor analysis is well suited for TDMs. An alternative might be to apply ecological momentary assessment methods to people across time and to then examine them person by person before seeking nomothetic generalizations.

The Relationship Between CCI-R Subscales and Symptoms

Additional research on the CCI-R was subsequently conducted by Frazier (2017) that involved examining the relationship between CCI-R subscales and clinical scales on the Personality Assessment Inventory (PAI). As shown in Table 3, many CCI-R subscales were significantly correlated with either the Anxiety or Anxiety-Related Disorders clinical scales on the PAI. The strongest associations ($r = .5$ or greater) were observed for Worry, Misappraisals, Threat Focus, and Rumination. The only CCI-R subscales that did not demonstrate any significant associations were Thought Control, Thought Suppression, and Externalizing.

The CCI-R subscales most strongly associated with the Depression clinical scale of the PAI were Internalizing Attributional Bias ($r = .49$), Worry ($r =. 44$), and Rumination ($r = .44$). These strong correlations are consistent with the literature linking repetitive negative thinking with depression and other emotional problems (Aldao & Nolen-Hoeksema, 2010; Mahoney, McEvoy, & Moulds, 2012).

Many CCI-R scales also correlated with the Borderline Personality Disorder subscale of the PAI. The strongest correlations were Emotion-Driven Behavior ($r = .55$), Rumination ($r = .42$), Misappraisals ($r = .36$), Internalizing ($r = .34$), Post-Event Processing ($r = .34$), and Emotional Avoidance ($r = .30$). Few CCI-R subscales correlated with the Somaticizing Disorders scale on the PAI, with only Interoceptive Avoidance ($r=.34$), Emotional Avoidance ($r = .25$), and Rumination ($r = .26$) demonstrating significant associations. This is consistent with many of the problematic behaviors that may be targeted in treatment of borderline personality disorder (Linehan, 1993 [text book, not skills manual]).

Overall, the CCI-R subscales that exhibited the highest correlations with the PAI were Worry, Rumination, Internalizing, and Post-Event Processing (all perseverative processes), Emotional Avoidance, Emotion-Driven Behavior, and Interoceptive Avoidance (all avoidance-based mechanisms), and Misappraisals.

Table 3. Correlations Between CCI-R Subscales and Clinical Scales on the PAI

CCR-I Subscale	Anxiety r	Anxiety p	Anxiety-Related Disorders r	Anxiety-Related Disorders p	Depression r	Depression p	Borderline Personality Disorder r	Borderline Personality Disorder p	Somaticizing Disorders r	Somaticizing Disorders p
Safety Seeking	.30	.001	.35	.000			.25	.006		
Reassurance Seeking	.28	.002					.26	.004		
Compulsion			.28	.002						
Situational Avoidance	.37	.000	.35	.000						
Thought Control										
Thought Suppression							.25	.007		
Worry	.58	.000	.46	.000	.44	.000	.27	.003		
Interoceptive Avoidance	.30	.001	.44	.000			.28	.002	.34	.000
Emotional Avoidance	.36	.000	.27	.004	.27	.003	.30	.001	.25	.007
Emotion-Driven Behavior	.26	.005	.28	.002	.34	.000	.55	.000		
Misappraisals	.59	.000	.43	.000	.34	.000	.36	.000		
Threat Focus	.54	.000	.42	.000	.36	.000				
Externalizing		.000		.000						
Internalizing	.47		.44		.49	.000	.34	.000		
Rumination	.50	.000	.56	.000	.44	.000	.42	.000	.26	.003
Post-Event Processing	.46	.000	.47	.000	.30	.001	.34	.000		

In order to examine change over time with the CCI-R and clinical outcomes, Frazier (2017) collected pre- and post-treatment scores using the CCI-R and the Depression, Anxiety, and Stress Scale (DASS; Lovibond & Lovibond, 1995) on 72 patients at a low-fee cognitive behavioral clinic in Berkeley, California. Assessments were taken at the beginning and then again at the end of a course of psychotherapy at the clinic. A correlational analysis performed for this cohort revealed fairly strong relationships between the DASS symptom scales (depression, anxiety, and stress) and multiple CCI-R subscales at post-test. The correlations reported in Table 4 are all at the $p < .01$ level.

Table 4. Correlations Between CCI-R Subscales and the DASS

DASS Symptom	CCI-R Subscale	r
Depression	Worry	.57
	Threat Focus	.54
	Rumination	.51
	Emotion-Driven Behavior	.50
	Situational Avoidance	.45
	Emotional Avoidance	.45
	Post-Event Processing	.45
	Internalizing	.44
	Misappraisal	.42
Anxiety	Safety Seeking	.42
	Compulsions	.43
	Misappraisals	.43
	Interoceptive Avoidance	.41
	Situational Avoidance	.40
	Threat Focus	.40
	Rumination	.39
	Emotional Avoidance	.38
Stress	Rumination	.48
	Emotion-Driven Behavior	.46
	Misappraisals	.45
	Post-Event Processing	.45
	Worry	.44
	Threat focus	.41
	Internalizing	.38

As shown in Table 4, depression was strongly linked to TDMs involving perseverative processes (worry, threat focus, rumination, post-event processing, and internalizing attributional bias). It was also associated with avoidance (situational avoidance, emotional avoidance, and emotion-driven behaviors). Misappraisals ranked relatively low among TDMs significantly associated with depression.

Anxiety was linked to TDMs involving avoidance (safety behaviors, compulsions, situational avoidance, interoceptive avoidance, and emotional avoidance), perseverative processes (rumination, threat focus), and misappraisals. Surprisingly, worry had a relatively low correlation (r = .34) in this sample.

Stress, as measured by the DASS, reflects difficulty relaxing and chronic nonspecific arousal such as agitation and irritability (Lovibond & Lovibond, 1995). These items correlated with perseverative processes (rumination, worry, threat focus, internalizing, and post-event processing), emotion-driven behavior (a form of avoidance), and misappraisals.

Overall, perseverative thinking (primarily worry) and avoidance processes (primarily emotion-driven behavior, followed by situational and emotional avoidance) were most associated with symptom pain in our sample.

Table 5 shows the variance accounted for in pre-post changes in depression, anxiety, and stress by pre-post changes in CCI-R subscales. Significant correlations ($p < .01$) are in bold. The CCI-R subscales are ranked by effect size in the table, with Worry at the top (Cohen's $d = .71$).

Reductions in worry and emotional avoidance correlated broadly with overall symptom mitigation. Lowered endorsements of misappraisals, reassurance seeking, interoceptive avoidance, and thought suppression (a form of cognitive avoidance) were primarily associated with reductions in anxiety scores. Reductions in CCI-R subscales had very little correlation with reductions in depression scores, with only worry and emotional avoidance accounting for 9% of the variance each. Interestingly, in this sample, significant reductions in rumination had almost no relation to depression. Changes in perseverative thinking (worry, internalizing, and rumination) plus emotional and situational avoidance and emotion-driven behavior were associated with the most change in stress. While directionality cannot be assumed, these processes may thus make the most salient process-based treatment targets in contributing to patient well-being.

Table 5. Variance Accounted for by the CCI-R in Pre-Post Changes in Depression, Anxiety, and Stress

CCI-R	Cohen's d	R^2 Depression	Anxiety	Stress
Worry	0.71	**9%**	**19%**	**17%**
Rumination	0.66	2%	**9%**	**12%**
Process	0.59	3%	5%	3%
Emotion-Driven Behaviors	0.53	7%	3%	**9%**
Misappraisals	0.53	1%	**10%**	3%
Internalizing	0.53	3%	5%	**11%**
Threat Focus	0.41	1%	**8%**	5%
Emotional Avoidance	0.35	**9%**	**10%**	**17%**
Situational Avoidance	0.34	6%	7%	**9%**
Reassurance Seeking	0.30	1%	**12%**	6%
Externalizing	0.26	0%	2%	3%
Thought Suppression	0.22	1%	**11%**	5%
Interoceptive Avoidance	0.20	0%	**10%**	3%
Compulsion	0.09	0%	0%	1%
Safety Seeking	0.02	1%	0%	0%
Thought Control	0.00	5%	0%	1%

TDM-Targeted Treatment Planning

Although more research is clearly needed to validate the CCI-R for this purpose, what we offer here is an example of how once TDMs have been identified, the therapist and patient can start understanding how specific vulnerabilities and coping responses interact with situational stressors to fuel and maintain presenting problems. In our use of the CCI-R, we have found that analyzing and discussing examples of how mechanisms create problems in daily living provides a lens into the functional and historical contexts in which TDMs play a central role in patients' efforts to avoid and cope with pain. It provides empirical support for initial mechanism hypotheses, which can then be used to help select treatment targets and clinical interventions.

A key aspect of treatment planning involves crystallizing global outcome goals—that is, how patients want their lives to be different when therapy concludes. These then provide concrete benchmarks (such as completing school, improving work performance, or no longer avoiding social events) that can be used to assess whether treatment is working. While a comprehensive program of research is needed to fully understand how TDMs must change in order to facilitate achievement of treatment goals, we can use the results of TDM measures and scales to inform the selection of interventions. Some interventions are well-established by decades of research, such as interoceptive exposure for panic-related intolerance of uncertainty and avoidance (Barlow, 2002), and emotional exposure and augmentation of distress tolerance skills for emotion dysregulation (Linehan, 1993). New interventions will likely be developed as research increasingly narrows the focus on TDMs as logical treatment targets. Periodic assessment with instruments such as the CCI-R will let both the therapist and the patient know whether those interventions are working.

Finally, patient-specific characteristics—such as cultural considerations, strengths, limitations, situational stressors, and motivational stages as individuals move through treatment—will further refine treatment planning. Depending on those characteristics, including the identification of specific problems over the course of therapy and the trajectory of patients' progress, interventions may serve different functions in facilitating achievement of global outcome and mechanism change goals at different points in time. These include: (a) enhancing understanding and motivation; (b) facilitating stepping back from the problem; (c) providing core strategies for cognitive, behavioral, and emotional change; and (d) providing adjunctive skills training for specific problems (Frank & Davidson, 2014; see appendix for this chapter). Knowing how we want specific interventions to be utilized at various points in therapy can help therapists select and tailor interventions to best meet patient needs.

How TDM Classification and Measurement Will Change CBT

By replacing the DSM with a transdiagnostic classification system, we can begin to delineate a range of changes that will likely follow. We will cast these changes in terms of process-based CBT (Hayes & Hofmann, 2018) since it is an approach that fits with the core arguments of this chapter. In our view, the following changes can be expected:

1. Process-based CBT will ultimately be married to a transdiagnostic classification system. Each TDM (both vulnerability and response mechanisms) will be targeted by evidence-based procedures or interventions that have been shown to alter that TDM.

2. Research will focus on new and more effective treatment modules or kernels for each TDM. Interventions will be more targeted, aiming at specific mechanisms rather than symptom classification.

3. Comprehensive protocols or packages for particular DSM categories will become obsolete. Component analysis of these packages will also no longer be useful or necessary because each process or intervention will singularly focus on a TDM, with a body of research to show efficacy.

4. Each patient will have an individually tailored treatment plan that includes *only* the treatment procedures or interventions appropriate for their profile of elevated TDMs.

5. Named therapies will disappear and will be replaced by process-based treatments for specific TDMs that are evidence-based and that can be tailored to individual patient needs.

6. Rigid, multicomponent protocols, with interventions that are unnecessary or inappropriate for a specific patient, and components that may be both untested and untargeted, will become extinct as research focuses on discrete interventions aimed at patient vulnerability and response mechanisms.

No one can say how long it will take for these various changes to occur, but the transition from the DSM to an era of process-based diagnosis and intervention is already strongly underway. The era of "protocols for syndromes" is over. It is time to pursue a new vision—one that is clearer in identifying the drivers of presenting problems, sharper in its ability to target those psychological processes, and more efficient and efficacious in reducing patients' suffering and improving their overall functioning and quality of living.

Appendix

Functional Categorization of Interventions

© 2014 Frank & Davidson

Interventions That Enhance Understanding and Motivation

- Psychoeducation
- Conversations about ambivalence and motivation to change
- Cost-benefit analysis
- Identifying values

Interventions That Facilitate Stepping Back from the Problem

- Problem deconstruction and analysis
- Self-monitoring
- Mindfulness (formal/informal practice)
- Detached mindfulness (meta-awareness)
- Acceptance and validation
- Cognitive defusion
- Pause/interrupt/slow down

Core Strategies for Change

- Behavioral activation
- Behavioral contingencies
- Acceptance-based responses
- Self-compassion training and imagery rescripting
- Cognitive restructuring
- Schema change
- Behavioral experiments
- Exposure (behavioral, cognitive, emotional, interoceptive)
- Attention training techniques
- Situational attention retraining
- Postponement strategies
- Distress tolerance skills
- Emotion regulation skills
- Interpersonal effectiveness and assertiveness skills

Adjunctive Skills Training
- Breathing retraining/calming breaths
- Progressive muscle relaxation
- Applied relaxation
- Guided imagery
- Self-soothing
- Anger management
- Problem solving
- Organization and planning
- Time management
- Sleep management
- Strategies for eating problems
- Strategies for body-focused repetitive behaviors

References

Aldao, A., & Nolen-Hoeksema, S. (2010). Specificity of cognitive emotion regulation strategies: A transdiagnostic examination. *Behaviour Research and Therapy, 48,* 974–983.

American Psychiatric Association. (2013). *Diagnostic and statistical manual of mental disorders.* (5th ed.). Arlington, VA: Author.

Barlow, D. H. (2002). *Anxiety and its disorders (2nd ed.).* New York: Guilford.

Barlow, D. H. (1981). On the relation of clinical research to clinical practice: Current issues, new directions. *Journal of Consulting and Clinical Psychology, 49*(2), 147–155.

Barlow, D. H., Farchione, T. J., Sauer-Zavala, S., Latin, H. M., Ellard, K. K., Bullis, J. R., ... Cassiello-Robbins, C. (2018). *Unified protocol for the treatment of emotional disorders* (2nd ed.). New York: Oxford University Press.

Barlow, D. H., Levitt, J. T., & Bufka, L. F. (1999). The dissemination of empirically supported treatments: A view to the future. *Behaviour Research and Therapy, 37,* S147–S162.

Barlow, D. H., & Knock, M. K. (2009). Why can't we be more idiographic in our research? *Perspectives on Psychological Science, 4*(1), 19–21.

Birnbaum, A. P. (2015). *Approaching transdiagnostically: A validation study of the Comprehensive Coping Inventory* (Unpublished doctoral dissertation). The Wright Institute: Berkeley, CA.

Borkovec, T. D., Alcaine, O. M., & Behar, E. (2004). Avoidance theory of worry and generalized anxiety disorder. In R. G. Heimberg, C. L. Turk, & D. S. Mennin (Eds.), *Generalized anxiety disorder: Advances in research and practice* (pp. 77–108). New York: Guilford Press.

Cattell R.B. (1988) The Meaning and Strategic Use of Factor Analysis. In: Nesselroade J.R., Cattell R.B. (eds) *Handbook of Multivariate Experimental Psychology. Perspectives on Individual Differences.* Springer, Boston, MA.

Choudri, N. (2018). *Developing a transdiagnostic vulnerability measure: A validation study of the General Vulnerabilities Questionnaire* (Unpublished doctoral dissertation). The Wright Institute: Berkeley, CA.

Dattilio, F. M., Edwards, D. J. A., & Fishman, D. B. (2010). Case studies within a mixed methods paradigm: Toward a resolution of the alienation between researcher and practitioner in psychotherapy research. *Psychotherapy, 47*(4), 427–441.

Dattilio, F. M., Piercy, F., & Davis, S. D. (2014). The divide between "evidence-based" approaches and practitioners of traditional theories of family therapy. *Journal of Marital and Family Therapy, 40*(1), 5–16.

Egan, S. J., Wade, T. D., & Shafran, R. (2012). The transdiagnostic process of perfectionism. *Revista de Psicopatologia y Psicologia Clinica, 17*(3), 279–294.

Egan, S. J., Wade, T. D., Shafran, R., & Antony, M. M. (2014). *Cognitive-behavioral treatment of perfectionism.* New York: Guilford Press.

Fishman, D. B., Messer, S. B., Edwards, D. J. A., & Dattilio, F. M. (2017). *Case studies within psychotherapy trials: Integrating qualitative and quantitative methods.* New York: Oxford University Press.

Frank, R. I., & Davidson, J. (2014). *The transdiagnostic road map to case formulation and treatment planning: Practical guidance for clinical decision making.* Oakland, CA: New Harbinger.

Frazier, J. (2017). *Comprehensive Coping Inventory: A study of concurrent validity and clinical utility* (Unpublished doctoral dissertation). The Wright Institute: Berkeley, CA.

Harvey, A. G., Watkins, E. R., Mansell, W., & Shafran, R. (2004). *Cognitive behavioural processes across psychological disorders: A transdiagnostic approach to research and treatment.* Oxford, UK: Oxford University Press.

Hayes, S. C., & Hofmann, S. G. (Eds.). 2018. *Process-based CBT: The science and core clinical competencies of cognitive behavioral therapy.* Oakland, CA: Context Press/New Harbinger.

Hayes, S. C., Wilson, K. W., Gifford, E. V., Follette, V. M., & Strosahl, K. (1996). Experiential avoidance and behavioral disorders: A functional dimensional approach to diagnosis and treatment. *Journal of Consulting and Clinical Psychology, 64*(6), 1152–1168.

Insel, T., Cuthbert, B., Garvey, M., Heinssen, R., Pine, D., Quinn, D. S., ... Wang, P. (2010). Research Domain Criteria (RDoC): Toward a new classification framework for research on mental disorders. *American Journal of Psychiatry, 167*(7), 748–751.

Kazantzis, N., Dattilio, F. M., & Dobson, K. S. (2017). *The therapeutic relationship in cognitive behavioral therapy: A clinician's guide.* New York: Guilford Press.

Leahy, R. L. (2002). A model of emotional schemas. *Cognitive and Behavioral Practice, 9*(3), 177–190.

Linehan, M. M. (1993). *Cognitive-behavioral treatment of borderline personality disorder.* New York: Guilford.

Lloyd, S., Schmidt, U., Khondoker, M., & Tchanturia, K. (2014). Can psychological interventions reduce perfectionism? A systematic review and meta-analysis. *Behavioural and Cognitive Psychotherapy, 43*(6), 705–731.

Lovibond, P. F., & Lovibond, S. H. (1995). The structure of negative emotional states: Comparison of the Depression Anxiety Stress Scales (DASS) with the Beck Depression and Anxiety Inventories. *Behaviour Research and Therapy, 33*(3), 335–343.

Mahoney, A. E. J., McEvoy, P. M., & Moulds, M. L. (2012). Psychometric properties of the Repetitive Thinking Questionnaire in a clinical sample. *Journal of Anxiety Disorders, 26,* 359–367.

McKay, M., Fanning, P., & Zurita Ona, P. (2011). *Mind and emotions: A universal treatment for emotional disorders.* Oakland, CA: New Harbinger.

Meidlinger, P. C., & Hope, D. A. (2017). The new transdiagnostic cognitive behavioral treatments: Commentary for clinicians and clinical researchers. *Journal of Anxiety Disorders, 46,* 101–109.

Molenaar, P. C. M. (2013). On the necessity to use person-specific data analysis approaches in psychology. *European Journal of Developmental Psychology, 10*(1), 29–39.

Nezu, A. M., Nezu, C. M., & D'Zurilla, T. J. (2013). *Problem-solving therapy: A treatment manual.* New York: Springer.

Nolen-Hoeksema, S., & Watkins, E. R. (2011). A heuristic for developing transdiagnostic models of psychopathology: Explaining multifinality and divergent trajectories. *Perspectives in Psychological Science, 6*(6), 589–609.

Norton, P. J. (2012). *Group cognitive-behavioral therapy of anxiety*. New York: Guilford Press.

Norton, P. J. (2017). Transdiagnostic approaches to the understanding and treatment of anxiety and related disorders. *Journal of Anxiety Disorders, 46*, 1–3.

Norton, P. J., & Paulus, D. J. (2017). Transdiagnostic models of anxiety disorder: Theoretical and empirical underpinnings. *Clinical Psychology Review, 56*, 122–137.

Persons, J. B. (2008). *The case formulation approach to cognitive-behavioral therapy*. New York: Guilford Press.

Riley, C., Lee, M., Cooper, Z., Fairburn, C. G., & Shafran, R. (2007). A randomized controlled trial of cognitive-behaviour therapy for clinical perfectionism: A preliminary study. *Behaviour Research and Therapy, 45*(9), 2221–2231.

Robichaud, M. (2013). Cognitive behavior therapy targeting intolerance of uncertainty. *Cognitive and Behavioral Practice, 20*(3), 251–263.

Silverman, W. (2001). Clinicians and researchers: A bridge to nowhere? *Psychotherapy: Theory, Research, Practice, Training, 38*(3), 249–251.

Sanislow, C. A., Pine, D. S., Quinn, K. J., Kozak, M. J., Garvey, M. A., Heinssen, R. K., … Cuthbert, B. N. (2010). Developing constructs for psychopathology research: Research Domain Criteria. *Journal of Abnormal Psychology, 119*(4), 631–639.

Steele, S. J., Farchione, T. J., Cassiello-Robbins, C., Ametaj, A., Sbi, S., Sauer-Zavala, S., & Barlow, D. H. (2018). Efficacy of the Unified Protocol for transdiagnostic treatment of comorbid psychopathology accompanying emotional disorders compared to treatments targeting single disorders. *Journal of Psychiatric Research, 104*, 211–216.

Watkins, E. R. (2016). *Rumination-focused cognitive-behavioral therapy for depression*. New York: Guilford Press.

Wells, A. (2009). *Metacognitive therapy for anxiety and depression*. New York: Guilford Press.

Zurita Ona, P. E. (2007). *Development and validation of a Comprehensive Coping Inventory* (Unpublished doctoral dissertation). The Wright Institute: Berkeley, CA.

CHAPTER 5

Expectations and Related Cognitive Domains
Implications for Classification and Therapy

Winfried Rief, PhD
The Philipps University of Marburg

Introduction

Over the last decade, the roles of expectations and predictions have become increasingly evident in the understanding of not only mental disorders in general, but also in the mechanisms of psychological interventions, treatment failures, or lack of improvements after mental problems have been established. This more sophisticated psychological understanding of disorders and treatment mechanisms is paralleled by a reformed understanding of the major functions of the human brain. Therefore, this chapter will focus on the role of expectations in characterizing and distinguishing mental disorders, as well as how to improve psychological interventions with a focus on expectations.

The Special Role of Expectations

Since the trendsetting work of pioneers such as Aaron T. Beck, Albert Ellis, and others, cognitions have become crucial to the understanding and treatment of mental disorders (Beck & Haigh, 2014). However, the concept of cognition has become even broader over the years, and the question has arisen regarding which parts of the cognitive system are determining mechanisms and which parts are mainly correlates of varying clinical conditions. Patient expectations are a pivotal part of the cognitive system and must be taken into account because they influence future well-being. Most people are able to cope with even very aversive events as long as they know these events are not long-lasting and will not result in persistent, negative effects. For example, tinnitus, localized pain, and other bodily discomforts are manageable if the affected person knows this unpleasant sensation will not last longer than a brief moment. However, if that person expects the same sensation to last several years or even for the remainder of their lifetime, then the very same unpleasant sensation can become a significant burden that proves to be a demoralizing factor.

Further support for the special role of expectations comes from the broad field of research on the placebo effect. Expectations in their broader sense are considered one of the main contributing factors to placebo and nocebo responses (Enck, Bingel, Schedlowski, & Rief, 2013; Rief, Bingel, Schedlowski, & Enck, 2011). For nearly every medical condition, it has been shown that placebo mechanisms can contribute to the success of the treatment. Moreover, all dimensions of treatment outcomes are prone to influence by expectations. The strongest effects of such influences have been shown for patient-reported outcomes, but observable behavioral aspects and biological parameters are also vulnerable to placebo influences (Schedlowski, Enck, Rief, & Bingel, 2015). Psychopharmacological treatments are associated with powerful placebo effects as well, and corresponding studies often have problems showing an advantage over strong placebo conditions (Kirsch, 2016; Shedden Mora, Nestoriuc, & Rief, 2011).

Explanations for the special role of expectations still need further elucidation, but examples of how expectations influence current and future mental states are easily observed. Expectations can explain, and even determine, the behavior that is shown after disorders have developed. For example, patients with cardiovascular problems who expect (and fear) a heart attack if they overtax the bodily system will significantly reduce their physical activity level, thereby contributing to a less favorable course of recovery. Similarly, patients who expect pain with certain movements will avoid any pain-provoking situations ("fear avoidance") (Vlaeyen & Linton, 2000).

Patient avoidance and security behaviors have been shown to significantly predict the persistence of mental and medical problems (Chou & Shekelle, 2010; Kroska, 2016; Porter & Chambless, 2015; Winer & Salem, 2016), but on an even more basic mechanistic level, expectations can determine attention and perception processes. For instance, if we expect some threat to appear in our left visual field, then we will focus our attention in this exact direction. And if we are subsequently presented with complex visual stimuli in this left visual field, then the parts of this stimuli that were expected will be processed more easily than others (Aue & Okon-Singer, 2015; Bouret & Sara, 2004; Kaiser, Vick, & Major, 2006; Summerfield & Egner, 2016). Likewise, if patients expect some side effect to develop from a medical treatment, then they will direct their attention to the corresponding body part associated with that side effect, causing them to amplify the perception of any unpleasant sensations (Rheker, Winkler, Doering, & Rief, 2017; Rief et al., 2009).

The significant psychological role of expectations is further underlined by a new understanding of the functions of our brain. Traditionally, the brain was considered a more passive information processing machine that waited to receive external stimulation, processed these perceptions, and then decided how to react. However, a more modern understanding of brain functionality considers the brain as an active prediction machine (Clark, 2013; Egner & Summerfield, 2013). This "predictive coding" theory maintains that the brain continuously generates predictions about what will happen next, and if the subsequent events are in the range of predicted outcomes, then stereotypical reactions can occur. On average, such a strategy is more economical compared to continuously processing the relevance of every single stimulus that appears. More sophisticated and effortful information processing is only necessary if prediction errors occur. Therefore, the concept of the brain as a prediction machine postulates that it is less energy-demanding if the brain continuously develops predictions, rather than making continuous, effortful transformations of external stimulation.

The brain as a prediction machine also proposes a highly relevant intermediate step: Predictions trigger anticipatory reactions. Even on a psychobiological level, examples have been shown. The expectation of physical effort serves to increase heart rate and activate other energy-providing mechanisms in the body. The expectation of fear-provoking situations results in tunnel vision, physiological activation, and motor preparedness. For some mental health problems, these anticipatory reactions can become more burdensome than the expected event itself, as in the case of anxiety disorders. Considering the new concepts of brain functioning and the role of expectations in clinical conditions, this brings our attention to the question of whether we can reconceptualize mental disorders as "expectation disorders." Examples will be highlighted in the next section.

Are Mental Disorders "Expectation Disorders"?

It can be argued that some psychiatric disorders, particularly anxiety disorders, are expectation disorders. Patients with anxiety disorders expect a harmful consequence to occur if they are confronted with anxiety-triggering stimuli. In this case, the major problem is not being confronted with the feared stimuli itself, which rarely happens, but the *expected* consequences of being confronted with the feared stimuli. Thus, focusing on conditioning and associative learning is insufficient in explaining the full phenomenon of anxiety: Why do patients continue to expect negative consequences even after being exposed to countless triggering situations that do not lead to a catastrophe? Patients with panic disorder can experience and survive hundreds of panic attacks, but they still expect the next one to result in a life-threatening cardiac event. Therefore, we must consider additional processes beyond associative learning to better understand the persistence of negative expectations in anxiety disorders.

Compared to anxiety disorders, the role of expectations in the detection and classification of affective disorders, such as depression, is less obvious. However, even in depression, uncorrected negative expectations can be considered a major mechanism for the persistence of the disorder (Winer & Salem, 2016). Depression-specific expectations, such as "Nothing will pull me up" and "Tomorrow will be as bad as today," are further supported by negative expectations about social interactions ("Nobody will notice me at the party tonight"). In other words, we suggest that there are depression-specific expectations that are potential mechanisms for the maintenance of the disorder. Furthermore, we suggest that there are expectation-violation situations for psychological treatments that make expectation-violation situations more powerful than before (Kube, D'Astolfo, Glombiewski, Doering, & Rief, 2017a; Kube, Rief, & Glombiewski, 2017b).

Table 1. Examples of Disorder-Specific Expectations

(from Rief & Glombiewski, 2016)

Depression
I will not be able to enjoy anything.
Others will not be interested in making contact with me.
Others will not treat me like a valuable person.

I will bring misfortune to others.

Others will hurt me.

I will not be able to bear it if others reject me.

Post-Traumatic Stress Disorder

I cannot stand to be reminded about this awful event.

I will never be able to experience life like a normal person.

People who look like the offender (e.g., sex, stature, clothes) are as dangerous as the offender.

Others will treat me like a damaged and socially excluded person or like a person who deserves no respect.

Complex Grief

If I start crying, then I will never be able to stop.

If I ever get as close to someone else as I was to my beloved person, then I am at risk of being left by the new partner as well.

I will not be able to manage my affairs alone.

I will lose control if I remember their death.

If I participate in everyday activities or parties, then I will lose touch with the memories of the person I lost.

Phobias, Panic Disorder

If I get in contact with [phobic stimuli], then this will result in catastrophe.

I will not survive the next panic attack.

If others were to see me in a state of anxiety, then they would reject me or never take me seriously again.

If I make mistakes, then others will think I am a loser.

I will not be able to stand it if I do something embarrassing.

Psychosis, Schizophrenia

Others will cause me harm.

Obsessive-Compulsive Disorder (OCD)

If I get into contact with [OCD-provoking stimuli], then catastrophe will result.

If I do not engage in [OCD behavior], then a catastrophe will happen.

Chronic Pain

If I don't move carefully, then I will damage my back.

I cannot function without my medicines.

My problems result from a fragile spine.

There are right and wrong movements.

Many other mental and biobehavioral disorders are characterized by specific expectations. For example, chronic pain conditions are driven by the expectation that certain movements (or the exposure to challenging bodily situations) could result in highly harmful consequences, and this fear avoidance is what results in the persistence of pain (Chou & Shekelle, 2010). Similarly, obsessive-compulsive disorder (OCD) is characterized by negative expectations that coming into contact with the triggering stimuli will result in catastrophe. Post-traumatic stress disorder is associated with violations to the expectation that the world is a safe place and that harmful events only happen to other people. Finally, paranoia is characterized by negative expectations about the behavior of others, which are presumed to involve harm. Table 1 shows more detailed examples of disorder-specific expectations. Disorders can only be successfully treated if these expectations are modified, which brings our focus to the treatment-relevant question of how existing expectations can be successfully changed.

A Psychological Model for the Development, Persistence, and Change of Expectations

It is crucial to understand that expectations mainly develop through experience. Therefore, processes such as "associative learning" are major mechanisms that allow the brain to develop neurophysiological predictions. Beyond personal experience, there are other factors that have a role in the development of expectations, including observational learning, verbal information (e.g. via the internet), and instructions of others. In addition to these well-defined processes, the accidental development of associations can also play a role, which can result in expectations that are difficult to modify.

From a clinical point of view, the original development of expectations is only of academic interest. During the clinical encounter, the focus switches from the development of expectations in the past to the maintenance and change of expectations in present. Typically, patients do not show up in clinical settings without any expectations. Instead, when patients meet physicians or psychotherapists, the disorder is already established—and so are some treatment-relevant expectations. Therefore, the goal of the therapeutic encounter is rarely to establish new expectations; it is to change existing and dysfunctional expectations.

A central process that leads to expectation change is being exposed to expectation-violation situations. Experts consider exposure to expectation-violation situations—and the subsequent changes in expectations that occur—to reflect "learning." Many therapeutic techniques have been developed that depend on expectation violation as a major principle, even if not formulated in detail. However, the question of how expectations change is only one part of the equation. The other part is: Why do expectations persist despite expectation-violation situations? To better understand these processes of expectation development, expectation maintenance, and expectation change, we developed the ViolEx-model (see Figure 5.1) (Rief et al., 2015).

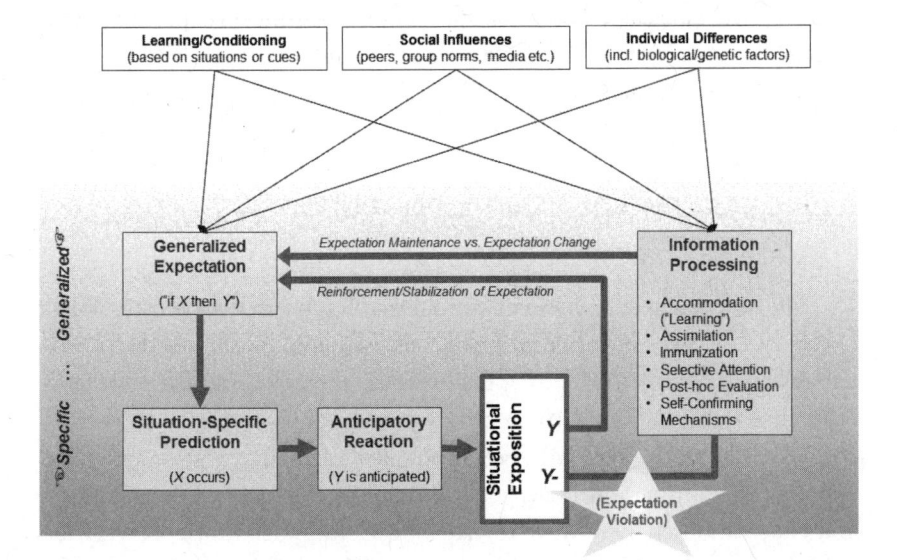

Figure 5.1. The ViolEx Model: A model of Persistence and Change of Expectations (from Rief et al., 2015)

Most patients have experienced hundreds or thousands of situations that violated illness-relevant expectations, but these situations did not lead to an expectation change. In these cases, we postulate that "cognitive immunization processes" are in action. Patients have developed strategies for how to neglect or reformulate the consequences of expectation-violation situations. An improved understanding of these cognitive immunization processes is key to being able to better comprehend the persistence of disorders and to being able to improve mechanisms of change in treatments. These immunization processes can be manifold: Patients can focus their attention on aspects of the situation that are not relevant to expectation violations; expectation violations can be reattributed ("This is the exception to the rule"); expectation violations can confirm preexisting expectations ("Although I survived this heart attack, it further damaged my heart, so the next heart attack will definitely be disastrous," in the case of panic disorder); or patients can reactivate past negative experiences to overwrite the current positive experience.

Most psychotherapeutic approaches have implicit or explicit assumptions about expectation change. However, the manner in which cognitive immunization processes work against expectation violations are typically underestimated or completely neglected. Thus, there is potential to further improve psychological interventions not only by focusing on expectation violations, but also by focusing on strategies to "immunize against cognitive immunization strategies."

Psychotherapy as an Intervention to Violate Expectations

The best example for an intervention that has been developed to violate expectations is exposure therapy. For people with anxiety disorders and anxiety-related disorders (such as OCD), exposure therapy is still the most powerful intervention. While traditional interpretations of exposure therapy considered habituation as the core mechanism of change, reformulations of exposure therapy put a stronger focus on inhibitory processes, expectations, and expectation changes (Craske, Treanor, Conway, Zbozinek, & Vervliet, 2014). Even earlier, Hofmann (2008) pointed out that harm expectation is the common core process that is addressed in extinction learning and exposure therapy. To strengthen the mechanism of expectation violation, it is recommended that practitioners explicitly ask about expectations before the exposure intervention and that they encourage patients to check whether these expectations come true during and after the exposure to feared situations. In a recent experimental study, we have shown that verbalizing expectations pre- and post-exposure amplifies the expectation-violation effect (d'Astolfo et al., in preparation). The expectation-violation effect can be further augmented by directing the patient's attention to situational cues that are crucial for the evaluation of specific predictions that result from more generalized expectations.

Considering the ViolEx-model described earlier, we can further speculate how to improve exposure therapy, not only by focusing on expectations, but also by addressing immunization strategies. Therapists should ask patients to verbalize their expectations before the exposure and give patients an a priori explanation of potential immunization strategies they should avoid using during the exposure. Verbalizing these potential immunization strategies *before they occur* could be a first step in preventing them from blocking treatment-induced changes. However, further interventions should be developed that focus on the exclusion of such immunization strategies that hinder treatment success.

Such an expectation-based understanding of exposure interventions can also be used for the treatment of other mental, biobehavioral, and even some medical problems. For example, in chronic pain, the majority of patients develop "fear avoidance," which is a tendency to avoid any situations or movements that could induce pain or that could result in catastrophic consequences. This avoidance behavior typically leads to selective movements, "learned misuse" of muscles, and reduction in daily activities, which can all contribute to the persistence of chronic pain. New exposure-based interventions have been developed that focus on changing this fear avoidance in chronic pain (Glombiewski et al., 2018), and these interventions have been shown to be more effective than standard cognitive behavioral interventions for chronic pain. Moreover, these positive effects can be achieved even with fewer treatment sessions than standard cognitive behavioral therapy (CBT), as has been shown in a randomized clinical trial (RCT) including more than one hundred chronic pain patients (Glombiewski et al., 2018).

Similarly, CBT for the treatment of depression has developed a tradition of using behavioral experiments, mainly with the aim to check and violate expectations, and these behavioral experiments could be improved if therapists focused not only on expectation violations, but also on potentially occurring cognitive immunization processes. For example, by applying the ViolEx-model to the range of cognitions that are discussed with depression, we have found depression-specific expectations that could be subject to expectation-violation approaches and behavioral experiments (Kube et al., 2017a, 2017b). Using the ViolEx-model to improve psychological interventions in patients with depression is just the beginning, and this is just one clinical example of how to generalize expectation-oriented interventions from anxiety-associated disorders to other mental disorders.

Other psychological interventions, such as psychodynamic therapies, could also be optimized to lead to better expectation-violation experiences. An old psychoanalytical concept says that psychotherapy should lead to "correcting experiences" (Alexander & French, 1946). Indeed, transference and countertransference work can be considered interventions that highlight typical interaction expectations and that eventually change them. Modern reformulations of this concept, such as in a cognitive behavioral analysis system of psychotherapy (McCullough, 2000), move the transference concept even closer to expectation-violation approaches. Together with the patient, the therapist formulates a "transference hypothesis" and continuously checks whether, in their role as a therapist, they are acting the way their patient expects them to behave. This transference hypothesis is eventually broadened to include other interaction partners as well. The associated interventions have the goal of showing patients that their expectations about the behavior of others have been developed with significant others in the past but may no longer prove valid with interaction partners in the present or in the future. Again, a more focused expectation-violation approach and a consideration of cognitive immunization strategies could help further improve these interventions.

There are similar examples of how existing psychological approaches could be optimized with a more rigorous consideration of expectation-violation principles (e.g., for systemic therapies, hypnotherapy), but these are not the subject of this chapter.

How to Modify Expectations: The Clinical Example of Heart Surgery Patients

While many studies have shown the specific role of patients' expectations in predicting treatment outcomes for both psychiatric disorders and medical problems, only a few studies have actively tried to optimize expectations to improve outcome (Kube, Glombiewski, & Rief, 2018). Therefore, we have developed an intervention program to optimize patient expectations, with a particular focus on patients undergoing heart surgery. In former studies, we have shown that even for this highly invasive intervention, pre-surgery expectations of patients can predict illness-induced disability and health-related quality of life several months after surgery (Rief et al., 2017).

Our pre-surgery intervention program to optimize expectations consists of two in-person sessions, two phone calls the week before surgery, and one booster session several weeks after surgery. The major content of the intervention is as follows:

1. *Optimization of outcome expectations:* providing full information about the expected improvements after surgery; linking the improvement process to potential activities patients will be able to do; and developing an activity plan for the sixth months after surgery.

2. *Personal control:* improving patient appraisal of personal control to support the recovery process after surgery; emphasizing the role of continuously increasing physical activity; and improving personal control over anticipated interactions with members of the health care system

3. *Side effect management:* improving patients' expectations of their ability to cope with side effects if they occur; discussing symptoms that could occur (such as swelling or insomnia); and discussing how the patient can deal with these symptoms (see Figure 5.2)

Common unpleasant sensations after the bypass operation.		My tool box against unpleasant sensations	
Appetite Possible side effects are a decreased appetite or a limited sense of taste. In some cases nausea can occur when smelling food. No need to be afraid as appetite and sense of taste will increase back to normal after a few weeks.		Unpleasant sensations/symptoms:	What I can do against them/Things that help me:
Swellings Swellings often arise when there is an incision in the leg. Helpful advice: Put your leg in a higher position. Wear your compression hosiery if you got them prescribed.			
Insomnia You may have difficulties to fall or to be asleep. Helpful advice: It will get better in a while. If pain is causing your sleeplessness you can take a painkiller before going to bed.			
Constipation Some patients suffer from constipation. Helpful advice: Purgatives (laxatives) or a specific diet: fruit, fibres, juice			
Mood Some patients report mood changes or feel depressed. Helpful advice: It passes by. Talking to your family and friends often helps. In addition, you can plan some pleasant activities.			
Swelling at the incision Some patients have a swelling above the incision. This is not a reason to get afraid because the swelling will get better after some time.			
Clicking noise During the first days after your operation, you might possibly hear a clicking noise from your chest. No need to be afraid! This is normal and should be getting better after a while.			

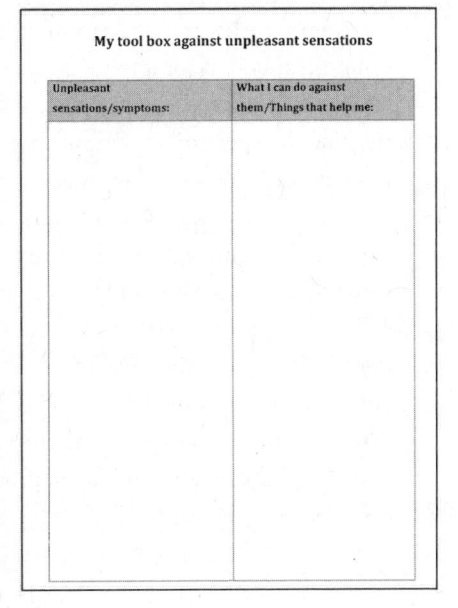

Figure 5.2. Optimizing Expectation about Side Effects and Coping Control

4. *Course and coping:* discussing the most likely course of the disorder after surgery and how patients can cope with the knowledge about their heart disease

Using an RCT design, we offered this pre-surgery intervention as one of three treatment conditions to patients undergoing heart surgery (expectation-optimization condition), with the other two groups being offered supportive therapy (psychological control condition) or standard medical care, in which the anesthesiologist offered typical information about the procedure and occasionally occurring problems (clinical control condition) (Rief et al., 2017). Patients in the expectation-optimization condition had the most pronounced improvements from baseline to six months after surgery. On more specific disability indices, such as working ability in hours per week, the expectation-optimization group had a significant incremental advantage compared to the clinical control group and the psychological control group. Both psychological pre-interventions also led to reduced biological stress responses after surgery (Salzmann et al., 2017).

These findings indicate that the expensive time spent on intensive care units could be reduced for patients participating in our psychological pre-surgery interventions (Auer et al., 2017). In fact, a similar approach was developed for women who underwent breast surgery after suffering from breast cancer and who were recommended to participate in a five-year drug treatment with aromatase inhibitors. While these drugs typically induce symptoms such as joint pain, patients in the expectation-optimization group reported fewer side effects and higher quality of life. The benefit from pre-treatment expectation optimization was most pronounced in women with more negative attitudes (Pan et al., 2018).

These two trials impressively show that the optimization of patients' expectations can significantly improve the outcome of even highly invasive medical interventions, and this type of intervention can also reduce negative side effects of psychological and medical treatments. Patients were very positive about these interventions, and acceptability scores were high (Laferton, Auer, Shedden-Mora, Moosdorf, & Rief, 2015). Further details of the intervention can be found elsewhere (Salzmann et al., 2018). These results encourage the use of similar approaches for other mental and biomedical disorders.

How Expectations Can Contribute to Nosology and Treatment Selection

Expectations fulfill RDoC criteria (Insel, 2014) in that they significantly impact how we describe and differentiate disorders, and they are linked with predictive coding theory, which is a corresponding neurophysiological process. Expectations are better descriptors of different disorders than psychiatric symptoms. For example, anxiety and depression are not unique entities, as they can occur in a range of mental disorders, such as psychosis, trauma-associated disorders, and various other conditions. Expectations, however, point to the crucial and disorder-characterizing mechanism.

Moreover, expectations offer clues that can inform the development of new and improved psychological intervention models. Significant improvement can only occur if disorder-specific expectations change. This requires that therapists better assess preexisting expectations; ask patients to verbalize their specific expectations before, during, and after interventions; and evaluate interventions according to their potential to reliably change expectations. Therefore, the core task of psychotherapists is to break down complex clinical and psychosocial problems to their basic expectations and to subject these expectations to expectation-violation situations. Different therapeutic traditions have developed strategies that directly (e.g., exposure) or indirectly attempt to change expectations. Thus, from an intervention perspective, there is no general need to develop new treatments from scratch. We can simply focus existing treatments on expectations and amplify their efficiency.

However, therapists frequently neglect to account for patients' tendency to block the effects of expectation violation by using cognitive immunization techniques. Therefore, when working with patients who have failed former treatments, who have chronic conditions, or who experience expectation-violation situations without resulting expectation changes, therapists should specifically assess for the presence of cognitive immunization strategies. If these strategies are evident, then the therapist can develop an approach in conjunction with the patient to evaluate these immunization strategies and to determine whether they are correct and helpful.

Finally, a stochastic understanding of prediction errors can further assist therapists in planning adequate interventions. Figure 5.3 shows that people who hold a generally positive attitude about their interpersonal interactions will classify a moderately positive experience as a confirmation of their expectation. In contrast, people who hold more negative attitudes about their interactions with others will classify the very same experience in a way that confirms their negative expectation. Therefore, to violate these negative expectations, people with negative attitudes will need much stronger experiences than the typical normal or moderately positive experiences of everyday life to change these negative expectations.

Prediction error model: "most people are quite friendly"

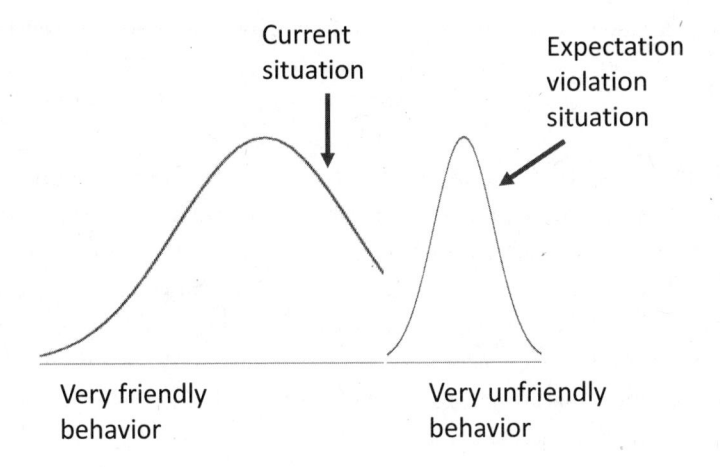

Current situation →

Expectation violation situation ←

Very friendly behavior

Very unfriendly behavior

Prediction error model: "most people are quite unfriendly"

Expectation violation situation →

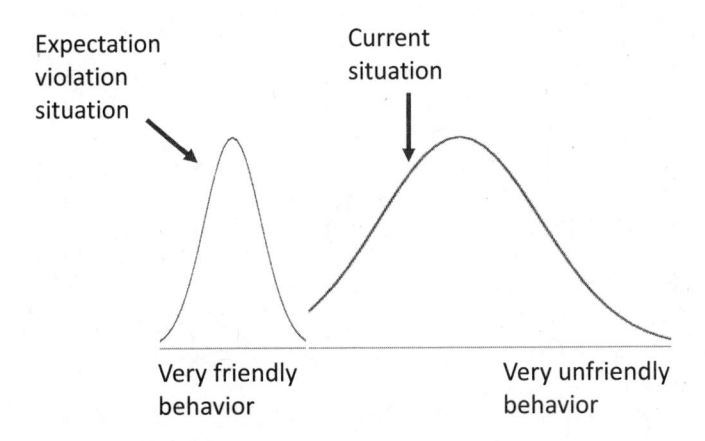

Current situation ↓

Very friendly behavior

Very unfriendly behavior

Figure 5.3. Why Expectation-Violation Interventions Usually Need Powerful Experiences

Conclusion

Expectations, which involve cognitions about future experiences, are crucial for an improved understanding and differentiation of mental disorders. Therefore, expectations should be used more rigorously for the definition and classification of disorders in diagnostic systems such as the DSM and the *International Classification of Diseases and Related Health Problems* (ICD). Indeed, while biological and psychological features notoriously do not discriminate between mental disorders or only do so to a weak amount, disorder-specific expectations do. They offer the critical discriminative information to diagnosticians in their decisions on which mental disorder to classify. Psychological interventions should not only focus on optimizing patients' expectations, but also on limiting the negative effects of cognitive immunization strategies. These expectation-focused interventions have the potential to trigger paradigmatic changes for the classification and treatment of disorders in psychology and medicine.

References

Alexander, F., & French, T. M. (1946). *The corrective emotional experience.* New York: Wiley (reprint 1974).

Aue, T., & Okon-Singer, H. (2015). Expectancy biases in fear and anxiety and their link to biases in attention. *Clinical Psychology Review, 42,* 83–95. doi: 10.1016/j.cpr.2015.08.005

Auer, C. J., Laferton, J. A. C., Shedden-Mora, M. C., Salzmann, S., Moosdorf, R., & Rief, W. (2017). Optimizing preoperative expectations leads to a shorter length of hospital stay in CABG patients: Further results of the randomized controlled PSYHEART trial. *Journal of Psychosomatic Research, 97,* 82–89. doi: 10.1016/j.jpsychores.2017.04.008

Beck, A. T, & Haigh, E. A. P. (2014). Advances in cognitive theory and therapy: The generic cognitive model. *Annual Review of Clinical Psychology, 10,* 1–24.

Bouret, S., & Sara, S. J. (2004). Reward expectation, orientation of attention and locus coeruleus-medial frontal cortex interplay during learning. *European Journal of Neuroscience, 20*(3), 791–802. doi: 10.1111/j.1460-9568.2004.03526.x

Chou, R., & Shekelle, P. (2010). Will this patient develop persistent disabling low back pain? *JAMA, 303*(13), 1295–1302. doi: 10.1001/jama.2010.344

Clark, A. (2013). Whatever next? Predictive brains, situated agents, and the future of cognitive science. *Behavioral and Brain Sciences, 36*(3), 181–204. doi: 10.1017/s0140525x12000477

Craske, M. G., Treanor, M., Conway, C. C., Zbozinek, T., & Vervliet, B. (2014). Maximizing exposure therapy: An inhibitory learning approach. *Behaviour Research and Therapy, 58,* 10–23. doi: 10.1016/j.brat.2014.04.006

D'Astolfo, L., Kircher, L., & Rief, W. (subm.). *Verbalising Expectations of Social Rejection Facilitates Expectation Change in Individuals with High Social Anxiety Traits.*

Egner, T., & Summerfield, C. (2013). Grounding predictive coding models in empirical neuroscience research. *Behavioral and Brain Sciences, 36*(3), 210–211. doi: 10.1017/s0140525x1200218x

Enck, P., Bingel, U., Schedlowski, M., & Rief, W. (2013). The placebo response in medicine: Minimize, maximize or personalize? *Nature Reviews Drug Discovery, 12*(3), 191–204. doi: 10.1038/nrd3923

Glombiewski, J. A., Jeroen, J., Vlaeyen, J., Riecke, J., Holzapfel, S., & Rief, W. (2018). Exposure and CBT for chronic back pain: An RCT on differential efficacy and optimal length of treatment. *Journal of Consulting and Clinical Psychology, 86*(6), 533–545.

Hofmann, S. G. (2008). Cognitive processes during fear acquisition and extinction in animals and humans: Implications for exposure therapy of anxiety disorders. *Clinical psychology review, 28*(2), 199–210.

Insel, T. R. (2014). The NIMH Research Domain Criteria (RDoC) project: Precision medicine for psychiatry. *American Journal of Psychiatry, 171*(4), 395–397.

Kaiser, C. R., Vick, S. B., & Major, B. (2006). Prejudice expectations moderate preconscious attention to cues that are threatening to social identity. *Psychological Science, 17*(4), 332–338. doi: 10.1111/j.1467-9280.2006.01707.x

Kirsch, I. (2016). The placebo effect in the treatment of depression. *Verhaltenstherapie, 26*(1), 55–61. doi: 10.1159/000443542

Kroska, E. B. (2016). A meta-analysis of fear-avoidance and pain intensity: The paradox of chronic pain. *Scandinavian Journal of Pain, 13,* 43–58. doi: 10.1016/j.sjpain.2016.06.011

Kube, T., D'Astolfo, L., Glombiewski, J. A., Doering, B. K., & Rief, W. (2017a). Focusing on situation-specific expectations in major depression as basis for behavioural experiments—Development of the Depressive Expectations Scale. *Psychology and Psychotherapy, 90*(3), 336–352. doi: 10.1111/papt.12114

Kube, T., Glombiewski, J. A., & Rief, W. (2018). Using different expectation mechanisms to optimize treatment of patients with medical conditions: A systematic review. *Psychosomatic Medicine, 80*(6), 535–543.

Kube, T., Rief, W., & Glombiewski, J. A. (2017b). On the maintenance of expectations in major depression—Investigating a neglected phenomenon. *Frontiers in Psychology, 8,* 1–7. doi: 10.3389/fpsyg.2017.00009

Laferton, J. A. C., Auer, C. J., Shedden-Mora, M. C., Moosdorf, R., & Rief, W. (2015). Optimizing preoperative expectations in cardiac surgery patients is moderated by level of disability: The successful development of a brief psychological intervention. *Psychology, Health & Medicine, 21*(3), 272–285. doi: 10.1080/13548506.2015.1051063

McCullough, J. P. (2000). *Treatment for chronic depression: Cognitive behavioral analysis system of psychotherapy.* New York: Guilford Press.

Pan, Y. Q., Heisig, S. R., von Blanckenburg, P., Albert, U. S., Hadji, P., Rief, W., & Nestoriuc, Y. (2018). Facilitating adherence to endocrine therapy in breast cancer: stability and predictive power of treatment expectations in a 2-year prospective study. *Breast Cancer Research and Treatment, 168*(3), 667–677.

Porter, E., & Chambless, D. L. (2015). A systematic review of predictors and moderators of improvement in cognitive-behavioral therapy for panic disorder and agoraphobia. *Clinical Psychology Review, 42,* 179–192. doi: 10.1016/j.cpr.2015.09.004

Rheker, J., Winkler, A., Doering, B. K., & Rief, W. (2017). Learning to experience side effects after antidepressant intake—Results from a randomized, controlled, double-blind study. *Psychopharmacology, 234,* 329–338.

Rief, W., Bingel, U., Schedlowski, M., & Enck, P. (2011). Mechanisms involved in placebo and nocebo responses and implications for drug trials. *Clinical Pharmacology & Therapeutics, 90*(5), 722–726. doi: 10.1038/clpt.2011.204

Rief, W., & Glombiewski, J. A. (2016). Expectation-focused psychological intervention (EFPI). *Verhaltenstherapie, 26*(1), 47–54.

Rief, W., Glombiewski, J. A., Gollwitzer, M., Schubö, A., Schwarting, R., & Thorwart, A. (2015). Expectations as core features of mental disorders. *Current Opinion in Psychiatry, 28,* 378–385.

Rief, W., Shedden-Mora, M., Laferton, J. A. C., Auer, C., Petrie, K.J., Salzmann, S., ... Moosdorf, R. (2017). Preoperative optimization of patient expectations improves long-term outcome in heart surgery patients: Results of the randomized controlled PSY-HEART trial. *BMC Medicine, 15,* 4.

Rief, W., von Lilienfeld-Toal, A., Nestoriuc, Y., Hofmann, S. G., Barsky, A., & Avorn, J. (2009). Differences in adverse effect reporting in placebo groups in SSRI and tricyclic antidepressant trials. A systematic review and meta-analysis. *Drug Safety, 32,* 1041–1056.

Salzmann, S., Euteneuer, F., Laferton, J. A. C., Auer, C. J., Shedden-Mora, M. C., Schedlowski, M., Moosdorf, R., & Rief, W. (2017). Effects of preoperative psychological interventions on catecholamine and cortisol levels after surgery in coronary artery bypass graft patients: The randomized controlled PSY-HEART trial. *Psychosomatic Medicine, 79*(7), 806-814.

Salzmann, S., Laferton, J., Auer, C., Shedden-Mora, M., Wambach, K., & Rief, W. (2018). Optimizing patients' expectations: Description of a brief preoperative intervention for patients undergoing coronary artery bypass graft surgery. *Verhaltenstherapie, 28,* 157–165.

Schedlowski, M., Enck, P., Rief, W., & Bingel, U. (2015). Neuro-bio-behavioral mechanisms of placebo and nocebo responses: Implications for clinical trials and clinical practice. *Pharmacological Reviews, 67,* 697–730.

Shedden Mora, M. C., Nestoriuc, Y., & Rief, W. (2011). Lessons learned from placebo groups in antidepressant trials. *Philosophical Transactions of the Royal Society B-Biological Sciences, 366*(1572), 1879–1888. doi: 10.1098/rstb.2010.0394

Summerfield, C., & Egner, T. (2016). Feature-based attention and feature-based expectation. *Trends in Cognitive Sciences, 20*(6), 401–404. doi: 10.1016/j.tics.2016.03.008

Vlaeyen, J. W. S., & Linton, S. J. (2000). Fear-avoidance and its consequences in chronic musculoskeletal pain: A state of the art. *PAIN, 85,* 317–332.

Winer, E. S., & Salem, T. (2016). Reward devaluation: Dot-probe meta-analytic evidence of avoidance of positive information in depressed persons. *Psychological Bulletin, 142*(1), 18–78. doi: 10.1037/bul0000022

CHAPTER 6

Learning, Language, and Derived Behaviors
Some Implications for a Process-Based Approach to Psychological Suffering

Dermot Barnes-Holmes, PhD,
Yvonne Barnes-Holmes, PhD, and
Ciara McEnteggart, PhD
Ghent University

The increasing focus on psychological processes in the post-*Diagnostical and Statistical Manual* (DSM) era, as exemplified in the current volume, connects rather oddly with a fifty-year line of research that emerged in behavior analysis (which we will refer to more generally as "behavioral science"). Behavioral science has always concerned itself with the behavioral processes of learning, adaptation, and so on, but until the late 1960s or early 1970s, a widely held assumption was that behavioral processes, broadly speaking, were common to both nonhuman and human animals.

This assumption was reflected in the earliest translational research associated with behavioral psychology. A clear-cut example is the famous study by Watson and Rayner (1920), in which they created and "treated" a phobia in a young child using the processes of classical conditioning and extinction that had been identified and studied by Pavlov using dogs (1897/1902). Other examples of learning principles identified in nonhumans being extended to human psychopathology abound in the literature, including studies of learned helplessness (Seligman, 1974), inhibition (Wolpe, 1958), and fear generalization (Lashley & Wade, 1946). In an evolutionary sense, the continuity assumption is that new adaptations include previous ones, but as it came to be applied in behavioral science, the continuity assumption was taken to mean that human functioning could best be explained based on psychological processes identified with nonhuman animals. Even in that distorted form, it has not been without value, but it remains an assumption, not an empirical fact.

This widely held assumption began to be challenged around fifty years ago in behavioral science, when B. F. Skinner proposed the concepts of instructional control and rule-governed behavior as a way in which humans could solve problems without direct contact with reinforcement contingencies (Skinner, 1966, 1969). A few years later, another major figure in behavioral science, Murray Sidman, identified a phenomenon that he labeled "stimulus equivalence" (Sidman, 1971), which appeared to provide a behavioral process underlying instructional control itself. This work, in turn, led to relational frame theory (RFT; Hayes & Brownstein, 1985), which is a modern behavioral science attempt to deal with the psychological processes that appear largely unique to the human species.

Within behavioral science, the connections amongst instructional control, rule-governed behavior, stimulus equivalence, and RFT—and understanding and treating the processes involved in human psychological suffering—are well-known. Outside of behavioral science, though, knowledge of this work is either limited or absent. A central purpose of the current chapter is to highlight the modern behavioral science approach to the study of human psychological processes and the implications these processes have for understanding and treating human suffering. A major reason to do so is that as intervention moves in a process-based direction, differences between various wings, waves, or traditions are diminished, and there can be a fresh look at the value of different ways of thinking about particular processes. In cognitive behavioral therapy (CBT), cognition has been a central focus, but the models of cognition generated therein rarely, if ever, consider modern work in behavioral science. Much of the CBT work has, of course, been clinically based, but to the extent that applied models have appealed to a basic account, they tend to rely on associationistic theorizing drawn directly from research with nonhuman animals.

Many basic scientists assume there are differences between human and nonhuman psychological processes (e.g., Premack, 2007), but within clinical psychology, it is not uncommon for highly regarded, cutting-edge process-oriented research to fail to grapple meaningfully with these differences. An example is provided by the recent work of Craske and colleagues on an inhibitory learning approach to maximizing the impact of exposure therapy

(Craske, Treanor, Conway, Zbozinek, & Vervliet, 2014). This work draws heavily on basic research conducted with nonhumans (e.g., Bouton, 1993). The underlying assumption is that psychotherapy should be based on, and needs to target, inhibitory learning processes that are common to both human and nonhuman species. In pointing to the work of Craske, we are not questioning its quality or effectiveness, and indeed we applaud Craske's focus on processes in developing therapeutic interventions. But we believe that a more complete process-based approach to human psychological suffering and its treatment should be informed by behavioral research that has sought to understand the lines of fracture that separate nonhuman animal and human psychological processes. The current chapter will attempt to present an overview of this work. (For a broadly similar argument, but from a different theoretical position, see LeDoux, Brown, Pine, & Hofmann, 2018; LeDoux & Hofmann, 2018.)

Skinner, Instructional Control, and Semantic Relations

The continuity assumption could be seen as an important context for the first serious behavioral attempt to provide an account of human language. Skinner's (1957) controversial book on human language, *Verbal Behavior*, drew heavily on a body of work that had been conducted with nonhumans. The book itself interpreted much of human language in terms of what were described as "verbal operants." For example, the concept of the "tact" referred to instances in which a speaker had learned to emit the correct name of an object, based on a history of generalized, conditioned reinforcement provided by a listener in the wider verbal community. Although the tact may have been reinforced socially (i.e., by a listener), the key process was an operant, which in principle could be observed in nonhuman species. Less than ten years after the publication of *Verbal Behavior*, however, Skinner (1966) offered an account of problem solving in terms of instructional control or rule-governed behavior, which suggested a clear break in the continuity between human and nonhuman learning. Specifically, he suggested that humans could solve problems by following rules or instructions (what he termed "contingency specifying stimuli") without having to contact reinforcement contingencies directly. Insofar as only human language provided the basis for (complex) instructional control, the bedrock of the continuity assumption within behavioral psychology had started to crack.

Only five years later, seminal research by Sidman (1971) laid the foundation for seriously undermining the central role of the continuity assumption in behavioral psychology. Specifically, Sidman identified a process he called "stimulus equivalence," which referred to the emergence of untaught or unreinforced behaviors that could not be readily explained using established behavioral principles previously wrought from animal research. The basic effect involved training participants to match arbitrary stimuli to each other (e.g., A-B and B-C) and then observing the emergence of untaught matching responses (e.g., B-A and C-A). The challenge to the continuity assumption became completely apparent with repeated failures to demonstrate even the simplest emergent matching responses in nonhumans, including higher primates (Barnes & Holmes, 1991; Dougher, Twohig, & Madden, 2014; Dugdale & Lowe, 2000; Zentall, 1998). The circle was then closed when Sidman (1994) used the concept of stimulus equivalence to provide a behavioral account of semantic or symbolic relations in human language that helped explain how humans could construct, understand, and follow simple instructions.

Sidman suggested that rules have their impact on behavior because the words contained within rules entered into "equivalence relations" with the stimuli and events specified in those rules. Thus, equivalence as an outcome began to provide the foundation for an account of how instructions could "specify" contingencies. However, equivalence itself needed to be explained: either it was a behavioral primitive or emerged via other behavioral processes.

Sidman's insight and contribution were particularly timely for a line of research in behavioral psychology that had begun to draw heavily on the concept of rule-governed behavior in the clinical domain. Specifically, Hayes and colleagues (e.g., Hayes, 1989; Hayes, Brownstein, Zettle, Rosenfarb, & Korn, 1986; Zettle & Hayes, 1982) had begun to argue that human psychological suffering resulted, in part, from excessive rule-following in some contexts at the expense of more contingency-sensitive behavior. As a simple example, imagine a person with chronic pain who rigidly follows the rule "Exercise will only make my pain worse." Such a person may never learn that exercise often has the opposite effect on pain. Cognitive effects of this kind were exactly what the emerging area of CBT was focused on, and many, but not all, cognitive methods were argued to make sense in light of the emerging evidence on rule-governance (Zettle & Hayes, 1982).

Although the focus on rules in the clinical domain looked promising, in terms of basic behavioral processes, exactly how humans came to form equivalence classes or learned to understand, construct, and follow such rules remained unclear. The need to address this issue was instrumental in generating the account of human language and cognition, known as RFT (Hayes & Brownstein, 1985; Hayes & Hayes, 1989; see Hayes, Barnes-Holmes, & Roche, 2001 for the first book-length treatment). This theory constituted a direct challenge to the continuity assumption in behavioral science in aiming to provide an account of human psychology that focused on psychological processes that appeared to be uniquely human. It also soon led to process-based extensions into human psychological suffering, beginning with acceptance and commitment therapy (ACT; Hayes, 1987). Because of this early intertwining of issues (e.g., Hayes, 1984), historical reviews see RFT and ACT as having co-evolved (McEnteggart, 2018; Zettle, 2005).

Relational Frame Theory

From an RFT point of view, stimulus equivalence was an example of a larger class of operant behavior: *arbitrarily applicable relational responding* (AARR; Hayes & Hayes, 1989). According to this extension of Sidman's seminal work, a history of reinforced relating between and among stimuli established particular patterns of overarching or generalized relational operants, referred to as relational frames (Barnes-Holmes, Barnes-Holmes, & Cullinan, 2000). For example, imagine a young child who learns to point to the family dog upon hearing the word "dog" and to say "dog" when someone else points to the dog. The child might also learn to say "Rover" when asked, "What is the dog's name?" Each of these naming or relational responses would be explicitly prompted, shaped, and reinforced initially by the verbal community. Across many such exemplars involving other stimuli in other contexts, the operant class of coordinating stimuli in this way becomes abstracted, such that direct reinforcement for all of the individual components of naming are no longer required when a novel stimulus is encountered. So if a child was shown a picture of an aardvark and the written word, and was told its name, then the child may later say, "That's an aardvark" when presented with a relevant picture or the word, without any prompting or direct reinforcement for doing so. In other words, the generalized relational operant of coordinating pictures, spoken words, and written words is established, and directly reinforcing a subset of the relating behaviors (spoken word-picture and spoken word-written word) "spontaneously" generates the complete set (e.g., picture-written word).

When a pattern of generalized relating is established, that class of behavior is defined as always being under some form of contextual control. Contextual cues are thus seen as discriminative for different patterns of relational responding or different relational frames. The cues acquire their functions through the types of histories described above. Thus, for example, the phrase "That is a"—as in *"That is a dog"*—would be established across exemplars as a contextual cue for the complete pattern of relational responding (e.g., coordinating the word "dog" with actual dogs). Once the relational functions of such contextual cues are established in the behavioral repertoire of a young child, the number of stimuli that may enter into such relational response classes becomes almost infinite (Hayes et al., 2001).

The core analytic concept of the relational frame proposed by Hayes and Hayes (1989) involved three common properties: (a) mutual entailment, (b) combinatorial entailment, (c) and the transformation of stimulus functions. First, mutual entailment refers to the relation between two stimuli. For example, if you are told A *is the same as* B, then you will derive that B *is the same as* A. That is, the specified A *is the same as* B relation mutually entails the (symmetrical) B *is the same as* A relation. Second, combinatorial entailment refers to the relations among three or more stimuli. For example, if you are told A *is more than* B and B *is more than* C, then you will derive that A *is more than* C and C *is less than* A. That is, the A-B and B-C relations combinatorially entail the A-C and C-A relations. Third, the transformation of stimulus functions refers to the "psychological content" involved in any instance of derived relational responding. For example, if A *is less than* B, and a reinforcing function is attached to A, then B will acquire a greater reinforcing function than A, even though the function was directly attached to A and not B.

Whereas Sidman's work on equivalence relations focused on what may be considered the most basic type of symbolic relation, RFT developed and expanded the conceptual analysis in an effort to cover the richness and complexity of human language and cognition in whole cloth. It was soon shown empirically that equivalence relations were just one type of symbolic relation and that numerous others could be established by multiple exemplar training (Steele & Hayes, 1991). From the early 1990s until the present day, these patterns of relational responding (e.g., coordination, opposition, distinction, comparison, spatial frames, temporal frames, deictic relations, and hierarchical relations) have been analyzed across numerous experimental studies and across a variety of procedures. Some research has also explored the transformation of functions (see Hughes & Barnes-Holmes, 2016a, for a recent review). In addition, empirical evidence has supported the core RFT postulate that exposure to multiple exemplars during early language development is required to establish these relational frames (see Hughes & Barnes-Holmes, 2016b). Therefore, the argument that relational framing may be thought of as overarching or generalized relational operants has gained considerable empirical traction.

Although RFT remains a work in progress as a behavioral account of the core processes involved in human language and cognition, the research it has generated appears to have broad-ranging implications for understanding and treating psychological suffering. To appreciate these implications, we will provide examples of how behavioral processes identified by RFT have been used in the clinical domain.

Transformations of Functions

The concept of transformation of functions has often been invoked in order to explain the development and maintenance of irrational fears and phobias (e.g., Augustson & Dougher, 1997; Dougher, Augustson, Markham, Greenway, & Wulfert, 1994). Imagine a young boy who experienced a bad fall from a horse while horseback riding for the first time and subsequently feared horses. Here, the fear of horses was directly conditioned. Now imagine that the boy develops a fear of cows even though he has not experienced any negative event with a cow. Such a *transformation* of functions, wherein cows are now fear-inducing, could be based, at least in part, on the fact that horses and cows participate in a frame of coordination in the context of "large farm animals." Because of this coordination, it is possible that the boy in time may show distress on a trip to the zoo because the fear-inducing function of large farm animals now spreads through "symbolic generalization" (i.e., the frame of coordination) to all large four-legged animals.

On the face of it, this example might be criticized because large animals bear some formal resemblance, and thus the more traditional step of explaining human psychopathology by appealing to learning processes demonstrable with nonhumans is readily available (e.g., the boy's fear expanded to the cow via stimulus generalization). The value of the concept of transformation of functions becomes more evident, however, when complex examples of human psychological suffering are examined. Imagine a woman who has begun to feel trapped in various areas of her life (e.g., work, relationships, and family). Her use of the word "trapped" in these contexts results in bouts of claustrophobia and panic when she enters enclosed spaces, such as elevators, subways, and shopping malls. The emergence of claustrophobia and panic may have little to do with actual aversive experiences in any of these contexts and is instead based on the transformation of functions of those contexts because they are coordinated via the term "trapped" to the relational networks that describe work, relationships, and family responsibilities. Unlike the earlier example, there are no formal properties that are shared between, say, relationship difficulties and an elevator. In this case, relating entire relational networks to other relational networks is involved in highly abstract transformations of functions.

As empirical methods were developed to understand how symbolic relations could lead to such behavioral effects, it was argued that simpler examples of the spread of psychopathology, such as the boy's fear of cows, could be partly due to relational learning. In addition, as human psychological suffering was interpreted or explained in terms of derived relational responses and the transformation of functions, it became possible to use RFT ideas to focus on the role of such symbolic relations in psychotherapy. In the case of the woman who developed claustrophobia and panic in the context of feeling trapped in several domains in her life, it may be useful in therapy to explore the word "trapped" itself. For instance, the therapist might explore the functional properties of "being trapped" by gently holding the client's wrists and asking her to describe how it feels to be trapped by someone else. Engaging in this physical metaphor may help the client see the connections among her claustrophobia, panic, and the wider unhappy features of her life. She can then explore her reactions to these contexts in ways that are defined as values-driven rather than values-disabling (e.g., she can consider changing jobs, sharing her fears with her partner, etc.).

Rule-Governed Behavior

From an early age, we learn to follow rules that are given to us by others and that provide us with useful strategies for controlling our behavior and predicting the behavior of others. For example, parents pass onto their children rules about poisonous foods (e.g., do not eat yellow berries) in order to avoid serious illness without the children having to make direct contact with the natural contingencies. In some contexts, however, rule-governed behavior may be relatively insensitive to contingencies, which in turn *promotes* psychological suffering rather than protecting us from potentially harmful events in the environment (McAuliffe, Hughes, & Barnes-Holmes, 2014, p. 2). Therefore, excessive reliance upon rules in daily life can become problematic. Consider a man who follows rules such as: "I must always appear strong," "People can never see me upset," "Men shouldn't cry," and so on. Following such rules may work well in his professional life as the CEO of a company. In a different context, though, such as his relationship with his partner, following these rules may be problematic because he does not share things that upset him or that appear to make him vulnerable, thereby leading to a lack of intimacy in the relationship.

In the context of therapy, undermining inflexible or excessive rule-following can be achieved by helping the client identify instances of rule-following and by exploring the *workability* of these rules in various contexts. Using the previous example, the man may identify the rule "People can never see me upset" as controlling his behavior, so the therapist might then ask questions such as, "Can you give me some examples of when you might use this rule?" The therapist can then begin to target the behavioral control functions of the rule by asking questions such as "Is it possible this might actually be pushing your partner away from you?" These questions can offer an alternative perspective from which the client can view his own behavior in the context of the rule. The therapist might then try to encourage the man to engage in contingency-sensitive (rather than rule-consistent) behaviors, such as talking openly to his partner about his feelings.

These examples would hardly be unique to therapies generated within a behavioral approach, but in the context of process-based therapy, that is the point. As practitioners begin to focus on basic behavioral process accounts of cognition, such as those as identified within RFT, a wider range of practical change methods becomes available, but they are always based on a close link between basic principles and application.

It is already evident that process-based therapy reduces the artificial barriers between traditional cognitive and behavioral accounts of therapy and their underlying mechanisms or processes of action (e.g., Hayes & Hofmann, 2018). In that context, it is not a large step for therapists interested in cognitive models of psychopathology and its alleviation to consider the implications of a basic behavioral account of cognition and symbolic meaning itself. Practically speaking, this is not a mere matter of terminology—the importance of a basic process account is felt in the precision, range, and impact of the applied methods it suggests. In the next sections, we will provide two extended examples.

Metaphor: The Relating of Relations

An area in which RFT can be applied to therapy is in its account of analogy and metaphor, in which relating relations lies at the core (Stewart & Barnes-Holmes, 2001). Consider the simple analogy "Peach is to pear as cat is to dog," in which one coordination relation (peach-pear) is related to another coordination relation (cat-dog). One coordination relation relates two stimuli in the context of fruit, while the other coordination relation relates two stimuli in the context of domestic animals. The phrase "is to" is the coordination relation that relates the two relations with each other. Critically, the four stimuli (peach, pear, cat, dog) do not collapse into a single relational network in which they all become equivalent or coordinated. Rather, the network consists of two separate relations that are related to each other *as relations*.

One of the key functions of analogy and metaphor in natural language is to help listeners use established knowledge in one domain to understand information in another domain. For example, the analogy "The heart is like a pump" is often used in anatomy. Relating relations, as the basis of analogy and metaphor, can also be used to help clients see their situation in a new or different way that may facilitate clinical change (see Foody et al., 2014). Consider one of the stock analogies often used in ACT: "Struggling with anxiety is like struggling in quicksand." This analogy contains three elements: (a) two coordination relations (struggling with anxiety-panic and struggling in quicksand-drowning), (b) a coordination relation between these relations (struggling with anxiety *is like* struggling in quicksand), and

(c) seeing the behavior of "struggling" as part of the problem. More technically, the analogy is designed so that the dominant functions of the vehicle in the metaphor (the dangers of struggling in quicksand) are transferred via the coordination-coordination relation to the target of the metaphor (the possible costs of struggling with anxiety). Thus, just as an unwise attempt to escape quicksand could lead to more rapid drowning, unnecessary struggles with anxiety may lead to being overwhelmed by panic. This type of analogy could be especially useful in therapy if a client had not previously noticed that the struggle to control anxiety might actually increase the likelihood of panic. Asking the client to consider the analogy may thus encourage the client to respond differently to the experience of anxiety when it occurs. Relating relations, in the context of this analogy, thus suggest that it may be useful to expose oneself to anxiety in much the same way as one survives in quicksand by lying out flat on its surface.

An advantage of having a basic account of therapeutic metaphor is the guidance that this account can provide clinically. For example, when attempting to use metaphors in therapy, it is important that the therapist does so along with a functional assessment of the client's key problem and its dominant felt sense. For example, if the client's anxiety does not involve a sense of being overwhelmed by panic, or if they have never heard of quicksand, then the coordination with drowning in quicksand will likely fail. The closer the analogy matches the relevant relational networks for the client, the more likely it will produce the desired behavior change. This match is based both on the shared functions between the vehicle and target (e.g., the physiological arousal of a physical struggle and that of overwhelming anxiety) and by the functions that are dominant in the vehicle (e.g., the life-and-death need to increase surface area when in contact with quicksand) but are relatively absent in the target (e.g., the importance of exposure and emotional openness when addressing panic). Understanding these features may help the practitioner select an apt clinical metaphor and present it in ways that maximize the hoped-for transformation of stimulus functions. For example, the feeling of physical exertion might be described in terms that fit the client's experience of panic as the metaphor is presented. If the client experiences cardiac symptoms and difficulty breathing as part of the panic episode, then the clinician might present the metaphor with terms that accentuate that very connection—for example, "*You gasp for breath* trying to pull one foot and then the other out of the quicksand, and *your heart thunders and skips beats* as, to your horror, you sink deeper and deeper."

Deictic Stimulus Relations and the Verbal Self

The emergence of a stable sense of self is a critical feature of human development and is an assumed prerequisite for complex verbal behavior and psychological well-being (Dymond & Barnes 1997; Hayes 1984). Indeed, clinical researchers have proposed that fractured development of the self may be associated with psychological suffering (e.g., Ingram 1990; McEnteggart, Barnes-Holmes, Dillon, Egger, & Oliver, 2017). For RFT, the verbal self (sometimes referred to as the "deictic-I") involves three functionally distinct deictic relational units: (a) the interpersonal I-YOU relations, (b) the spatial HERE-THERE relations, and (c) the temporal NOW-THEN relations (Barnes-Holmes, 2001). According to RFT, the verbal community teaches a young child across time to distinguish themselves from others and to locate the verbal self in space and time. For example, young children are frequently asked questions such as, "What are you doing now?", "What did you do then?", "Where are you going tomorrow?", and "Did you go there with your dad or your mom?" As a child learns to respond appropriately to these questions, the verbal self, located in time and space and in relation to others, emerges out of the social-verbal contingencies within which the child is raised.

Some authors have argued that the verbal self may be central to psychological suffering (e.g., Barnes-Holmes et al., 2018), especially when the self participates in instances of what might be called excessive rule-following. For example, consider the rule or relational network "Only bad people end up alone." This may facilitate a negative evaluation of the verbal self in the context of, for example, a divorce. In more technical terms, excessive rule-following in this case produces a transformation of negative evaluative functions of the self, which are based on coordinating the verbal self with "alone" and coordinating "alone" with "badness." In ACT, this effect may be referred to as fusion with negative thoughts and with feelings about the self. Critically, these negative self-evaluations, which reflect instances of excessive rule-following, reduce the likelihood that future behavior will bring the individual into contact with contingencies that could potentially undermine the problematic rule-following. For example, engaging in new social activities following a divorce may be less likely if the individual believes they deserve to be alone because they are a bad, unlovable person.

The Relationship Between the Verbal Self and Others

The development of the relationship between the verbal self and others also appears to be critical in psychological suffering (Barnes-Holmes et al., 2018; McEnteggart et al., 2017). Imagine a young boy who is subjected to emotional abuse by a parent over a period of years. The parent will perhaps abuse the child in one moment, and in the next say, "You know that I love you." The fact that the parent emits relational networks or rules pertaining to the child's verbal self (i.e., that he is loved) in a way that is incoherent with how the wider verbal community responds to such networks (most people do not routinely abuse people they love) may undermine the child's ability to connect in a healthy way with others in adulthood. Specifically, this individual may find it challenging in later life to form a close and intimate relationship with someone who is not abusive toward him. In extreme cases, the levels of relational incoherence created by this highly abusive parenting may alter the development of a coherent or stable verbal self, resulting in severe psychological manifestations such as auditory hallucinations, dissociation, or paranoia (McEnteggart et al., 2017).

To the extent that relational processes of this kind are key to psychopathology and its treatment, the psychological processes established in nonhuman learning may be of less value in understanding human psychological suffering. Said more simply, if human cognition is central to human mental and behavioral problems and yet involves unique psychological processes, an account of psychopathology and its treatment will ultimately need to deal with these processes. Unpacking existing cognitive models in relational learning terms will require increasingly refined analyses of the symbolic processes that are unique to the human species. RFT remains a work in progress, and some recent conceptual developments in this area appear to have important implications for understanding the dynamics of the behavioral processes involved in human psychological suffering.

A multidimensional, multilevel framework (MDML) has recently been proposed as a means of conceptualizing the dynamics of relational processes. In the next section, we will briefly review this framework. (For a detailed treatment, see Barnes-Holmes, Barnes-Holmes, Luciano, & McEnteggart, 2017.)

A Multidimensional, Multilevel Framework

The MDML framework does not introduce any new process-based concepts to RFT, but rather attempts to bring some order to the myriad ways in which RFT researchers have analyzed human language and cognition in both laboratory and applied settings. In doing so, the framework identifies what are described as twenty experimental units of analysis that, at this time, appear to be central to analyzing the dynamical interactions involved in the core process of derived relational responding itself. To assist the reader in understanding the MDML framework, a visual representation of the framework is provided in Table 1.

Table 1. A Multidimensional, Multilevel (MDML) Framework Consisting of Twenty Intersections Between the Dimensions and Levels of Arbitrarily Applicable Relational Responding

Levels	Dimensions			
	Coherence	Complexity	Derivation	Flexibility
Mutually Entailing	Analytic Unit 1	Analytic Unit 2	Analytic Unit 3	Analytic Unit 4
Relational Framing	...	...	...	...
Relational Networking	...	...	...	...
Relating Relations	...	...	...	...
Relating Relational Networks	...	...	...	Analytic Unit 20

According to the MDML framework, there are five levels of relational responding: (a) mutual entailing (bidirectional relations between two stimuli), (b) relational framing (simplest relational network), (c) relational networking, (d) relating relations, and (e) relating relational networks. The framework conceptualizes each of these levels as having four dimensions: *derivation, complexity, coherence,* and *flexibility*. Each level intersects with each dimension, yielding twenty units of analysis for conceptualizing the dynamics of relational responding. In brief, *derivation* refers to how many times a derived response has been emitted. The first response is, by definition, high in derivation because it is derived entirely from a trained relation(s). Subsequently, however, derived responses gradually acquire their own history and are thus derived less and less from the initially trained relation(s). *Complexity* refers to the detail or density of a pattern of relational responding, such as the number of relations or the different types of relations in a given network. *Coherence* refers to the extent to which relational responding is generally predictable or consistent with previously established patterns of relational responding (whether directly trained or derived). *Flexibility* refers to the extent to which patterns of derived relational responding may be altered or impacted by various contextual variables (e.g., how readily a pattern of equivalence responding may change when the trained baseline relations are reversed).

We can examine a short clinical interaction to consider how the MDML framework may connect in a fine-grained way to clinical dialogue. (To link the MDML framework to basic experimental research, consult Barnes-Holmes et al., 2017.) Imagine a client who comes into therapy, and during the first session, the following exchange occurs:

Client: "I am a useless person."

Therapist: "Do you really believe that you're useless?"

Client: "Without a doubt, I truly am useless. "

Therapist: "How long have you felt useless?"

Client: "Oh, for many, many years."

Therapist: "What makes you think you're so useless?"

Client: "It's hard to say really, I just know that I am."

Therapist: "I find it hard to believe that you're totally useless."

Client: [defensively] "But you don't know me. If you did, then you'd know how useless I really am."

How might we conceptualize this therapeutic interaction in the language of the MDML? First, when the client says, "I am a useless person," this may be defined as mutually entailing the verbal self with "useless." Second, when the client states, "Without a doubt, I truly am useless," the mutual entailing may be defined as high in coherence (i.e., it is highly consistent with the client's other self-descriptive statements). Third, when the client reports thinking this "for many, many years," the mutually entailing is defined as low in derivation (i.e., the client has been thinking this almost habitually). Fourth, when the client says, "I just know that I am" as an explanation for being useless, the mutual entailing is defined as relatively *simple* (i.e., it is low in complexity) at that point in the therapeutic exchange. Finally, when the client reacts negatively to the therapist's suggestion that the client does not seem like a useless person, the mutually entailing may be defined as highly *inflexible.*

The MDML framework can be used to conceptualize relatively subtle differences in the type of therapeutic exchange presented above. Imagine, for example, that the client provided a long list of reasons for qualifying as useless (rather than simply saying, "I just am"). For example, he might say, "I'm a failed husband, I'm a useless father, and I keep getting fired." This "reason-giving" may be categorized as relational networking or relating relational networks. In terms of dimensions, the client's responding might be defined as *low* in coherence if the response to the therapist's question, "What makes you think you're so useless?" was, "I don't know really, and sometimes I can see ways in which I am not completely useless." If the client indicated having only recently self-identified as useless (rather than thinking this for years), then the network might be considered relatively *high* in derivation (i.e., as a verbal response that had only emerged recently in the client's cognitive repertoire). Because the client replied with a list of reasons why he is useless, the networking may be defined as *high* in complexity, particularly if the reasons are also supplemented with extended narratives around each reason. When challenged by the therapist, had the client replied with, "Maybe you're right, I'm probably not useless at everything," then this may have indicated a higher level of *flexibility* than that presented in the example above.

The MDML framework is relatively new in the literature on derived relational responding, but it seems useful to present it here because it makes a larger point that is relevant to an attempt to construct process-based accounts that can be an alternative to the DSM approach to human misery. Efforts to identify and understand therapeutic change processes need to go hand in hand with efforts to systematize and refine the experimental and conceptual analyses of the basic processes involved in cognition, emotion, sense of self, attention, motivation, and the like. Basic behavioral processes have important implications for understanding human psychological suffering.

Indeed, in this context, it seems important to note that the MDML framework itself has recently been developed to include a specific focus on two generic classes of transformation of functions: orienting and evoking functions. This development generates a highly dynamic conceptual unit of analysis for RFT involving relating, orienting, and evoking, referred to as ROEing (Barnes-Holmes, 2018; Barnes-Holmes et al., 2019). The concept of ROEing allows RFT to analyze core psychological processes—such as attention, perception, emotion, motivation, language, and cognition—as dimensional, dynamical, and nonlinear behavioral interactants rather than as separate systems or components of human mental life. The MDML framework has thus become hyperdimensional (i.e., the HDML) and has been used recently to create basic behavioral process accounts of human psychological suffering (see Barnes-Holmes, 2019; Barnes-Holmes, McEnteggart, & Barnes-Holmes, in press).

The emphasis on behavioral dynamics and change that are so clearly inherent in the MDML (now HDML) framework is reflected in the definition of therapeutic change processes articulated by Hofmann and Hayes (2019):

> *Therapeutic processes* are the underlying change mechanisms that lead to the attainment of a desirable treatment goal. We define a therapeutic process as a set of theory-based, dynamic, progressive, and multilevel changes that occur in predictable empirically established sequences oriented toward the desirable outcomes. These processes are *theory-based* and associated with falsifiable and testable predictions, they are *dynamic,* because processes may involve feedback loops and nonlinear changes, they are *progressive* in the long term in order to be able to reach the treatment goal, and they form a *multilevel system* because some processes supersede others. Finally, these processes are oriented toward both immediate and long-term goals (p. 38).

Processes of this kind are inherently idiographic (Hayes et al., 2019), and understanding them will require basic theoretical accounts that are similarly dynamic, multidimensional, nonlinear, nested, multilevel, and idiographically applicable. The HDML approach to symbolic cognitive processes fits all of those descriptors. Process-based CBT moves the CBT tradition in a behavioral science direction, and thus, there seem to be few reasons not to consider the hundreds of studies available on relational framing as integrated in the HDML when attempting to understand processes of change in psychological intervention.

Conclusion

Any attempt to provide a transdiagnostic framework for psychological suffering will need to grapple with the fact that human learning processes appear so much more complex than those that have been studied in nonhuman animals. In this chapter, we have attempted to show that the tradition of behavioral science that is perhaps most closely associated with the continuity assumption has, ironically, seriously challenged that assumption—empirically and conceptually—for almost half a century. Indeed, behavioral science continues to grapple with what is perhaps the most significant challenge facing the post-DSM era and perhaps even psychology as a science: the need to work out an experimental and conceptual analysis of human cognition that can feed directly into a better understanding of the processes involved in psychological suffering and its successful treatment. Without serious progress in this regard, we seem destined to repeat some of the errors of the past in the new era of a process-based nosology and treatment approach. Thus, it is important to the long-term success of a process-based approach that applied and basic scientists work together to identify processes of change that are themselves understood at a basic process level.

References

Augustson, E. M., & Dougher, M. J. (1997). The transfer of avoidance evoking functions through stimulus equivalence classes. *Journal of Behavior Therapy and Experimental Psychiatry, 28*(3), 181–191.

Barnes, D., & Holmes, Y. (1991). Radical behaviorism, stimulus equivalence, and human cognition. *The Psychological Record, 41,* 19–30.

Barnes-Holmes, D. (2018, May). *Relational frame theory: Past, present, and future.* Paper presented at the Annual Convention of the Association for Behavior Analysis, International, San Diego, CA.

Barnes-Holmes, D. (2019, February 15). *The double edged sword of human language and cognition: Shall we be Olympians or fallen angels?* [Blog post]. Retrieved from https://science.abainternational.org/the-double-edged-sword-of-human-language-and-cognition-shall-we-be-olympians-or-fallen-angels/rrehfeldtabainternational-org/

Barnes-Holmes, Y. (2001). *Analysing relational frames: Studying language and cognition in young children* (Unpublished doctoral thesis). National University of Ireland Maynooth.

Barnes-Holmes, D., Barnes-Holmes, Y., & Cullinan, V. (2000). Relational frame theory and Skinner's verbal behavior: A possible synthesis. *The Behavior Analyst, 23,* 69–84.

Barnes-Holmes, D., Barnes-Holmes, Y., Finn, M., Harte, C., Kavanagh, D., Leech, A., … Quak, M. (2019). *The dynamics of arbitrarily applicable relational responding and an updated version of relational frame theory.* Manuscript submitted for publication.

Barnes-Holmes, D., Barnes-Holmes, Y., Luciano. C., & McEnteggart, C. (2017). From the IRAP and REC model to a multi-dimensional multi-level framework for analyzing the dynamics of arbitrarily applicable relational responding. *Journal of Contextual Behavioral Science, 6*(4), 434–445.

Barnes-Holmes, Y., Boorman, J., Oliver, J., Thompson, M., McEnteggart, C., & Coulter, C. (2018). Using conceptual developments in RFT to direct case formulation and clinical intervention: Two case summaries [Special section]. *Journal of Contextual Behavioral Science, 7,* 89–96.

Barnes-Holmes, Y., McEnteggart, C., & Barnes-Holmes, D. (in press). Recent conceptual and empirical advances in RFT: Implications for developing process-based assessments and interventions. Chapter to appear in M. E. Levin, M. P. Twohig, & J. Krafft (Eds.), *Recent innovations in ACT.* Oakland, CA: New Harbinger Publications.

Bouton, M. E. (1993). Context, time, and memory retrieval in the interference paradigms of Pavlovian learning. *Psychological Bulletin, 114*(1), 80–99.

Craske, M. G., Treanor, M., Conway, C. C., Zbozinek, T., & Vervliet, B. (2014). Maximizing exposure therapy: An inhibitory learning approach. *Behaviour Research and Therapy, 58,* 10–23.

Dougher, M. J., Augustson, E., Markham, M. R., Greenway, D. E., & Wulfert, E. (1994). The transfer of respondent eliciting and extinction functions through stimulus equivalence classes. *Journal of the Experimental Analysis of Behavior, 62*(3), 331–351.

Dougher, M., Twohig, M. P., & Madden, G. (Eds.). (2014). Editorial: Basic and translational research on stimulus-stimulus relations. *Journal of the Experimental Analysis of Behavior, 101*(1), 1–9.

Dugdale, M., & Lowe, C. F. (2000). Testing for symmetry in the conditional discriminations of language-trained chimpanzees. *Journal of the Experimental Analysis of Behavior, 73*(1), 5–22.

Dymond, S., & Barnes, D. (1997). Behavior-analytic approaches to self-awareness. *The Psychological Record, 47*(2), 181–200.

Foody, M., Barnes-Holmes, Y., Barnes-Holmes, D., Törneke, N., Luciano, C., Stewart, I., & McEnteggart, C. (2014). RFT for clinical use: The example of metaphor. *Journal of Contextual Behavioral Science, 3*(4), 305–313.

Hayes, S. C. (1984). Making sense of spirituality. *Behaviorism, 12,* 99–110.

Hayes, S. C. (1987). A contextual approach to therapeutic change. In N. Jacobson (Ed.), *Psychotherapists in clinical practice: Cognitive and behavioral perspectives* (pp. 327–387). New York: Guilford Press.

Hayes, S. C. (1989). *Rule-governed behavior: Cognition, contingencies, and instructional control.* New York: Plenum Press.

Hayes, S. C., Barnes-Holmes, D., & Roche, B. (2001). *Relational frame theory: A post-Skinnerian account of human language and cognition.* New York: Plenum Press.

Hayes, S. C., & Brownstein, A. J. (1985, May). *Verbal behavior, equivalence classes, and rules: New definitions, data, and directions.* Invited address presented at the meeting of the Association for Behavior Analysis, Columbus, OH.

Hayes, S. C., Brownstein, A. J., Zettle, R. D., Rosenfarb, I., & Korn, Z. (1986). Rule-governed behavior and sensitivity to changing consequences of responding. *Journal of the Experimental Analysis of Behavior, 45,* 237–256.

Hayes, S. C., & Hayes, L. J. (1989). The verbal action of the listener as a basis for rule-governance. In S. C. Hayes (Ed.), *Rule-governed behavior: Cognition, contingencies, and instructional control* (pp. 153–190). New York: Plenum Press.

Hayes, S. C., & Hofmann, S. G. (Eds.). (2018). *Process-based CBT: The science and core clinical competencies of cognitive behavioral therapy.* Oakland, CA: Context Press/New Harbinger Publications.

Hayes, S. C., Hofmann, S. G., Stanton, C. E., Carpenter, J. K., Sanford, B. T., Curtiss, J. E., & Ciarrochi, J. (2019). The role of the individual in the coming era of process-based therapy. *Behaviour Research and Therapy, 117,* 40–52. doi: 10.1016/j.brat.2018.10.005

Hofmann, S. G., & Hayes, S. C. (2019). The future of intervention science: Process-based therapy. *Clinical Psychological Science, 7*(1), 37–50. doi: 10.1177/2167702618772296

Hughes, S., & Barnes-Holmes, D. (2016a). Relational frame theory: The basic account. In R. D. Zettle, S. C. Hayes, D. Barnes-Holmes, & A. Biglan (Eds.), *The Wiley handbook of contextual behavioral science* (pp. 129–178). West Sussex, UK: Wiley-Blackwell.

Hughes., S., & Barnes-Holmes, D. (2016b). Relational frame theory: Implications for the study of human language and cognition. In R. D. Zettle, S. C. Hayes, D. Barnes-Holmes, & A. Biglan (Eds.), *The Wiley handbook of contextual behavioral science* (pp. 179–226). West Sussex, UK: Wiley-Blackwell.

Ingram, R. E. (1990). Self-focused attention in clinical disorders: Review and a conceptual model. *Psychological Bulletin, 107*(2), 156–176.

Lashley, K. S., & Wade, M. (1946). The Pavlovian theory of generalization. *Psychological Review, 53,* 72–87.

LeDoux, J. E., Brown, R., Pine, D., & Hofmann, S. G. (2018). Know thyself: Well-being and subjective experience. In *Cerebrum.* New York: The Dana Foundation.

LeDoux, J. E., & Hofmann, S. G. (2018). The subjective experience of emotion: A fearful view. *Current Opinion in Behavioral Sciences, 19,* 67–72. doi: 10.1016/j.cobeha.2017.09.011.

McAuliffe, D., Hughes, S., & Barnes-Holmes, D. (2014). The dark-side of rule governed behavior: An experimental analysis of problematic rule-following in an adolescent population with depressive symptomatology. *Behavior Modification, 38*(4), 587–613.

McEnteggart, C. (2018). A Brief Tutorial on Acceptance and Commitment Therapy as Seen through the Lens of Derived Stimulus Relations. *Perspectives on Behavioral Science (Special Issue on Derived Relations), 41*(1), 215–227.

McEnteggart, C., Barnes-Holmes, Y., Dillon, J., Egger, J., & Oliver, J. E. (2017). Hearing voices, dissociation, and the self: A functional-analytic perspective. *Journal of Trauma & Dissociation, 18*(4), 575–594.

Pavlov, I. P. (1897/1902). *The work of the digestive glands.* London: Griffin.

Premack, D. (2007). Human and animal cognition: Continuity and discontinuity. *Proceedings of the National Academy of Sciences, 104*(35), 13861–13867.

Seligman, M. E. P. (1974). Depression and learned helplessness. In R. J. Friedman & M. M. Katz, (Eds.), *The psychology of depression: Contemporary theory and research* (pp. 83–126). Washington, DC: Winston-Wiley.

Sidman, M. (1971). Reading and auditory-visual equivalences. *Journal of Speech, Language, and Hearing Research, 14*(1), 5–13.

Sidman, M. (1994). *Equivalence relations and behavior: A research story.* Boston: Authors Cooperative.

Skinner, B. F. (1957). *Verbal behavior.* New York: Appleton-Century-Crofts.

Skinner, B. F. (1966). An operant analysis of problem-solving. In B. Kleinmuntz (Ed.), *Problem solving: Research, method, teaching* (pp. 225–257). New York: Wiley.

Skinner, B. F. (1969). *Contingencies of reinforcement: A theoretical analysis.* New York: Appleton-Century-Crofts.

Steele, D. L., & Hayes, S. C. (1991). Stimulus equivalence and arbitrarily applicable relational responding. *Journal of the Experimental Analysis of Behavior, 56,* 519–555. doi: 10.1901/jeab.1991.56-519

Stewart, I., & Barnes-Holmes, D. (2001). Understanding metaphor: A relational frame perspective. *The Behavior Analyst, 24,* 191–199.

Watson, J. B., & Rayner, R. (1920). Conditioned emotional reactions. *Journal of Experimental Psychology, 3,* 1–14.

Wolpe, J. (1958). *Psychotherapy by reciprocal inhibition.* Stanford, CA: Stanford University Press.

Zentall, T. R. (1998). Symbolic representation in animals: Emergent stimulus relations in conditional discrimination learning. *Animal Learning & Behavior, 26*(4), 363–377.

Zettle, R. (2005). The evolution of a contextual approach to therapy: From comprehensive distancing to ACT. *International Journal of Behavioral and Consultation Therapy, 1,* 77–89.

Zettle, R. D., & Hayes, S. C. (1982). Rulegoverned behavior: A potential theoretical framework for cognitivebehavior therapy. In P. C. Kendall (Ed.), *Advances in cognitivebehavioral research and therapy* (pp. 73–118). New York: Academic Press.

CHAPTER 7

Cultural and Social Influences on Individual Variation in Emotion Processes

Shruthi M. Venkatesh

Stacey N. Doan, PhD
Claremont McKenna College

Abigail L. Barthel

Stefan G. Hofmann, PhD
Boston University

In the *Natya Shastra*, the oldest treatise on performing arts in India, the following nine emotions (the *navarasas*) are described: *shringar* (love), *adhbhut* (surprise), *bheebatsam* (disgust), *veeram* (bravery), *hasyam* (laughter), *roudram* (anger), *sogum* (sadness), *karuna* (compassion), and *shantam* (peace). Written more than two thousand years ago, the treatise explicitly details how each emotion is to be expressed using nonverbal facial and bodily movements. Despite its great age and basis in Indian culture, when Hejmadi, Davidson, and Rosin (2000) asked modern Indian and American participants to label emotions as displayed by a trained Indian classical dancer using methods specified by the *Natya Shastra,* participants from both countries were able to label the emotions accurately about sixty percent of the time. While there was not complete agreement between participants, this study is one of many to find that— akin to Ekman's (1972) basic emotions theory—emotions are, at some level, universally perceived and expressed. Consistent with this perspective, many emotion theorists view emotions as reactions to stimuli that activate certain brain circuits and psychobiological responses. Accordingly, emotions can be thought of as universal experiences that are cross-culturally portrayed through similar facial expressions (Ekman, Friesen, & Ellsworth, 1972).

At the same time, however, these researchers ignored the fact that even in simple labeling of emotion faces, agreement is never one hundred percent. Moreover, the human experience of emotion goes beyond simple perception. Human emotions are complex phenomena with both biological and psychological correlates. Although they may begin as a biological process, they occur in a social and cultural context and are experienced interpersonally, through and with others. Importantly, the nature and experience of emotions changes across development (Hofmann & Doan, 2018), involving the interaction of culture and biology (Richerson & Boyd, 2005) and the development of the self across time (Hofmann & Doan, 2018). Moreover, emotions are molded by cultural and social influences, such that humans become "active constructionists" of their emotional experiences (Barrett, 2017; Barrett & Russell, 2014; Hofmann & Doan, 2018).

Thus, while there may be overlap in how emotions are experienced, there is large individual variation in how people experience emotions, which is influenced by each person's innate temperamental predispositions, family upbringing, and cultural background, to name a few. In the current chapter, we will focus on the specific temperamental, social, and cultural factors that shape this variation. We will examine the developmental origins of emotion, the role of culture in emotional expression, and the social regulation of emotions. We will end with clinical implications, arguing that any process-based and functional approach to diagnosis needs to address emotion regulation as a process that unfolds over time and development.

Temperament and Individual Variability in Emotion

There is evidence to suggest that emotions emerge very early in development. Even before birth, there is evidence of fetal crying (Gingras, Mitchell, & Grattan, 2005). Because maternal emotions and moods influence basic physiological responses that are associated with multiple child developmental outcomes (see Zijlmans, Riksen-Walraven & de Weerth, 2015 for a review), we cannot definitively rule out the impact of social and environmental factors on emotional experience even before birth, but it seems likely that these influences are small in affecting individual variability in infancy. More dominant during this developmental stage are individual characteristics, such as childhood temperament, including aspects of reactivity and regulation (Rothbart & Derryberry, 1981), that shape how infants react to and experience the world—and, in turn, the frequency and intensity of their emotions.

Early studies on infant temperament have laid out nine dimensions of temperament, including activity level, approach-withdrawal, intensity, threshold, adaptability, rhythmicity, mood, attention span-persistence, and distractibility (Thomas & Chess, 1977). These dimensions have since been reduced due to their overlapping nature and their failure to account for individual variability in temperament later in life. For example, Rothbart and Bates (1998) proposed a shorter list of temperament dimensions composed of fear, irritability or frustration, positive affect and approach, attentional persistence, and activity level. Further revisions have identified three broad temperament dimensions involving effortful control, negative affectivity, and extraversion/surgency (Rothbart, 2007; Rothbart, Ahadi, Hershey, & Fisher, 2001).

Genetic and environmental influences both contribute to infant temperament (Gjone & Stevenson, 1997; Sheese, Voelker, Rothbart & Posner, 2007), which in turn affect children's emotional lives. When it comes to temperament, infants can be characterized as high or low in reactivity and self-regulation. Children who have higher levels of negative emotionality (one aspect of reactivity) are more likely to experience emotions more intensely, leading to more difficulties in regulating behavior and mood, while those who score lower on negative emotionality and higher on attentional control (a measure of self-regulation) are likely to have better adjustment and less externalizing problems (Eisenberg et al., 2000). Moreover, individual variability in infant temperament is associated with prosocial behavior, classroom behaviors later on in childhood, and maternal parenting styles (Coplan, Reichel, & Rowan, 2009; Fox & Henderson, 1999; Rimm-Kaufman & Kagan, 2005).

Social Influences

Children do not develop in isolation but are part of an intimate social world. Caregivers in particular play an integral role in the emotion-socialization process of children. For example, parents have their own philosophical perspectives on emotions, and they pass this perspective on to their children through the ways they model their own emotional expression and how they respond to their child's emotions. In particular, parents' perspectives regarding the value, functions, and importance of emotions—or parents' meta-emotion philosophy—influence their emotion coaching and socialization behaviors toward their children (Katz, Maliken, & Stettler, 2012). Parents who have an emotion-coaching outlook encourage the expression of emotion, discuss their child's emotions, and use emotions as teaching opportunities for their children. In contrast, parents with an emotion-dismissing outlook belittle the value of emotions and encourage emotion suppression and minimization, especially for negative emotions (Cleary & Katz, 2008).

These types of philosophies, in turn, influence how parents behave. Particularly in the context of children's displays of negative emotions, parents who validate, provide support, and offer coping strategies augment their children's capacity to regulate and understand negative emotions (Eisenberg, Cumberland, & Spinrad, 1998; McElwain, Halberstadt, & Volling, 2007). Similarly, parents' philosophy about emotions is also likely to influence how they respond to children's positive emotions; the extent to which parents encourage or allow children to express and experience positive emotions also influences their child's moods and emotions (Fredrick, Mancini, & Luebbe, 2019; Moran, Root, Vizy, Wilson, & Gentzler, 2019; Nelis, Bastin, Raes, & Bijttebier, 2019).

In addition to emotion-socialization process, cognitive processes—such as the use of mental state language and the ability to accurately interpret children's psychological states—lay the foundation for individual variability in emotion later in life. Mental state language (Symons, 2004) refers to the terms used to describe internal physical and emotional states (e.g., want, desire, sad, cry). Language directs attention to these internal states and highlights their importance. The use of mental state language helps children talk through contradictory emotions they experience both interpersonally and intrapersonally (Doan & Wang, 2010), and it helps them determine the significance of those feelings (Rudek & Haden, 2005). Moreover, longitudinal studies have established that utilizing mental state language enhances children's later understanding of emotions (e.g., Doan, Lee, & Wang, 2019; Ensor & Hughes, 2008; Hughes, Marks, Ensor, & Lecce, 2010).

However, references to mental states are only likely to be beneficial if caregivers are accurate in labeling and interpreting children's emotions.

Reflective functioning—the accuracy with which mothers can identify and label their child's internal psychological states (Slade, 2005)—is linked to the child's understanding of their own and others' emotion (Meins et al., 2002; Taumoepeau & Ruffman, 2008). For example, infants who are nurtured by a caregiver who is attuned to their emotional states and who is sensitive to their needs exhibit greater connectedness and regulation later in childhood (Feldman, 2007; Hove & Risen, 2009). In addition, by mirroring and exaggerating certain child emotions, mothers reinforce particular emotion experiences (Malatesta & Haviland, 1982). These findings highlight how individual variations in caregiving styles affect children's emotion processes and begin to support the evolution of individual variability in one's emotional self (Schore, 1994). In addition, as children develop, their social world grows to include siblings, peers, and other adults, all of whom are also likely to shape their emotions.

In sum, fundamental social forces, particularly caregiver behaviors, shape children's social world and emotional experience. In addition to these early processes that shape individual variability in emotional experiences, the cultural background is also likely to play a role.

Cultural Influences

Culture refers to the experiences that are shared by a group of people and that are passed on intergenerationally. As a concept, culture consists of objective aspects, such as food and clothing (Triandis, 1980), as well as subjective aspects, such as beliefs, values, religiosity, communication practices, and cognitive styles (Betancourt & López, 1993; Hughes, Seidman, & Williams, 1993; Rohner, 1984). In addition, culture shapes emotional expression, emotional experience, and the social construction of the self.

Appraisal theory predicts that when people from different cultures appraise a scenario in a similar manner, the corresponding emotion will also be similar (Scherer, 1997), but some research has suggested that appraisal biases are themselves shaped by culture, which in turn influence emotional experiences (Scherer & Brosch, 2009). Social constructivists view emotions as constructions of reality, the framework of which is provided by culture (Gergen, 1985). One important cultural factor that influences how individuals vary in their emotional experience is self-construal, particularly the extent to which the self is related to a collective orientation or an individual orientation (Markus & Kitayama, 1991). At birth, infants across cultures experience similar emotions because, at this stage of life, emotion is more based on physiological underpinnings than a sense of self. With time and socialization, though, the social self gets shaped and accentuated, bringing forth individual variations in emotional responses (Hofmann & Doan, 2018). Our view is that people can be thought of as having multiple selves that play a dynamic role in the experience of emotion depending on which self is prominent in particular contexts.

Individualism and collectivism are two ends of a continuum (Hofstede, 1980), with individual desires and motives driving behavior in individualistic cultures, and larger societal context influencing behavior in collectivistic cultures (Choi, Nisbett, & Norenzayan, 1999). These culturally established differences in self-orientation are known to impact motivation (Oyserman & Lee, 2008; Markus & Kitayama, 1991), and they even influence the emotions that individuals in such cultures commonly experience. For example, people from individualistic cultures tend to report more positive emotions than those from collectivistic cultures (Basabe et al., 2002; Lu, 2008).

Self-construal affects multiple aspects of the emotional experience, including arousal, localization, and the extent to which emotions are context dependent (Hofmann & Doan, 2018). It has been found that those from collectivistic cultures report lower levels of arousal and perceive arousal differently (Matsumoto, 1990, 1993; Matsumoto & Ekman, 1989; Scherer & Wallbott, 1994), perhaps because the self as broadly understood is less tied to physiological responses. In line with this view, those from collectivistic cultures are more likely to have varying expression of the self that differs according to context (Suh, 2002).

Another example of the effects of self-construal is on the localization of emotions. In individualistic cultures, emotions are considered to be individualized, private mental states (Lutz, 1982) that directly manifest onto facial expressions (Carroll & Russell, 1996). In individualistic cultures, one's self-orientation establishes emotions as personal, basic, independent, and directive. This is in contrast to more collectivistic cultures, where relational, contextual, and hierarchical factors play a more salient role. In such cultures, emotions are interdependent, contextual, and obligatory. For example, in Hispanic and Japanese cultures, emotions are more context dependent (Oishi, Diener, Napa Scollon, & Biswas-Diener, 2004), and facial expressions may not be an accurate indicator of internal states (Rothbaum, Pott, Azuma, Miyake, & Weisz, 2000).

In addition, emotional expressivity differs across cultures, as individuals from collectivistic cultures are more heavily influenced by sociocultural norms that dictate how they are expected to behave (Suh, Diener, Oishi, & Triandis, 1998). For example, individuals from East Asian cultures are more likely to down-regulate positive emotions compared to people from other cultures (Miyamoto & Ma, 2011; Sang, Deng, & Luan, 2014). This is in contrast to individualistic cultures and cultures with stable democracies, which are more likely to encourage the expression of emotions, specifically with regard to positive emotions (Matsumoto, Yoo, & Nakagawa, 2008; van Hemert, Poortinga, & van de Vijver, 2007). Indeed, studies have shown that Americans and Europeans display more positive emotions than their Turkish and Chinese American counterparts (Matsumoto et al., 2008; Tsai, Levenson, & McCoy, 2006). Furthermore, self-conscious emotions, such as pride and guilt, differ in their expression across cultures. In individualistic cultures, there are stricter norms for expression of self-conscious emotions, but in collectivistic cultures, failure is seen as a letdown of family and culture, so the notion of losing face and paying respect to others is more pronounced (Chang & Holt, 1994). These examples all demonstrate how cultural orientation shapes emotional expressivity.

These cultural orientations have translated to parenting practices too. American parents have been found to support their child's verbalizations and expressions of emotions, while Asian parents emphasize constricted emotional expression (Rothbaum, Weisz, Pott, Miyake, & Morelli, 2000). Moreover, Chinese parents have a higher tendency to engage in behavior-oriented conversations with their children rather than focusing on internal states (Doan & Wang, 2010), which lowers child-emotion understanding (Wang, 2003; Wang, Hutt, Kulkofsky, McDermott, & Wei, 2006). Empirical studies have also shown that Chinese mothers emphasize connectedness and physical proximity more than their Canadian counterparts, who encourage autonomy (Liu et al., 2005). However, for minority children, parents' "unsupportive reactions" toward negative emotions may serve as a socialization tool that helps children learn when it is appropriate to express certain emotional experiences (Lugo-Candelas, Harvey, & Breaux, 2015; Smith & Walden, 2001).

Cultural values also influence the ways emotions are expressed, suppressed, or experienced (Matsumoto, 2006; Miyamoto & Ma, 2011; Miyamoto & Ryff, 2011). For example, emotional expression is more restricted in Asian cultures, where showing emotion is considered a weakness (Cheung, Lau, &

Waldmann, 1981). In fact, Japanese parents often seek to control their child's emotions (Denham, Caal, Bassett, Benga, & Geangu, 2004). In addition, those from Western cultures view positive emotions as more important and desirable (Bastian et al., 2012), while those from Asian cultures are more likely to accept negative emotions, like sadness, or even mixed emotions (Miyamoto, Uchida, & Ellsworth, 2010; Spencer-Rodgers, Peng, Wang, & Hou, 2004). Thus, while we acknowledge that it is difficult to parse out the exact cultural factors that lead to differences in emotion, there is an undeniable influence of self-construal, cultural norms, orientation, and values on individual variability in the experience of emotion.

Social Regulation of Emotion

Emotion regulation is influenced by internal (e.g., cognitive processes) and external factors (e.g., parenting), and it is a dynamic process that evolves across the lifespan. Despite certain intrinsic antecedents that influence the development of emotion regulation (Calkins & Hill, 2007; Morris, Silk, Steinberg, Myers, & Robinson, 2007), children develop their capacity to self-regulate in the context of their relationship with their caregivers, and it is unlikely that interpersonal influences disappear in adulthood (Diamond & Aspinwall, 2003).

Until recently, research on emotion regulation in adults has primarily focused on *intrapersonal* processes that influence a variety of emotional states, including anxiety (Hofmann, Sawyer, Fang, & Asnaani, 2012; Hofmann, Heering, Sawyer, & Asnaani, 2009; Wirtz, Hofmann, Riper, & Berking, 2014), trauma (Hinton, Hofmann, Pollack, & Otto, 2009; Nickerson et al., 2016, 2017), depression (Berking, Ebert, Cuijpers, & Hofmann, 2013; Berking, Wirtz, Svaldi, & Hofmann, 2014), and anger (Szasz, Hofmann, Heilman, & Curtiss, 2016; Szasz, Szentagotai, & Hofmann, 2011). Intrapersonal processes have also been the focus of research in the field of motivation (Riediger, Schmiedek, Wagner, & Lindenberger, 2009; Szasz, Szentagotai, & Hofmann, 2012). It is only recently that *interpersonal* emotion regulation—that is, an individual's ability to regulate other people's emotions, as well as to use others as a way to regulate their own emotions—has caught the attention of the research community (e.g., Hofmann, 2014; Hofmann & Doan, 2018; Marroquín, 2011). There is also a dearth of literature regarding adolescents in this area, who are beginning to develop self-regulatory abilities but whose emotional development is still heavily influenced by their family environment (Hooper, Luciana, Conklin, & Yarger, 2004; Yap, Allen, & Ladouceur, 2008).

Research in the adult field has primarily focused on the effects of two intrapersonal regulatory processes: suppression and reappraisal. Suppression is an emotion regulation strategy that involves inhibiting the expression of emotions, whereas reappraisal involves modifying one's interpretation of a situation to alter its emotional impact (Gross, 1998). Suppression leads to undesirable, often long-term consequences, such as elevated stress response, poorer eating behaviors, and lower social well-being (Chervonsky & Hunt, 2017; Ferrer, Green, Oh, Hennessy, & Dwyer, 2017). In contrast, a third self-regulatory strategy—acceptance—is associated with more desirable consequences. Acceptance involves taking a nonjudgmental, compassionate, and kind stance toward one's emotions, and research has found that this strategy is more effective than reappraisal in mitigating symptoms of depression (Diedrich et al., 2014, 2016). Indeed, the utility of acceptance and compassion-oriented strategies for emotion regulation is in line with newer forms of therapies (Hofmann, Grossman, & Hinton, 2011; Hofmann et al., 2015).

One limitation of this research on self-regulatory strategies is that most studies have examined the effects of these strategies on a group level, but few have considered individual variability and processes underlying changes in a given individual. This ties into process-based therapy and the importance of the idiographic and functional analytic approach (Hofmann & Hayes, 2019; Hayes & Hofmann, 2017, 2018; Hayes et al., 2019). *Process-Based Therapy* refers to evidence-based, biopsychosocial processes that focus on helping and promoting the prosperity of the individual (Hayes & Hofmann, 2017). This relies on idiographic approaches to research and treatment, which facilitate identification of reliable change processes that are often lost in traditional group-level, nomothetic approaches (Hofmann & Hayes, 2019; Hayes et al., 2019). Emotion regulation, among other cognitive and behavioral processes, is considered to be a core instigator of change in treatment, and thus should be monitored and addressed through interventions.

Form a cultural and social context, we expect that temperament, family, and cultural factors are likely to shape the extent to which individuals may be more or less likely to engage these self-regulatory strategies, as well as the consequences of these strategies. For example, due to the effects of socialization, children in Asian cultures are more likely to suppress negative emotions, such as anger, sadness, and pain (Novin, Rieffe, Banerjee, Miers, &

Cheung, 2011; Wilson, Raval, Salvina, Raval, & Panchal, 2012). Moreover, culture has been found to moderate the consequences of emotion suppression, such that suppression is associated with more adverse effects in Western cultures compared to Eastern cultures, including displays of interpersonal hostility and negative emotion, impaired psychological functioning, and increases in blood pressure (Butler, Lee, & Gross, 2007, 2009; Soto, Perez, Kim, Lee, & Minnick, 2011).

Related to suppression is the idea of experiential avoidance, which refers to the efforts one puts into controlling and escaping from unwanted negative thoughts and feelings (Hayes, 1994). The act of trying to inhibit these negative thoughts and experiences ironically increases those same symptoms, such that experiential avoidance is associated with symptoms of anxiety and panic (Hofmann et al., 2012; Feldner, Zvolensky, Eifert, & Spira, 2003; Roemer, Salters, Raffa, & Orsillo, 2005). Furthermore, experiential avoidance has been found to mediate suppression and reappraisal strategies on daily hedonic functioning (Kashdan, Barrios, Forsyth, & Steger, 2006).

Beyond these individual, or intrapersonal, regulatory strategies, recent research has shifted from a focus on the individual to a focus on interpersonal emotion regulation (Hofmann, 2014; Hofmann, Carpenter, & Curtiss, 2016). In line with Social Baseline Theory, which suggests that the human brain is wired for a communal existence (Coan & Sbarra, 2015), interpersonal emotion regulation perspectives argue that social regulation is likely to be more primary than individual regulatory processes. For example, sharing emotions after a negative event, hand-holding, and regulation in daily interactions all buffer against the impacts of stress and negative experiences (Lakey & Orehek, 2011; Rimé, 2009). Furthermore, capitalization, or the interpersonal sharing of positive emotion events with a reciprocative receiver, aids in well-being (Gable, Gonzaga, & Strachman, 2006; Gable, Reis, Impett, & Asher, 2004).

More recently, researchers have underscored the importance of being able to flexibly use a variety of emotion regulation strategies. Emotional flexibility refers to the understanding that successful adaptation occurs when one can suppress or enhance emotional expression based on contextual demands (Bonanno, Papa, Lalande, Westphal, & Coifman, 2004). For example, emotional flexibility has been found to help individuals adjust in the aftermath of 9/11 (Bonanno et al., 2004), although those experiencing complicated grief are less likely to flexibly regulate their emotions following such an aversive event (Gupta & Bonanno, 2011). Nonetheless, it is clear that individual variability in regulatory flexibility influences how individuals vary in their emotional responses to differing situations (Bonanno & Burton, 2013).

There are also a myriad of contextual and social factors that are likely to affect individual variability in these emotion regulatory processes. First and foremost are caregiver responses. In particular, caregivers' own ability to self-regulate, as well as their sensitivity and reactions to the child's emotions, all influence the child's navigation of this process (Eisenberg, Spinrad, & Eggum, 2010; Posner & Rothbart, 2000; Power, 2004). Parenting styles also play a role, as authoritative parenting styles provide a supportive environment in which parents can effectively model how to express emotions (Morris et al., 2007). In contrast, authoritarian parenting is associated with more negative emotional outcomes, including decreased psychological flexibility (Williams, Ciarrochi, & Heaven, 2012). In addition to parents, sibling relationships impact individual variability in emotion regulation, as siblings co-regulate one other's emotions (Bedford & Volling, 2004) and emotionally support each other (Howe, Aquan-Assee, Bukowski, Lehoux, & Rinaldi, 2001). Interestingly, while parents model emotion strategies, peers empathize with these strategies, which highlights the importance of both support systems (Burleson & Kunkel, 2002).

In addition to these family-level variables, macro-level processes, such as socioeconomic status and religion, are likely to shape emotion regulatory processes. For example, research suggests that those from socioeconomically disadvantaged backgrounds are more likely to be supportive and cognizant of the emotional needs of others (Kraus, Piff, Mendoza-Denton, Rheinschmidt, & Keltner, 2012). At the same time, poverty negatively affects parenting styles, responsive caregiving, and stress, which leads to more emotional dysregulation in children (Hajat et al., 2010). Finally, religion may also have self-regulatory benefits, as research has found that the belief in a higher power can buffer against the effects of health-related stressors and can reduce mortality risk (Siegel, Anderman, & Schrimshaw, 2001).

In sum, the experience of emotion is heavily influence by regulatory processes. Importantly, there are a variety of methods that individuals have at their disposal to either enhance or diminish specific emotions. At the same time, both micro- and macro-level processes impact the extent to which we use these strategies as well as their effectiveness. In the last section, we discuss some of the consequences of this variability in the clinical context.

Clinical Implications

Clinically speaking, research on emotion processes has long provided expansive evidence for the role of emotions in the etiology and maintenance of psychopathology across the lifespan (for a review, see Barthel, Hay, Doan, & Hofmann, 2018; Hofmann & Doan, 2018). As we have discussed, individual variability in emotion processes is influenced by a range of individual and social factors. This variability, in turn, has a wide range of clinical implications. In this section, we apply our discussion of temperament, social influences, and cultural factors on emotion processes related to psychopathology.

Individual Differences in Emotional Reactivity and Psychopathology

Early in life, infants exhibit individual differences in reactivity and regulation that have important implications for a range of clinical processes. One general framework is that children who are high in a reactive temperament factor known as "emotionality/neuroticism" and low in a regulative temperament factor known as "effortful control" are more susceptible to mental health problems later in life, particularly internalizing symptoms (for a review, see Muris & Ollendick, 2005). This is because emotionality/neuroticism is associated with an underlying tendency toward fear, anger, and sadness that is often involved in the origin and maintenance of psychological disorders. In contrast, effortful control reflects the ability to inhibit one's behavior and shift attention if necessary, so individuals low on this trait are unable to adequately manage their emotional and behavioral responses, which can lead to the development of psychopathology (Muris & Ollendick, 2005). At the same time, these temperamental characteristics merely increase susceptibility to psychopathology, but they are not a direct cause, as it is the interaction of life events and one's temperamental characteristics that predict outcomes (Monroe & Simons, 1991).

Nigg (2006) has also proposed a model to illustrate potential pathways of temperament that can be linked to psychopathology, specifically with regard to conduct disorder, attention deficit/hyperactivity disorder, and anxiety disorders in children. This model combines the trait aspects of temperament—including the traits of approach (which is related to extraversion or the readiness to take on reward and reinforcement) and withdrawal (which is related to neuroticism or the tendency to withdraw in unrewarding circumstances)—to regulatory processes. According to this view, children's reactivity and regulatory skills influence their vulnerability to psychopathology.

Since the effects of temperament on childhood outcomes are usually indirect and moderated by various contextual factors, Frick (2004) argues that the fields of developmental psychology and clinical psychology should be integrated in order to aid in the identification of early risk factors for disorders in childhood. Additionally, since early temperament forms the basis for personality, psychopathology and adult personality are linked in part through these broad temperament dimensions (Clark, 2005).

Finally, it is important to note that the extent to which temperamental characteristics, such as negative emotionality and effortful control, are beneficial or maladaptive depends very much on context. Recent research suggests that exhibiting high effortful control in certain contexts comes at a health cost, while negative emotionality might actually buffer against some of the effects of adversity in risky environments (see Doan, Dich & Evans, 2016; Dich, Doan & Evans, 2017)

Social Influences and Psychopathology

A broad range of social factors affect emotion, including both parenting and other macro-level factors. Parenting and child temperament interact to shape trajectories of well-being and maladjustment, and this microcosm exists within a larger sociocultural structure. For example, interpersonal factors—like level of peer or familial support, social withdrawal, abuse or neglect, and victimization—all play key roles in contributing to suicidal behaviors in teenagers (King & Merchant, 2008). And at the extreme, evidence suggests that prior abuse as a child may negatively impact emotion regulation and interpersonal skills in the future, as well as contribute to the development of post-traumatic stress disorder (Cloitre, Miranda, Stovall-McClough, & Han, 2005). In this section, we discuss how these social factors may play out in the clinical context.

Early in development, parent-child interactions lay the foundation for the quality of the parent-child relationship. These early interactions have differential effects on future child behaviors, as a developmental history of insecure attachment can lead to the emergence of problem behaviors, including passive-withdrawal and aggression (Malatesta et al., 1989; Renken,

Egeland, Marvinney, Mangelsdorf, & Sroufe, 1989). More broadly, however, parent-child interactions lay the foundation for how social others may affect dysregulation and adaptation. To illustrate, several models on anxiety and related disorders highlight the role of social others in emotion regulation and emotional well-being.

For example, in his interpersonal emotion regulation model of mood and anxiety disorders, Hofmann (2014) details the ways in which interpersonal relationships contribute to the creation and maintenance of psychopathology. For instance, close others often provide individuals with a sense of safety, which may cause them to associate that person with a sense of reduced distress, in turn creating a safety behavior and form of experiential avoidance. Over the long term, reassurance seeking can become maladaptive, as it maintains symptoms and reinforces dependency on someone else for relief (Hofmann, 2014). Individuals must learn to reduce and eliminate safety behaviors if they are to expose themselves fully to anxiety-provoking situations and learn to tolerate potential negative emotions that may occur. Therefore, interventions for anxiety and related disorders should address interpersonal factors, such as communication patterns, countering avoidance, safety behaviors, and reassurance seeking, when examining the ways in which emotional, social, and cultural experiences interact.

Social factors also play a pivotal in interpersonal emotion regulation. For example, laboratory studies have found that being in the presence of a trusted other, or being physically touched by this trusted other, can reduce negative affect and cortisol levels under conditions of threat (Coan, Schaefer, & Davidson, 2006; Flores & Berenbaum, 2012; Jakubiak & Feeney, 2018). Even calling upon a mental representation of this trusted other can have these same buffering effects (Bourassa, Ruiz, & Sbarra, 2019). The positive effects of interpersonal emotion regulation are also seen in studies finding that romantic touch between partners is associated with increased positive affect and better psychological functioning (Debrot, Schoebi, Perrez, & Horn, 2013). More recent evidence from the field of social neuroscience shows that romantic partnerships characterized by cognitive empathy (Levy-Gigi & Shamay-Tsoory, 2017) and perceived mutual social support (Coan, Kasle, Jackson, Schaefer, & Davidson, 2013; Coan et al., 2017) can help reduce distress and negative affect.

At the same time, the regulating function of these social factors is affected by individual difference variables that reflect each person's unique upbringing and experiences in intimate relationships. As our early relationships set up working models for how we interact with others, parents who are harsh and unsupportive are more likely to have children who grow up unable to trust and rely on others. For example, the combination of low maternal support and high maternal problem solving has been found to increase the risk of borderline personality disorder (Dixon-Gordon, Whalen, Scotts, Cummins, & Stepp, 2016). Other research supports the notion that interpersonal difficulties relate strongly to symptom presentations in borderline personality disorder, such as a general distrust in others, interpersonal problems related to forming and maintaining relationships, and fear of abandonment, which makes interpersonal emotion regulation a key treatment target, especially in dialectical behavior therapy.

Cultural Influences and Psychopathology

Differences in cultural factors may also have a significant impact on psychopathology and its manifestations, as well as on basic emotion processes that have clinical implications. For example, research has demonstrated that the impact of intra-emotion regulatory strategies varies across cultures (Butler et al., 2009), suggesting that certain antecedents of maladaptation are not universal. Moreover, culture is also likely to shape types of disorders, as well as their manifestations.

To illustrate, we can consider the existence of culture-bound syndromes, which are created by culture-specific values and beliefs (Yap, 1967). Two examples of such syndromes include *taijin kyfusho* and *ataque de nervios*, which are specific to Japanese and Latino cultures, respectively (e.g., Hofmann, Asnaani, & Hinton, 2010), and are likely tied to culture self-conceptualizations. *Taijin kyfusho* is essentially a form of social anxiety that is likely driven by a culture where social networks are key to survival, whereas an *ataque de nervios* reflects symptoms such as uncontrollable crying, shouting, and possibly physical aggression that are driven by disruptions in social networks (Guarnaccia, Lewis-Fernández, & Marano, 2003; Hofmann et al., 2010). It is particularly interesting to consider how these responses to social disruption are different. Because Asian cultures value emotion control, it makes sense that one sees more of an internalizing pattern of behavior in these cultures.

Moreover, in the clinical context, the extent to which patients are able to openly discuss their symptoms and emotions may be affected by culture. For example, somatic complaints and alexithymia (which is the inability to label one's emotional states) are higher in both Asia and Latin America (Kleinman, 1982). This may be due to cultural norms and values around psychological complaints and expression of distress. Not only do these characteristics impact the extent to which patients may be able to discuss their symptoms, but it also impacts their willingness to seek help. Indeed, research suggests that lower adherence to Asian values is associated with more positive help-seeking attitudes (Shea & Yeh, 2008).

In sum, our cultural context, values, norms, language, traditions, and beliefs all shape our lived experiences of emotions and have important clinical ramifications.

Conclusion

This chapter has explored the factors behind individual variability in emotion experiences and their clinical implications. Emotions are closely tied to the development of the self, which in turn is influenced by a range of biological and social factors. As the social self develops across the lifespan, so too does one's experience of emotions. Importantly, individual variability in temperamental, familial, and cultural factors shapes how one experiences emotions. These factors conglomerate and shape the dynamic process of emotions across the lifespan. For the sake of clarity, we have written this chapter in such a way that delineates these factors (temperament, social, culture) as if they are separate and unique bins, but this separation does not exist in reality. All of these factors coexist, interact, and develop together over the life course. They do not occur in a vacuum but are situated within environmental factors (e.g., exposure to life events) that ultimately impact individual experiences of emotion as well as their clinical implications. Given the social nature of emotion processes and the sociocultural factors that contribute to and maintain clinical symptoms, it is important to conceptualize each individual's symptoms in a personalized, contextual manner and use the idiographic approach of *Process-Based Therapy* to facilitate change and target specific goals in clients.

References

Barrett, L. F. (2017). The theory of constructed emotion: An active inference account of interoception and categorization. *Social Cognitive and Affective Neuroscience, 12*(1), 1–23. doi: 10.1093/scan/nsw154

Barrett, L. F., & Russell, J. A. (2014). *The psychological construction of emotion*. New York: Guilford Press.

Barthel, A. L., Hay, A., Doan, S. N., & Hofmann, S. G. (2018). Interpersonal emotion regulation: A review of social and developmental components. *Behaviour Change, 35,* 203–216. doi: 10.1017/bec.2018.19

Basabe, N., Paez, D., Valencia, J., Gonzalez, J. L., Rimé, B., & Diener, E. (2002). Cultural dimensions, socioeconomic development, climate, and emotional hedonic level. *Cognition and Emotion, 16*(1), 103–125. doi: 10.1080/02699930143000158

Bastian, B., Kuppens, P., Hornsey, M. J., Park, J., Koval, P., & Uchida, Y. (2012). Feeling bad about being sad: The role of social expectancies in amplifying negative mood. *Emotion, 12*(1), 69–80. doi: 10.1037/a0024755

Bedford, V. H., & Volling, B. L. (2004). A dynamic ecological systems perspective on emotion regulation development within the sibling relationship context. In F. R. Lang & K. L. Fingerman (Eds.), *Growing together: Personal relationships across the lifespan* (pp. 76–102). New York: Cambridge University Press.

Berking, M., Ebert, D., Cuijpers, P., & Hofmann, S. G. (2013). Emotion regulation skills training enhances the efficacy of inpatient cognitive behavioral therapy for major depressive disorder: A randomized controlled trial. *Psychotherapy and Psychosomatics, 82,* 234–245. doi: 10.1159/000348448

Berking, M., Wirtz, C. M., Svaldi, J., & Hofmann, S. G. (2014). Emotion regulation predicts symptoms of depression over five years. *Behaviour Research and Therapy, 57,* 13–20. doi: 10.1016/j.brat.2014.03.003.

Betancourt, H., & López, S. R. (1993). The study of culture, ethnicity, and race in American psychology. *American Psychologist, 48,* 629–637. doi: 10.1037/0003-066X.48.6.629

Bonanno, G. A., Papa, A., Lalande, K., Westphal, M., & Coifman, K. (2004). The importance of being flexible: The ability to both enhance and suppress emotional expression predicts long-term adjustment. *Psychological Science, 15*(7), 482–487.

Bonanno, G. A., & Burton, C. L. (2013). Regulatory flexibility: An individual differences perspective on coping and emotion regulation. *Perspectives on Psychological Science, 8*(6), 591–612.

Bourassa, K. J., Ruiz, J. M., & Sbarra, D. A. (2019). The impact of physical proximity and attachment working models on cardiovascular reactivity: Comparing mental activation and romantic partner presence. *Psychophysiology, 56*(5), e13324. doi: 10.1111/psyp.13324

Burleson, B. R., & Kunkel, A. (2002). Parental and peer contributions to the emotional support skills of the child: From whom do children learn to express support? *Journal of Family Communication, 2*(2), 81–97. doi: 10.1207/S15327698JFC0202_02

Butler, E. A., Lee, T. L., & Gross, J. J. (2007). Emotion regulation and culture: Are the social consequences of emotion suppression culture-specific? *Emotion, 7*(1), 30–48.

Butler, E. A., Lee, T. L., & Gross, J. J. (2009). Does expressing your emotions raise or lower your blood pressure? The answer depends on cultural context. *Journal of Cross-Cultural Psychology, 40*(3), 510–517.

Calkins, S. D., & Hill, A. (2007). Caregiver influences on emerging emotion regulation. In J. J. Gross (Ed.), *Handbook of emotion regulation* (pp. 229–248). New York: Guilford Press.

Carroll, J. M., & Russell, J. A. (1996). Do facial expressions signal specific emotions? Judging emotion from the face in context. *Journal of Personality and Social Psychology, 70,* 205–218. doi: 10.1037/0022-3514.70.2.205

Chang, H.-C., & Holt, G. R. (1994). A Chinese perspective on face as inter-relational concern. In S. Ting-Toomey (Ed.), *The challenge of facework: Cross-cultural and interpersonal issues* (pp. 95–132). Albany: SUNY Press.

Chervonsky, E., & Hunt, C. (2017). Suppression and expression of emotion in social and interpersonal outcomes: A meta-analysis. *Emotion, 17*(4), 669–683.

Cheung, F. M., Lau, B. W. K., & Waldmann, E. (1981). Somatization among Chinese depressives in general practice. *The International Journal of Psychiatry in Medicine, 10,* 361–374. doi: 10.2190/BVY5-YCCR-CT1V-20FR

Choi, I., Nisbett, R. E., & Norenzayan, A. (1999). Causal attribution across cultures: Variation and universality. *Psychological Bulletin, 125,* 47–63. doi: 10.1037/0033-2909.125.1.47

Clark, L. A. (2005). Temperament as a unifying basis for personality and psychopathology. *Journal of Abnormal Psychology, 114*(4), 505–521.

Cleary, R. P., & Katz, L. F. (2008). Family-level emotion socialization and children's comfort with emotional expressivity. *Family Psychologist, 24,* 7–13.

Cloitre, M., Miranda, R., Stovall-McClough, K. C., & Han, H. (2005). Beyond PTSD: Emotion regulation and interpersonal problems as predictors of functional impairment in survivors of childhood abuse. *Behavior Therapy, 36,* 119–124. doi: 10.1016/S0005-7894(05)80060-7

Coan, J. A., Beckes, L., Gonzalez, M. Z., Maresh, E. L., Brown, C. L., & Hasselmo, K. (2017). Relationship status and perceived support in the social regulation of neural responses to threat. *Social Cognitive and Affective Neuroscience, 12*(10), 1574–1583. doi: 10.1093/scan/nsx091

Coan, J. A., Kasle, S., Jackson, A., Schaefer, H. S., & Davidson, R. J. (2013). Mutuality and the social regulation of neural threat responding. *Attachment & Human Development, 15*(3), 303–315. doi: 10.1080/14616734.2013.782656

Coan, J. A., & Sbarra, D. A. (2015). Social baseline theory: The social regulation of risk and effort. *Current Opinion in Psychology, 1,* 87–91. doi: 10.1016/j.copsyc.2014.12.021

Coan, J. A., Schaefer, H. S., & Davidson, R. J. (2006). Lending a hand: Social regulation of the neural response to threat. *Psychological Science, 17*(12), 1032–1039.

Coplan, R. J., Reichel, M., & Rowan, K. (2009). Exploring the associations between maternal personality, child temperament, and parenting: A focus on emotions. *Personality and Individual Differences, 46*(2), 241–246.

Debrot, A., Schoebi, D., Perrez, M., & Horn, A. (2013). Touch as an interpersonal emotion regulation process in couples' daily lives: The mediating role of psychological intimacy. *Personality and Social Psychology Bulletin, 39*, 1373–1385. doi: 10.1177/0146167213497592

Denham, S. A., Caal, S., Bassett, H., Benga, O., & Geangu, E. (2004). Listening to parents: Cultural variations in the meaning of emotions and emotion socialization. *Cognition Brain Behavior, 8*, 321–350.

Diamond, L. M., & Aspinwall, L. G. (2003). Emotion regulation across the life span: An integrative perspective emphasizing self-regulation, positive affect, and dyadic processes. *Motivation and Emotion, 27*(2), 125–156. doi: 10.1023/A:1024521920068

Dich, N., Doan, S. N., & Evans, G. W. (2017). In risky environments, emotional children have more behavioral problems but lower allostatic load. *Health Psychology, 36*(5), 468–476.

Diedrich, A., Grant, M., Hofmann, S. G., Hiller, W., & Berking, M. (2014). Self-compassion as an emotion regulation strategy in major depressive disorder. *Behaviour Research and Therapy, 58*, 43–51. doi: 10.1016/j.brat.2014.05.006

Diedrich, A., Hofmann, S. G., Cuijpers, P., & Berking, M. (2016). Self-compassion enhances the efficacy of explicit cognitive reappraisal as an emotion regulation strategy in individuals with major depressive disorder. *Behaviour Research and Therapy, 82*, 1–10. doi: 10.1016/j.brat.2016.04.003

Dixon-Gordon, K. L., Whalen, D. J., Scott, L. N., Cummins, N. D., & Stepp, S. D. (2016). The main and interactive effects of maternal interpersonal emotion regulation and negative affect on adolescent girls' borderline personality disorder symptoms. *Cognitive Therapy and Research, 40*, 381–393. doi: 10.1007/s10608-015-9706-4

Doan, S. N., Dich, N., & Evans, G. W. (2016). Stress of stoicism: Low emotionality and high control lead to increases in allostatic load. *Applied Developmental Science, 20*(4), 310–317.

Doan, S. N., Lee, H. Y., & Wang, Q. (2019). Maternal mental state language is associated with trajectories of Chinese immigrant children's emotion situation knowledge. *International Journal of Behavioral Development, 43*(1), 43–52.

Doan, S. N., & Wang, Q. (2010). Maternal discussions of mental states and behaviors: Relations to emotion situation knowledge in European American and Immigrant Chinese children. *Child Development, 81*, 1490–1503. doi: 10.1111/j.1467-8624.2010.01487.x

Eisenberg, N., Cumberland, A., & Spinrad, T. L. (1998). Parental socialization of emotion. *Psychological Inquiry, 9*, 241–273.

Eisenberg, N., Spinrad, T. L., & Eggum, N. D. (2010). Emotion-related self-regulation and its relation to children's maladjustment. *Annual Review of Clinical Psychology, 6*, 495–525.

Eisenberg, N., Guthrie, I. K., Fabes, R. A., Shepard, S., Losoya, S., Murphy, B., ... Reiser, M. (2000). Prediction of elementary school children's externalizing problem behaviors from attentional and behavioral regulation and negative emotionality. *Child Development, 71*(5), 1367–1382.

Ekman, P. (1972). Universal and cultural differences in facial expressions of emotions. In J. Cole (Ed.), *Nebraska symposium of motivation* (pp. 207–283). Lincoln, NE: University of Nebraska Press.

Ekman, P., Friesen, W. V., & Ellsworth, P. (1972). *Emotion in the human face: Guidelines for research and a review of findings.* New York: Permagon Press.

Ensor, R., & Hughes, C. (2008). Content or connectedness? Mother-child talk and early social understanding. *Child Development, 79*(1), 201–216.

Feldman, R. (2007). Parent-infant synchrony and the construction of shared timing; Physiological precursors, developmental outcomes, and risk conditions. *Journal of Child Psychology and Psychiatry, 48,* 329–354.

Feldner, M. T., Zvolensky, M. J., Eifert, G. H., & Spira, A. P. (2003). Emotional avoidance: An experimental test of individual differences and response suppression using biological challenge. *Behaviour Research and Therapy, 41*(4), 403–411.

Ferrer, R. A., Green, P. A., Oh, A. Y., Hennessy, E., & Dwyer, L. A. (2017). Emotion suppression, emotional eating, and eating behavior among parent-adolescent dyads. *Emotion, 17*(7), 1052–1065.

Flores, L. E., & Berenbaum, H. (2012). Desire for emotional closeness moderates the effectiveness of the social regulation of emotion. *Personality and Individual Differences, 53*(8), 952–957. doi: 10.1016/j.paid.2012.07.009

Fox, N. A., & Henderson, H. A. (1999). Does infancy matter? Predicting social behavior from infant temperament. *Infant Behavior and Development, 22*(4), 445–455.

Fredrick, J. W., Mancini, K. J., & Luebbe, A. M. (2019). Maternal enhancing responses to adolescents' positive affect: Associations with adolescents' positive affect regulation and depression. *Social Development, 28*(2), 290–305. doi: 10.1111/sode.12326

Frick, P. J. (2004). Integrating research on temperament and childhood psychopathology: Its pitfalls and promise. *Journal of Clinical Child and Adolescent Psychology, 33*(1), 2–7.

Gable, S. L., Gonzaga, G. C., & Strachman, A. (2006). Will you be there for me when things go right? Supportive responses to positive event disclosures. *Journal of Personality and Social Psychology, 91,* 904–917. doi: 10.1037/0022-3514.91.5.904

Gable, S. L., Reis, H. T., Impett, E. A., & Asher, E. R. (2004). What do you do when things go right? The intrapersonal and interpersonal benefits of sharing positive events. *Journal of Personality and Social Psychology, 87,* 228–245. doi: 10.1037/0022-3514.87.2.228

Gergen, K. J. (1985). The social constructionist movement in modern psychology. *American Psychologist, 40,* 266–275. doi: 10.1037/0003-066X.40.3.266

Gingras, J. L., Mitchell, E. A., & Grattan, K. E. (2005). Fetal homologue of infant crying. *Archives of Disease in Childhood-Fetal and Neonatal Edition, 90*(5), F415–F418.

Gjone, H., & Stevenson, J. (1997). A longitudinal twin study of temperament and behavior problems: Common genetic or environmental influences? *Journal of the American Academy of Child & Adolescent Psychiatry, 36*(10), 1448–1456.

Gross, J. J. (1998). The emerging field of emotion regulation: An integrative review. *Review of General Psychology, 2*(3), 271–299.

Guarnaccia, P. J., Lewis-Fernández, R., & Marano, M. R. (2003). Toward a Puerto Rican popular nosology: *Nervios* and *ataque de nervios. Culture, Medicine and Psychiatry, 27*(3), 339–366.

Gupta, S., & Bonanno, G. A. (2011). Complicated grief and deficits in emotional expressive flexibility. *Journal of Abnormal Psychology, 120*(3), 635–643.

Hajat, A., Diez-Roux, A., Franklin, T. G., Seeman, T., Shrager, S., Ranjit, N., ... Kirschbaum, C. (2010). Socioeconomic and race/ethnic differences in daily salivary cortisol profiles: The Multi-Ethnic Study of Atherosclerosis. *Psychoneuroendocrinology, 35,* 932–943. doi: 10.1016/j.psyneuen.2009.12.009

Hayes, S. C. (1994). Content, context, and the types of psychological acceptance. *Acceptance and change: Content and Context in psychotherapy,* 13–32.

Hayes, S. C., & Hofmann, S. G. (2017). The third wave of CBT and the rise of process-based care. *World Psychiatry, 16,* 245–246. doi: 10.102/wps.20442

Hayes, S. C., & Hofmann, S. G. (Eds.). (2018). *Process-based CBT: The science and core clinical competencies of cognitive behavioral therapy.* Oakland, CA: Context Press/New Harbinger Publications.

Hayes, S. C., Hofmann, S. G., Stanton, C. E., Carpenter, J. K., Sanford, B. T., Curtiss, J. E., & Ciarrochi, J. (2019). The role of the individual in the coming era of process-based therapy. *Behaviour Research and Therapy, 117,* 40–53. doi: 10.1016/j.brat.2018.10.005.

Hejmadi, A., Davidson, R. J., & Rozin, P. (2000). Exploring Hindu Indian emotion expressions: Evidence for accurate recognition by Americans and Indians. *Psychological Science, 11*(3), 183–187.

Hinton, D. E., Hofmann, S. G., Pollack, M. H., & Otto, M. W. (2009). Mechanisms of efficacy of CBT for Cambodian refugees with PTSD: Improvement in emotion regulation and orthostatic blood pressure response. *CNS Neuroscience & Therapeutics, 15,* 255–263. doi: 10.1111/j.1755-5949.2009.00100.x

Hofmann, S. G. (2014). Interpersonal emotion regulation model of mood and anxiety disorders. *Cognitive Therapy and Research, 38,* 483–492. doi: 10.1007/s10608-014-9620-1

Hofmann, S. G., Asnaani, A., & Hinton, D. E. (2010). Cultural aspects in social anxiety and social anxiety disorder. *Depression and Anxiety, 27*(12), 1117–1127.

Hofmann, S. G., Carpenter, J. K., & Curtiss, J. (2016). Interpersonal Emotion Regulation Questionnaire (IERQ): Scale development and psychometric characteristics. *Cognitive Therapy and Research, 40,* 341–356. doi: 10.1007/s10608-016-9756-2

Hofmann, S. G., & Doan, S. N. (2018). *The social foundations of emotion: Developmental, cultural, and clinical dimensions.* Washington DC: American Psychological Association.

Hofmann, S. G., Grossman, P., & Hinton, D. E. (2011). Loving-kindness and compassion meditation: Potential for psychological interventions. *Clinical Psychology Review, 31,* 1126–1132. doi: 10.1016/j.cpr.2011.07.003ofmnHH

Hofmann, S. G., & Hayes, S. C. (2019). The future of intervention science: Process-based therapy. *Clinical Psychological Science, 7*(1), 37–50. doi: 10.1177/2167702618772296

Hofmann, S. G., Heering, S., Sawyer, A. T., & Asnaani, A. (2009). How to handle anxiety: The effects of reappraisal, acceptance, and suppression strategies on anxious arousal. *Behaviour Research and Therapy, 47,* 389–394. doi: 10.1016/j.brat.2009.02.010

Hofmann, S. G., Petrocchi, N., Steinberg, J., Lin, M., Arimitsu, K., Kind, S., ... Stangier, U. (2015). Loving-kindness meditation to target affect in mood disorders: A proof-of-concept study. *Evidence-Based Complementary and Alternative Medicine*, 269126, 1–11. doi: dx.doi.org/10.1155/2015/269126

Hofmann, S. G., Sawyer, A. T., Fang, A., & Asnaani, A. (2012). Emotion dysregulation model of mood and anxiety disorders. *Depression and Anxiety, 29*, 409–416. doi: 10.1002/da.21888.

Hofstede, G. (1980). Motivation, leadership, and organization: Do American theories apply abroad? *Organizational Dynamics, 9*(1), 42–63. doi: 10.1016/0090-2616(80)90013-3

Hooper, C. J., Luciana, M., Conklin, H. M., & Yarger, R. S. (2004). Adolescents' performance on the Iowa Gambling Task: Implications for the development of decision making and ventromedial prefrontal cortex. *Developmental Psychology, 40*, 1148–1158. doi: 10.1037/0012-1649.40.6.1148

Hove, M. J., & Risen, J. L. (2009). It's all in the timing: Interpersonal synchrony increases affiliation. *Social Cognition, 27*, 949–960.

Howe, N., Aquan-Assee, J., Bukowski, W. M., Lehoux, P. M., & Rinaldi, C. M. (2001). Siblings as confidants: Emotional understanding, relationship warmth, and sibling self-disclosure. *Social Development, 10*, 439–454. doi: 10.1111/1467-9507.00174

Hughes, C., Marks, A., Ensor, R., & Lecce, S. (2010). A longitudinal study of conflict and inner state talk in children's conversations with mothers and younger siblings. *Social Development, 19*, 822–837. doi: 10.1111/j.1467-9507.2009.00561

Hughes, D., Seidman, E., & Williams, N. (1993). Cultural phenomena and the research enterprise: Toward a culturally anchored methodology. *American Journal of Community Psychology, 21*, 687–703. doi: 10.1007/BF00942243

Jakubiak, B. K., & Feeney, B. C. (2018). Interpersonal touch as a resource to facilitate positive personal and relational outcomes during stress discussions. *Journal of Social and Personal Relationships, 36*(9), 2918–2936. doi: 10.1177/0265407518804666

Kashdan, T. B., Barrios, V., Forsyth, J. P., & Steger, M. F. (2006). Experiential avoidance as a generalized psychological vulnerability: Comparisons with coping and emotion regulation strategies. *Behaviour Research and Therapy, 44*(9), 1301–1320.

Katz, L. F., Maliken, A. C., & Stettler, N. M. (2012). Parental meta-emotion philosophy: A review of research and theoretical framework. *Child Development Perspectives, 6*(4), 417–422.

King, C. A., & Merchant, C. R. (2008). Social and interpersonal factors relating to adolescent suicidality: A review of the literature. *Archives of Suicide Research, 12*, 181–196. doi: 10.1080/13811110802101203

Kleinman, A. (1982). Neurasthenia and depression: A study of somatization and culture in China. *Culture, Medicine and Psychiatry, 6*(2), 117–190.

Kraus, M. W., Piff, P. K., Mendoza-Denton, R., Rheinschmidt, M. L., & Keltner, D. (2012). Social class, solipsism, and contextualism: How the rich are different from the poor. *Psychological Review, 119*, 546–572. doi: 10.1037/a0028756

Lakey, B., & Orehek, E. (2011). Relational regulation theory: A new approach to explain the link between perceived social support and mental health. *Psychological Review, 118*, 482–495.

Levy-Gigi, E., & Shamay-Tsoory, S. G. (2017). Help me if you can: Evaluating the effectiveness of interpersonal compared to intrapersonal emotion regulation in reducing distress. *Journal of Behavior Therapy and Experimental Psychiatry, 55,* 33–40. doi: 10.1016/j.jbtep.2016.11.008

Liu, M., Chen, X., Rubin, K. H., Zheng, S., Cui, L., Li, D., ... Wang, L. (2005). Autonomy vs. connectedness-oriented parenting behaviours in Chinese and Canadian mothers. *International Journal of Behavioral Development, 29*(6), 489–495.

Lu, L. (2008). The individual-oriented and social-oriented Chinese bicultural self: Testing the theory. *The Journal of Social Psychology, 148,* 347–374. doi: 10.3200/SOCP.148.3.347-374.

Lugo-Candelas, C. I., Harvey, E. A., & Breaux, R. P. (2015). Emotion socialization practices in Latina and European-American mothers of preschoolers with behavior problems. *Journal of Family Studies, 21*(2), 144–162. doi: 10.1080/13229400.2015.1020982

Lutz, C. (1982). The domain of emotion words on Ifaluk. *American Ethnologist, 9*(1), 113–128. doi: 10.1525/ae.1982.9.1.02a00070

Malatesta, C. Z., Culver, C., Tesman, J. R., Shepard, B., Fogel, A., Reimers, M., & Zivin, G. (1989). The development of emotion expression during the first two years of life. *Monographs of the Society for Research in Child Development, 54,* i–136. doi: 10.2307/1166153

Malatesta, C. Z., & Haviland, J. M. (1982). Learning display rules: The socialization of emotion expression in infancy. *Child Development, 53,* 991–1003.

Markus, H. R., & Kitayama, S. (1991). Culture and the self: Implications for cognition, emotion, and motivation. *Psychological Review, 98,* 224–253.

Marroquín, B. (2011). Interpersonal emotion regulation as a mechanism of social support in depression. *Clinical Psychology Review, 31,* 1276–1290. doi: 10.1016/j.cpr.2011.09.005

Matsumoto, D. (1990). Cultural similarities and differences in display rules. *Motivation and Emotion, 14*(3), 195–214. doi: 10.1007/BF00995569

Matsumoto, D. (1993). Ethnic differences in affect intensity, emotion judgments, display rule attitudes, and self-reported emotional expression in an American sample. *Motivation and Emotion, 17*(2), 107–123. doi: 10.1007/BF00995188

Matsumoto, D. (2006). Culture and cultural worldviews: Do verbal descriptions about culture reflect anything other than verbal descriptions of culture? *Culture & Psychology, 12*(1), 33–62. doi: 10.1177/1354067X06061592

Matsumoto, D., & Ekman, P. (1989). American-Japanese cultural differences in intensity ratings of facial expressions of emotion. *Motivation and Emotion, 13*(2), 143–157. doi: 10.1007/BF00992959

Matsumoto, D., Yoo, S. H., & Nakagawa, S. (2008). Culture, emotion regulation, and adjustment. *Journal of Personality and Social Psychology, 94,* 925–937. doi: 10.1037/0022-3514.94.6.925

McElwain, N. L., Halberstadt, A. G., & Volling, B. L. (2007). Mother- and father-reported reactions to children's negative emotions: Relations to young children's emotional understanding and friendship quality. *Child Development, 78,* 1407–1425. doi: 10.1111/j.1467-8624.2007.01074.x

Meins, E., Fernyhough, C., Wainwright, R., Das Gupta, M., Fradley, E., & Tuckey, M. (2002). Maternal mind-mindedness and attachment security as predictors of theory of mind understanding. *Child Development, 73*(6), 1715–1726.

Miyamoto, Y., & Ma, X. (2011). Dampening or savoring positive emotions: A dialectical cultural script guides emotion regulation. *Emotion, 11*, 1346–1357. doi: 10.1037/a0025135

Miyamoto, Y., & Ryff, C. D. (2011). Cultural differences in the dialectical and non-dialectical emotional styles and their implications for health. *Cognition and Emotion, 25*(1), 22–39. doi: 10.1080/02699931003612114

Miyamoto, Y., Uchida, Y., & Ellsworth, P. C. (2010). Culture and mixed emotions: Co-occurrence of positive and negative emotions in Japan and the United States. *Emotion, 10*, 404–415. doi: 10.1037/a0018430

Monroe, S. M., & Simons, A. D. (1991). Diathesis-stress theories in the context of life stress research: Implications for the depressive disorders. *Psychological Bulletin, 110*(3), 406–425. doi: 10.1037/0033-2909.110.3.406

Moran, K. M., Root, A. E., Vizy, B. K., Wilson, T. K., & Gentzler, A. L. (2019). Maternal socialization of children's positive affect regulation: Associations with children's savoring, dampening, and depressive symptoms. *Social Development, 28*(2), 306–322. doi: 10.1111/sode.12338

Morris, A. S., Silk, J. S., Steinberg, L., Myers, S. S., & Robinson, L. R. (2007). The role of the family context in the development of emotion regulation. *Social Development, 16*(2), 361–388. doi: 10.1111/j.1467-9507.2007.00389.x

Muris, P., & Ollendick, T. H. (2005). The role of temperament in the etiology of child psychopathology. *Clinical Child and Family Psychology Review, 8*(4), 271–289.

Nelis, S., Bastin, M., Raes, F., & Bijttebier, P. (2019). How do my parents react when I feel happy? Longitudinal associations with adolescent depressive symptoms, anhedonia, and positive affect regulation. *Social Development, 28*(2), 255–273. doi: 10.1111/sode.12318

Nigg, J. T. (2006). Temperament and developmental psychopathology. *Journal of Child Psychology and Psychiatry, 47*(3–4), 395–422.

Nickerson, A., Garber, B., Ahmed, O., Asnaani, A., Cheung, J., Hofmann, S. G., ... Bryant, R. A. (2016). Emotional suppression in torture survivors: Relationship to posttraumatic stress symptoms and trauma-related negative affect. *Psychiatry Research, 242*, 233–239. doi: 10.1016/jpsychres.2016.05.048

Nickerson, A., Garber, B., Liddell, B. J., Litz, B. T., Hofmann, S. G., Asnaani, A., ... Bryant, R. A. (2017). Impact of cognitive reappraisal on negative affect, heart rate, and intrusive memories in traumatized refugees. *Clinical Psychological Science, 5*, 497–512. doi: 10.1177/2167702617690857.

Novin, S., Rieffe, C., Banerjee, R., Miers, A. C., & Cheung, J. (2011). Anger response styles in Chinese and Dutch children: A socio-cultural perspective on anger regulation: Anger response styles in Chinese and Dutch children. *British Journal of Developmental Psychology, 29*, 806–822. doi: 10.1348/2044-835X.002010

Oishi, S., Diener, E., Napa Scollon, C., & Biswas-Diener, R. (2004). Cross-situational consistency of affective experiences across cultures. *Journal of Personality and Social Psychology, 86*, 460–472. doi: 10.1037/0022-3514.86.3.460

Oyserman, D., & Lee, S. W. S. (2008). Does culture influence what and how we think? Effects of priming individualism and collectivism. *Psychological Bulletin, 134,* 311–342. doi: 10.1037/0033-2909.134.2.311

Posner, M. I., & Rothbart, M. K. (2000). Developing mechanisms of self-regulation. *Development and Psychopathology, 12,* 427–441.

Power, T. G. (2004). Stress and coping in childhood: The parents' role. *Parenting, 4*(4), 271–317. doi: 10.1207/s15327922par0404_1

Renken, B., Egeland, B., Marvinney, D., Mangelsdorf, S., & Sroufe, L. A. (1989). Early childhood antecedents of aggression and passive-withdrawal in early elementary school. *Journal of Personality, 57,* 257–281. doi: 10.1111/j.1467-6494.1989.tb00483.x

Richerson, P. J., & Boyd, R. (2005). *Not by genes alone: How culture transformed human evolution.* Chicago: University of Chicago Press.

Riediger, M., Schmiedek, F., Wagner, G. G., & Lindenberger, U. (2009). Seeking pleasure and seeking pain: Differences in prohedonic and contra-hedonic motivation from adolescence to old age. *Psychological Science, 20,* 1529–1535. doi: 10.1111/j.1467-9280.2009.02473.x

Rimé, B. (2009). Emotion elicits the social sharing of emotion: Theory and empirical review. *Emotion Review, 1*(1), 60–85. doi: 10.1177/1754073908097189

Rimm-Kaufman, S. E., & Kagan, J. (2005). Infant predictors of kindergarten behavior: The contribution of inhibited and uninhibited temperament types. *Behavioral Disorders, 30*(4), 331–347.

Rohner, R. P. (1984). Toward a conception of culture for cross-cultural psychology. *Journal of Cross-Cultural Psychology, 15*(2), 111–138. doi: 10.1177/0022002184015002002

Roemer, L., Salters, K., Raffa, S. D., & Orsillo, S. M. (2005). Fear and avoidance of internal experiences in GAD: Preliminary tests of a conceptual model. *Cognitive Therapy and Research, 29*(1), 71–88.

Rothbart, M. K. (2007). Temperament, development, and personality. *Current Directions in Psychological Science, 16*(4), 207–212.

Rothbart, M. K., Ahadi, S. A., Hershey, K., & Fisher, P. (2001). Investigations of temperament at three to seven years: The Children's Behavior Questionnaire. *Child Development, 72,* 1394–1408.

Rothbart, M. K., & Bates, J. E. (1998). Temperament. In W. Damon & N. Eisenberg (Eds.), *Handbook of child psychology: Social, emotional and personality development* (5th ed., Vol. 3, pp. 105–176). New York: Wiley.

Rothbart, M. K., & Derryberry, D. (1981). Development of individual differences in temperament. In M. E. Lamb & A. L. Brown (Eds.), *Advances in developmental psychology* (pp. 37–86). Hillsdale, NJ: Lawrence Erlbaum Associates.

Rothbaum, F., Pott, M., Azuma, H., Miyake, K., & Weisz, J. (2000). The development of close relationships in Japan and the United States: Paths of symbiotic harmony and generative tension. *Child Development, 71,* 1121–1142. doi: 10.1111/1467-8624.00214

Rothbaum, F., Weisz, J., Pott, M., Miyake, K., & Morelli, G. (2000). Attachment and culture: Security in the United States and Japan. *American Psychologist, 55,* 1093–1104. doi: 10.1037/0003-066X.55.10.1093

Rudek, D., & Haden, C. (2005). Mothers' and preschoolers' mental state language during reminiscing over time. *Merrill-Palmer Quarterly, 51*(4), 523–549.

Sang, B., Deng, X., & Luan, Z. (2014). Which emotional regulatory strategy makes Chinese adolescents happier? A longitudinal study. *International Journal of Psychology, 49,* 513–518. doi: 10.1002/ijop.12067

Scherer, K. (1997). Profiles of emotion-antecedent appraisal: Testing theoretical predictions across cultures. *Cognition & Emotion, 11*(2), 113–150.

Scherer, K. R., & Brosch, T. (2009). Culture-specific appraisal biases contribute to emotion dispositions. *European Journal of Personality, 23,* 265–288.

Scherer, K. R., & Wallbott, H. G. (1994). Evidence for universality and cultural variation of differential emotion response patterning. *Journal of Personality and Social Psychology, 66,* 310–328.

Schore, A. N. (1994). *Affect regulation and the origin of self.* Hillsdale, NJ: Lawrence Erlbaum Associates.

Shea, M., & Yeh, C. (2008). Asian American students' cultural values, stigma, and relational self-construal: Correlates of attitudes toward professional help seeking. *Journal of Mental Health Counseling, 30*(2), 157–172.

Sheese, B. E., Voelker, P. M., Rothbart, M. K., & Posner, M. I. (2007). Parenting quality interacts with genetic variation in dopamine receptor D4 to influence temperament in early childhood. *Development and Psychopathology, 19*(4), 1039–1046.

Siegel, K., Anderman, S. J., & Schrimshaw, E. W. (2001). Religion and coping with health-related stress. *Psychology & Health, 16,* 631–653. doi: 10.1080/0887044010 8405864

Slade, A. (2005). Parental reflective functioning: An introduction. *Attachment & Human Development, 7*(3), 269–281.

Smith, M., & Walden, T. (2001). An exploration of African American preschool-aged children's behavioral regulation in emotionally arousing situations. *Child Study Journal, 31,* 13–45.

Soto, J. A., Perez, C. R., Kim, Y. H., Lee, E. A., & Minnick, M. R. (2011). Is expressive suppression always associated with poorer psychological functioning? A cross-cultural comparison between European Americans and Hong Kong Chinese. *Emotion, 11*(6), 1450–1455.

Spencer-Rodgers, J., Peng, K., Wang, L., & Hou, Y. (2004). Dialectical self-esteem and east-west differences in psychological well-being. *Personality and Social Psychology Bulletin, 30,* 1416–1432. doi: 10.1177/0146167204264243

Suh, E. M. (2002). Culture, identity consistency, and subjective well-being. *Journal of Personality and Social Psychology, 83,* 1378–1391. doi: 10.1037/0022-3514.83.6.1378

Suh, E., Diener, E., Oishi, S., & Triandis, H. C. (1998). The shifting basis of life satisfaction judgments across cultures: Emotions versus norms. *Journal of Personality and Social Psychology, 74,* 482–493. doi: 10.1037/0022-3514.74.2.482

Symons, D. K. (2004). Mental state discourse, theory of mind, and the internalization of self–other understanding. *Developmental Review, 24*(2), 159–188.

Szasz, P. L., Hofmann, S. G., Heilman, R., & Curtiss, J. (2016). Effect of regulating anger and sadness on decision-making. *Cognitive Behaviour Therapy, 45,* 479–495. doi: 10.1080/16506073.2016.1203354

Szasz, P. L., Szentagotai, A., & Hofmann, S. G. (2011). The effect of emotion regulation strategies on anger. *Behaviour Research and Therapy, 49,* 114–119. doi: 10.1016/j.brat.2010.11.011

Szasz, P. L., Szentagotai, A., & Hofmann, S. G. (2012). Effects of emotion regulation strategies on smoking craving, attentional bias, and task persistence. *Behaviour Research and Therapy, 50,* 333–340. doi: 10.1016/j.brat.2012.02.010

Taumoepeau, M., & Ruffman, T. (2008). Stepping stones to others' minds: Maternal talk relates to child mental state language and emotion understanding at 15, 24, and 33 months. *Child Development, 79*(2), 284–302.

Thomas, A., & Chess, S. (1977). *Temperament and development.* New York: Bruner/Mazel.

Triandis, H. C. (1980). Reflections on trends in cross-cultural research. *Journal of Cross-Cultural Psychology, 11*(1), 35–58. doi: 10.1177/0022022180111003

Tsai, J. L., Levenson, R. W., & McCoy, K. (2006). Cultural and temperamental variation in emotional response. *Emotion, 6,* 484–497. doi: 10.1037/1528-3542.6.3.484

van Hemert, D. A., Poortinga, Y. H., & van de Vijver, F. J. R. (2007). Emotion and culture: A meta-analysis. *Cognition and Emotion, 21*(5), 913–943. doi: 10.1080/02699930701339293

Wang, Q. (2003). Emotion situation knowledge in American and Chinese preschool children and adults. *Cognition and Emotion, 17,* 725–746. doi: 10.1080/02699930302285

Wang, Q., Hutt, R., Kulkofsky, S., McDermott, M., & Wei, R. (2006). Emotion situation knowledge and autobiographical memory in Chinese, immigrant Chinese, and European American 3-year-olds. *Journal of Cognition and Development, 7*(1), 95–118. doi: 10.1207/s15327647jcd0701_5

Williams, K. E., Ciarrochi, J., & Heaven, P. C. (2012). Inflexible parents, inflexible kids: A 6-year longitudinal study of parenting style and the development of psychological flexibility in adolescents. *Journal of Youth and Adolescence, 41*(8), 1053–1066.

Wilson, S. L., Raval, V. V., Salvina, J., Raval, P. H., & Panchal, I. N. (2012). Emotional expression and control in school-age children in India and the United States. *Merrill-Palmer Quarterly, 58*(1), 50–76. doi: 10.1353/mpq.2012.0005

Wirtz, C. M., Hofmann, S. G., Riper, H., & Berking, M. (2014). Emotion regulation predicts anxiety over a five-year interval: A cross-lagged panel analysis. *Depression and Anxiety, 31,* 87–95. doi: 10.1002/da.22198

Yap, P. M. (1967). Classification of the culture-bound reactive syndromes. *Australian and New Zealand Journal of Psychiatry, 1*(4), 172–179.

Yap, M. B. H., Allen, N. B., & Ladouceur, C. D. (2008). Maternal socialization of positive affect: The impact of invalidation on adolescent emotion regulation and depressive symptomatology. *Child Development, 79,* 1415–1431. doi: 10.1111/j.1467-8624.2008.01196.x

Zijlmans, M. A. C., Riksen-Walraven, J. M., & de Weerth, C. (2015). Associations between maternal prenatal cortisol concentrations and child outcomes: A systematic review. *Neuroscience and Biobehavioral Reviews, 53,* 1–24.

CHAPTER 8

What a Complex Systems Perspective Can Contribute to Process-Based Assessment and Psychotherapy[2]

Adele M. Hayes, PhD and Leigh A. Andrews
University of Delaware

As science progresses, themes and overarching principles can be identified from a body of apparently disparate findings. With the proliferation of hundreds of brands of psychotherapy with empirical support, the time has come to take stock and identify principles and processes of change. Recent technological and statistical advances allow us to begin to model general human change processes in a way that is less constrained by the lenses of clinical diagnoses, theoretical orientations, or the search for single factors responsible for a given form of psychopathology and recovery from it.

The Traditional Approach to Psychotherapy Research and Development

Psychopathology and treatment research have been dominated by the biomedical model, disorder-oriented diagnostic systems, and entrenched theoretical orientations emphasizing one component of human functioning (cognitive, behavioral, emotional, interpersonal, physiological) over another

---

[2] Author Note: The work of A. M. Hayes related to this chapter was supported by grants from the National Institute of Mental Health (NIMH: R01-MH086558, R21-MH062662).

(A. M. Hayes & Alpert, 2017). To loosen these constraints, the National Institute of Mental Health (NIMH) introduced the Research Domain Criteria (RDoC) initiative to identify mechanisms of psychopathology (and potential treatment targets), focusing on such domains as negative and positive valence systems, cognitive systems, social processes, and arousal or modulatory systems (Cuthbert & Insel, 2013). More recent iterations of the RDoC approach (Kozak & Cuthbert, 2016; Sanislow, 2016) highlight the search for networks of biopsychosocial variables associated with the onset and maintenance of psychopathology. If misused, however, the RDoC approach can also reduce human functioning into ever smaller components studied in isolation, such as specific molecules, genes, and cells. In addition, psychotherapy research has been constrained by assumptions that change occurs linearly and is best captured by snapshots of symptoms at pre- and post-treatment and summarized by group averages. This traditional approach is giving way to more transtheoretical, multimodal, and personalized treatments and to research methods that consider the individual (Fisher, Reeves, Lawyer, Medaglia, & Rubel, 2017) and the nonlinear dynamics of therapeutic change (A. M. Hayes, Laurenceau, Feldman, Strauss, & Cardaciotto, 2007c; S. C. Hayes et al., 2018; Zilcha-Mano, 2018; Tschacher & Haken, 2019).

Psychotherapy process research, which is designed to identify different patterns of change and factors that predict treatment outcomes (A. M. Hayes, Laurenceau, & Cardaciotto, 2007b; Holmes et al., 2018; Kazdin, 2009), has a long history. Until recently, it had been eclipsed by comparative outcome trials on the various brands of psychotherapy. With renewed attention to processes and mechanisms of change (Holmes et al., 2018), we now not only have lists of empirically supported treatments for a range of clinical disorders (Cuijpers, 2017; McHugh & Barlow, 2012), but also lists of principles and processes of change common across clinical disorders (Castonguay & Beutler, 2006; Laska, Gurman, & Wampold, 2014; Norcross & Wampold, 2018). The NIMH experimental therapeutics approach (Insel, 2015), which is an initiative to identify mechanisms of therapeutic change in clinical trials, will likely add additional factors to the mix. It is encouraging that psychotherapy research and development has progressed to the point that such lists can be generated. The pressing question now is what to do with all of this information.

Toward a Process-Based Approach

A central task is to organize all of this information so clinicians can use the science to individualize treatment targets and interventions. The process-based approach that is the focus of this book is such an attempt. This approach considers general principles of change and also helps clinicians to identify processes that maintain psychopathology for a given person in context and to tailor interventions to those processes (Hofmann & Hayes, 2019).

As we broaden the perspective from a tight focus on symptoms, disorders, and techniques, it is important to consider the level of abstraction and scale that we target (Hofmann & Hayes, 2019). In the early days of process research and the psychotherapy integration movement, Goldfried (1980) argued that the way forward from competing theoretical orientations and treatment packages was to target a midlevel of abstraction. At the highest level of abstraction—theory—proponents of different theoretical orientations have long vied for dominance, while at the lowest level of abstraction—concrete techniques—interventions and packages have proliferated and been evaluated in numerous comparative outcome trials, often revealing similar outcomes. At the midlevel, researchers can identify general *principles and processes of change* that are common across theoretical orientations and techniques. For example, psychodynamic, behavioral, cognitive behavioral, and experiential treatments may differ in their theoretical framework and the form of their interventions, but they converge on the principle that it is important to expose clients to corrective experiences and to help them process this new information (Carey, 2011; Castonguay & Hill, 2012).

As we widen the lens, another key consideration involves scale; that is, whether to focus on the individual (idiographic), the group (nomothetic), or on broader contextual factors (Hofmann & Hayes, 2019). Each of these perspectives can reveal useful information. The process-based approach described in this book targets the "sweet spot"—principles and processes of change—and illustrates them at multiple scales, from the individual to the broad context of evolutionary science, which is applicable across living systems. In addition, the "functional periodic table" that S. C. Hayes and colleagues (2018) propose can be used to organize the multiple dimensions and levels of maladaptive and adaptive change processes identified in psychopathology and intervention research.

We add to this picture by exploring the nature of human change in the context of psychotherapy. We describe some general principles of pattern formation and change from complexity science, particularly dynamical systems theory, synergetics, and network theory, which can be used to optimally fit therapeutic process targets and intervention strategies to a particular client. We illustrate how this framework can be used to formulate therapeutic targets, the type of change to induce, and interventions that can mobilize that change. This framework also has exciting implications for psychotherapy research. This perspective naturally has connections with the principles from evolution science, as the frameworks are complementary and differ primarily in level of analysis and scale.

Principles of System Change: Resilience, Fluctuation, and Transition

An essential task of therapy is to disrupt entrenched maladaptive patterns and habits and to help clients develop more adaptive ways of functioning. This task is similar to moving any living system in nature from a less functional to a more functional state.

Sciences that study complex adaptive systems have shifted away from reductionistic analyses of component parts and linear cause-and-effect relationships toward the study of patterns of interconnected elements and feedback loops that often change in nonlinear ways. Using the common organizing framework of complex systems theory, sciences as varied as physics, ecology, neuroscience, economics, global health and infectious disease, and political science have identified some general principles of pattern development and change. At this midlevel of abstraction involving principles and processes of change (Goldfried, 1980; S. C. Hayes et al., 2018), we believe that psychotherapy researchers and clinicians can progress to a different way of thinking about how to relieve suffering and promote better adaptation. This framework can place our field more in line with other sciences that study complex dynamical systems and facilitate comparisons across different systems.

We summarize here key principles that can be used to conceptualize how human behavior settles into pathological patterns and how psychotherapy can facilitate adjustments or transitions into new patterns (for more detailed presentations in the context of psychopathology and treatment, see Gelo & Salvatore, 2016; Haken & Tschacher, 2017; Hofmann, Curtiss, & McNally, 2016; Mahoney, 1991; Nelson, McGorry, Wichers, Wigman, & Hartmann, 2017; Schiepek, Aichhorn, & Schöller, 2017; Tschacher & Haken, 2019). When the concepts of complexity science are applied to psychological constructs, they are often used in a metaphorical way to understand how systems lock in and change, but we also provide examples of research with high resolution time-series data that apply statistical tools from dynamical systems and network science.

Pattern Formation and Attractors

As we have summarized elsewhere (A. M. Hayes & Andrews, in press; A. M. Hayes, Yasinski, Barnes, & Bockting, 2015), a dynamical system is a set of interconnected elements that evolve over time into higher-order patterns that are preferred and relatively stable called *attractor states*. Attractors constrain system behavior such that it tends to return or be "pulled" back to these states when perturbed. To sustain itself, a system must be both resilient to perturbations and flexible enough to adapt to changing conditions (Hollenstein, Lichtwarck-Aschoff, & Potworowski, 2013).

Attractors that are well-established have elements that strongly influence each other, with reinforcing and inhibiting feedback loops that can increase or decrease the probability of activation across time and contexts (Vallacher, van Geert, & Nowak, 2015). Individual components of an attractor pattern can become increasingly synchronized and form higher-order functional units, as occurs with brain regions that coordinate to perform a task or muscle movements, such as walking (Kelso, Dumas, & Tognoli, 2013; Nowak, Vallacher, Zochowski, & Rychwalska, 2017). If attractor patterns become too entrenched, they can become rigid and relatively insensitive to challenges or new information. Entrenched attractors are highly resilient and therefore require a significant amount of perturbation or strong jolts to disrupt them; that is, they tend to bounce back to their dominant state when perturbed (Scheffer et al., 2018). Attractors that are less well-developed, or those that have been destabilized, have less of a hold, allowing the system to switch to alternative states. The likelihood of transition from one attractor to another depends not only on the type of perturbation, but also on the strength of the alternate attractor (Scheffer et al., 2018; Vallacher et al., 2015).

System Change: Early Warning Signals, Tipping Points, and Phase Transitions

At times, change in complex systems can be incremental, gradual, and continuous, with minor fluctuations and adjustments within the dominant pattern of functioning (attractor). This does not require system reorganization. Another type of change, which characterizes much of nature, is more abrupt and discontinuous, with periods of turbulence and critical fluctuations. With this type of change, attractors are destabilized, creating the potential for *phase transitions*, when systems can reorganize into qualitatively new patterns of functioning (Gelo & Salvatore, 2016; Tschacher & Haken, 2019). At or before these transition points, the factors that drive the change (control parameters) can be revealed and manipulated (Haken & Schiepek, 2006; Haken & Tschacher, 2017). Challenges to the system are a combination of deterministic (causal) and stochastic (random, chance) forces (Tschacher & Haken, 2019). To maintain cohesion, the system can adapt to, incorporate, or defend against challenges, but when a "tipping point" is reached, the dominant state can suddenly shift (Scheffer et al., 2018).

Scheffer and colleagues (2018) illustrate such nonlinear transitions in the context of human frailty. For example, after experiencing a fall and hip fracture, an elderly person in average health can deteriorate rapidly due to the cascade of complications from a jolt to the system that cannot be absorbed. Transition can involve movement from adaptive to maladaptive states or the converse. For example, Scheffer and Westley (2007) describe a number of "social traps" (e.g., poverty or cultural norms) that act as maladaptive attractors that constrain behavior and need to be disrupted before change can occur.

New patterns, whether newly developed or latent, are relatively weak unless they are strengthened with repeated activation across multiple contexts and unless feedback loops that maintain the new state are amplified. Therefore, there can be a period of vacillation or "flickering" (Dakos, van Nes, & Scheffer, 2013; Wang et al., 2012) between the old and new until one state is strong enough to capture the system. As the new attractor strengthens, it can compete with or inhibit the old attractor to prevent a return to that state, or, over time, it can become the preferred or default state (Kelso, 2012; Kelso, Ding, & Schöner, 1993; Scheffer et al., 2012; Thelen & Smith, 1996). This new attractor is not always more adaptive, as is the case when a person moves from a healthy state into psychopathology.

The principles of complex dynamical systems theory are often described metaphorically with attractor landscape diagrams, although with high resolution time-series data, it is possible to mathematically quantify and examine attractors, synchronization, and critical instabilities. A clear example of how this metaphor is being applied and quantified with real-life social problems is in the case of intractable conflict, which has been conceptualized as a highly resilient and destructive attractor with feedback loops that strengthen and maintain it (Coleman, 2018; Coleman, Vallacher, Bartoli, Nowak, & Bui-Wrzosinska, 2011). As these researchers note, patterns of extreme, negative intergroup attitudes, hatred, and violence can be so entrenched that they persist across individuals and even across generations (e.g., persistent conflicts in Israel-Palestine, Syria, and Sudan). Although the processes of system lock-in and transition from persistent conflict operate on a different scale, this research and its applications have clear implications for the tasks and processes of psychotherapy.

Nowak and colleagues (2010) have developed an attractor simulator program to depict conflict and peaceful relations attractors relevant to a given dispute, the variables that maintain the attractors, and the effects of manipulating the maintaining factors or introducing other interventions. They also use causal looping diagrams to capture the conflict network linkages and dynamics before initiating any attempts at actual conflict resolution. If possible, they identify relevant control parameters (e.g., police or security forces, sanctions, attacks) and their effects on the attractor landscape (e.g., inhibiting or increasing the probability of violence).

When thinking about how to change the connectivity of the elements of an attractor, Nowak and colleagues refer to concepts from network theory. They suggest identifying system parameters, strong conflict-maintaining feedback loops, and central hubs that can be used as "leverage points," where interventions can have maximum impact and propagate through the network (Coleman, 2018). This conflict mapping exercise and the attractor simulation program allow all parties to visualize and work interactively with the dynamics of conflict over time.

This research group also conducts simulations to mathematically examine the effects of variables identified in their qualitative, naturalistic, and lab-based studies. They have used the attractor simulator program and causal looping diagrams to work on the ground with particularly difficult problems, such as gang violence, urban poverty and violence, international conflict, and environmental disputes and conflicts. This program of work, although from a different field, provides a concrete example that might inspire similar scale projects in psychotherapy research.

From Metaphor to Measurement

As complex systems theory is applied across disciplines, including psychology, the science can advance with a standard set of indicators of system resilience, early warning signs of transition, and change to a new equilibrium. To this end, Scheffer and colleagues (2015, 2018) reviewed complex systems research across a range of sciences to identify three "indicators of dynamic resilience" that reliably quantify system stability. In response to perturbation, a system that is highly resilient shows (a) low variance in behavior (stability); (b) low temporal autocorrelation (the extent to which a measurement at one time predicts values of that variable at the next time point), such that temporary change in the system quickly returns to baseline; and (c) low cross-correlations between elements of the system, such that a challenge to one element does not easily change other elements in the system.

Transitions from one state to another occur as patterns develop and evolve, so we also must also be able to model change and the breakdown of resilience. System transition can have such important implications that researchers have tried to identify "early warning signs" (Scheffer et al., 2012, 2018) that herald such changes. Early warning signals can differ depending on the type of system being modeled and its history. Information on system resilience and how near it is to transition can guide efforts to reinforce resilience or to marshal prevention and intervention efforts. For instance, Scheffer and colleagues use these tools to identify ecosystems at risk for destruction and to develop interventions that decrease risk.

There are a number of indicators of impending transition that have been consistently documented in research across a range of systems in nature, including psychological constructs. A period of rising variability in system behavior called *critical fluctuations* (Haken & Tschacher, 2017; Kelso, 1995; Schiepek et al., 2017; Schiepek & Strunk, 2010) reflects the destabilization of attractors and can indicate an increase in flexibility and potential for new patterns to emerge. A period of *critical slowing* indicates resilience or a slower return to equilibrium in response to perturbations (Scheffer et al., 2012, 2018; van de Leemput et al., 2014; Wichers, Schreuder, Goekoop, & Groen,

2019). Changing *threshold sensitivity* can indicate that there is an increased probability of repeated pattern activation and that perturbations will have a larger effect (Cramer et al., 2016; Nelson et al., 2017; Schiepek, Schöller, Carl, Aichhorn, & Lichtwarck-Aschoff, 2019). Early warning signs highlight entry points when the system is on the verge of transition, which can be facilitated, slowed, or inhibited.

Scheffer and colleagues (2018) provide a useful, open-source toolbox for computing dynamic resilience and early warning signals (www.sparcscenter.org/resources/statistical-packages.html). In clinical psychology, Schiepek and his research group have developed the Synergetic Navigation System (SNS; Schiepek, Eckert, Aas, Wallot, & Wallot, 2015; Schiepek et al., 2016), a program that uses complexity-based assessment and analytic tools in treatment. The SNS can quantify and graphically depict the following in real time: repetitive patterns in the data stream and their stability (recurrence quantification analysis and plots), synchronization of the components (inter-item correlations over a sliding window of time), critical instabilities (dynamic complexity analyses considering the amplitude, frequency, and distribution of fluctuations), and transitions to new patterns (Schiepek et al., 2017). Dynamic complexity can also be calculated using a package available in R (https://fredhasselman.com/casnet/). Tschacher and Haken (2019) provide detailed descriptions and concrete examples of how the process of psychotherapy can be modeled mathematically, considering deterministic, stochastic, and contextual factors. These are exciting examples of cross-disciplinary collaboration with physicists and computer modelers to apply the concepts and methods of dynamical systems and self-organization theory (synergetics) to psychotherapy research.

GridWare (Hollenstein, 2013; Lamey, Hollenstein, Lewis, & Granic, 2004; http://www.statespacegrids.org/) is an example of a program developed by developmental psychologists to graphically depict and quantify system behavior over time across possible states in a state space grid. GridWare can quantify system stability, flexibility, and destabilization by calculating how frequently possible states are visited, the number of transitions between these states, dispersion across the grid, and the duration in each state (e.g., van Dijk et al., 2017).

The concept of an attractor suggests a pattern with strongly connected components and amplifying or inhibiting feedback loops. The analytic tools just described capture the stability and instability of patterns and their movement over time, but they do not reveal details about pattern structure. For this reason, network analysis tools and graph theory have been incorporated into complex systems research to zoom in on, depict, and quantify the structure, connectivity, and function of a network.

Technological and statistical advances have provided tools to conceptualize and monitor networks that contribute to psychopathology for a given sample or individual (for comprehensive descriptions of these methods, see Borsboom & Cramer, 2013; Costantini et al., 2019; Epskamp, Borsboom, & Fried, 2018; Robinaugh, Hoekstra, Toner, & Borsboom, 2019). Network analysis can be used to assess network properties such as density, the strength of the connections between components or nodes, and the centrality of the nodes and their thresholds of sensitivity. Networks can be modeled for a group (between-subject) or the individual (within-subject), and they can be modeled both cross-sectionally and longitudinally (Epskamp et al., 2018). The network structure and autoregressive feedback loops can be depicted visually and the network properties can be computed mathematically using the R statistical program (R Core Team, 2013) and freely available packages, such as qgraph and graphicalVAR (https://cran.r-project.org/web/packages/qgraph/index.html).

Fisher and colleagues (Fernandez, Fisher, & Chi, 2017; Fisher, 2015) have developed a system that creates personalized networks of symptoms that can be used to guide treatment selection for a specific person. The program uses their Dynamic Assessment Treatment Algorithm (DATA), which considers, for a specific person, the strength of cross-sectional covariance of symptoms from P-technique factor analyses, the time-lagged relationships in dynamic factor analyses, and the mean levels of symptom severity over the baseline time period. The factors that account for the most variance in the P-technique analyses and that have the strongest time-lagged effects are then matched with modules of cognitive behavioral therapies (e.g., cognitive reappraisal, emotion regulation). The modules with the best fit are identified, thus suggesting a sequencing of interventions that match the client's symptoms. Presumably, this method could also be used for pathological and adaptive networks and maintaining processes in addition to disorder-based symptoms.

Most of the network modeling studies in psychopathology and treatment research have examined symptoms as the components of the network, but it is also possible to model a range of constructs, such as health-, lifestyle-, and disease-related variables (e.g., Fried et al., 2017) and to use different types of measures in a single network, such as self-report, lab and behavioral tasks, and physiological measures (e.g., Heeren & McNally, 2016). Network modeling has also been extended to include sets of risk and protective factors in depression (Hoorelbeke, Marchetti, De Schryver, & Koster, 2016) and to test theoretical models of suicide risk (de Beurs, 2017). As we move from purely symptom-based networks to consider other variables, the insights and hypotheses that can be generated will grow commensurately.

Most of the early studies on clinical constructs examined network structure and connectivity cross-sectionally, but from a complex systems perspective, the goal is to model the dynamics of change over time and to capture nonlinear constructs, such as critical slowing and critical fluctuations. Indeed, the very purpose of psychotherapy is to induce change. Networks can be modeled over time, examining the extent to which one time point predicts the next, but there are some limitations. Costantini and colleagues (2019) describe combinations of autoregressive models and mixed models (Bringmann et al., 2013, 2016), or a network analysis and structural equation modeling approach (Epskamp, Rhemtulla, & Borsboom, 2017), to model change in longitudinal time-series data. However, as Piccirillo, Beck, and Rodebaugh (2019) caution, a limitation of most idiographic methods is that they cannot model nonlinear change, and they assume stationarity—that each variable over time demonstrates a similar mean, variance, and relationship with other variables and with itself. Variables can fluctuate temporally, but when they change systematically in response to another variable or the relationships between variables change, as occurs in therapy, then the assumption of stationarity is violated.

It is possible, however, to analyze data during time periods of approximate stationarity, such as at the beginning and end of treatment (e.g., Snippe et al., 2017). Another recent approach is network intervention analysis (NIA; Blanken et al., 2019), which adds treatment condition as a variable in network analyses and examines the sequencing of treatment effects on symptoms in three time windows: baseline, during a segment of treatment, and after treatment. This is related to the "moving" or "sliding windows" approach over the time-series data, such as summarizing the network structure in seven-day periods across the course of treatment, and then examining changes in network structure from window to window (e.g., Schiepek et al., 2019). Other approaches to address violations of stationarity include using residuals from ordinary least squares regression models or detrending the data (see Beltz & Gates, 2017; Fisher et al., 2017). More recent analytic strategies are also being developed to address the problems of non-stationarity using semi-parametric time-varying vector-autoregressive (TV-VAR) techniques (Bringmann, Ferrer, Hamaker, Borsboom, & Tuerlinckx, 2018) and methods to examine nonlinear jumps and regime (attractor) changes in networks (e.g., Cabrieto, Adolf, Tuerlinckx, Kuppens, Ceulemans, 2018).

In addition to analyzing network structure, it is possible to examine functional connectivity, which involves modeling dynamic networks of functional links in response to different tasks. This method, commonly used with functional magnetic resonance imaging (fMRI) and electrophysiology (EEG) data, quantifies synchronization dynamics and also functional unit assembly and disassembly, either statically or across time (dynamic functional connectivity analyses; Keilholz, Woolrich, Chang, & Miller, 2018). These functional connectivity methods have not yet been used in psychotherapy research because they require high resolution time-series data, but with recent advances in data collection methods, these analyses might be added to the toolbox for intervention science in the near future.

All of these tools can be used to study the process of change in psychotherapy as we move from simpler pre- to post-treatment measurement designs and linear change to more intensive time-series data and methods that can capture the dynamics and nonlinear process of change. It is also important to examine variables at both the within- and between-person levels, as findings from one level might not generalize to the other (Fisher, Medaglia, & Jeronimus, 2018). System dynamics can be modeled with data from naturalistic observations, archived datasets of populations, experimental manipulations of variables (perturbation experiments), and computer simulations.

Application: A Complex Systems Perspective on the Process of Change in Psychotherapy

The cross-disciplinary principles of change that we have examined have implications for what to target in psychotherapy, what type of change to induce, and how to conceptualize relapse. These principles can also be used to generate hypotheses on how change occurs in psychotherapy and to guide a new generation of research.

What to Target: From Diagnoses and Single Components to Dynamic Networks

A complex dynamical systems approach focuses on multicomponent patterns that can form attractors that a system settles into and returns to, unless perturbations overwhelm the regulatory systems maintaining that organization. Psychological treatments can be viewed as a way to destabilize recurrent, maladaptive patterns and to facilitate new learning and movement toward more adaptive patterns of functioning. From this perspective, the therapeutic targets are networks and processes that maintain clinical problems.

NETWORKS

A number of psychopathology models propose pathological patterns or associative networks of interrelated cognitive, affective, behavioral, and physiological components that can act like attractors that rigidly maintain pathology (Cramer et al., 2016; A. M. Hayes & Yasinski, 2015; A. M. Hayes et al., 2015; Hofmann et al., 2016; Robinaugh et al., 2019; Schiepek et al., 2017; van de Leemput et al., 2014). For instance, fear and trauma networks have been proposed as central in anxiety and stress-related disorders (Foa, Huppert, & Cahill, 2006), and multimodal networks, interlocks, schemas (Beck & Dozois, 2011; Teasdale, 1999) and emotional schemas (Greenberg & Watson, 2006) have been proposed in depression and personality disorders (Beck, Freeman, & Davis, 2004; Young, Klosko, & Weishaar, 2003). Borsboom and Cramer's (2013) network theory also conceptualizes psychopathology as a causal system of functionally interrelated symptoms that have settled into a pathological equilibrium.

Yet, many of our treatments still prioritize a single component of functioning that is part of a multimodal network, as with cognitive, behavioral, emotion-focused, and interpersonal therapies. Treatments have also been developed to target a specific process that maintains clinical disorders, such as rumination, anhedonia, or attentional control. Not surprisingly, research on the process of change also tends to examine one component in isolation, often finding that the single component out of context is not a strong predictor of outcome nor specific to the hypothesized treatment (Holmes et al., 2018; Lemmens et al., 2017).

In addition, relatively little attention has been paid to more adaptive networks of functioning, although there is increasing interest in the idea that new learning in treatment can compete with or inhibit the activation of pathological patterns (Brewin, 2006; Craske, Treanor, Conway, Zbozinek, & Vervliet, 2014). These single component or single process approaches have contributed significantly to the treatment of psychopathology, but as a next step, we recommend better aligning the assessment and treatment of psychopathology with current theories that propose multimodal networks with maintaining and inhibiting feedback loops. As Greene and Loscalzo (2017) argue in the context of medicine, it is time to move past reductionism and put the human back together.

We use the case of depression to illustrate how complex systems concepts can be applied to psychopathology and treatment, but the principles of pattern formation and system change should also apply across a range of clinical problems. We developed the *network destabilization and transition (NDT) model* (A. M. Hayes & Andrews, in press; A. M. Hayes et al., 2015) to integrate principles from dynamical systems, synergetics, and network theories with principles of change in psychotherapy and modern learning theory. This way of thinking broadens the scope from a focus on a single component of functioning or maintaining process to a focus on broader principles of system change. This model is also the foundation of a treatment for depression we have developed, exposure-based cognitive therapy (EBCT; A. M. Hayes et al., 2007a; A. M. Hayes, Ready, & Yasinski, 2014), which applies these principles. EBCT uses techniques from exposure therapies and schema-focused approaches to reduce the processes that maintain depression, destabilize a depressive network, and develop a more adaptive network. We use the NDT model and the associated treatment (i.e., EBCT) to illustrate how principles from complex systems science can be applied in a concrete way. The NDT model focuses on psychosocial variables and treatments, but because this is a theory of general system change, it might also apply to biological risk and maintaining factors and treatments.

Depression is a useful context to illustrate the principles of change in complex systems because it is a problem that tends to recur, with estimates of recurrence as high as ninety percent by the third episode (Cuijpers et al., 2014). Attractors in recurrent and chronic depression have a long history with repeated activation and increased sensitivity, so they can be particularly difficult to dislodge. Perturbations are likely to be assimilated or deflected by a powerful set of maintaining processes. Although they do not refer to complex systems principles, Holtzheimer and Mayberg (2011) urge researchers and clinicians to rethink depression as a recurrent tendency to become "stuck in a rut" rather than an episodic disorder. This stuckness involves persistent difficulty disengaging from negative mood states and impaired updating processes in the face of new information (Joormann & Tanovic, 2015; Koster, De Lissnyder, Derakshan, & De Raedt, 2011).

Indeed, a wide range of research suggests that depression involves rigidity across cognitive, behavioral, emotional, and biological domains (Rottenberg, 2017). Depressive networks are easily activated and can have a strong pull or "attractor" strength as they become the default mode of operation (Cramer et al., 2016; van de Leemput et al., 2014; Wichers, 2014). Thus, both psychopathology research and a complex systems approach suggest that treatments should disrupt multimodal patterns that contribute to depression.

PROCESSES: MAINTAINING AND INHIBITING FEEDBACK LOOPS

In addition to identifying the components of a pathological network, it is important to identify maintaining and inhibiting processes that form feedback loops. These are the processes associated with entering and staying in a depressive (or other pathological) state (Holtzheimer & Mayberg, 2011). It is here that the process-based approach to treatment (Hofmann & Hayes, 2019) might have the most to offer. Inhibiting feedback loops also come into play but are most relevant for relapse prevention, as is suggested by competing retrieval and inhibitory learning theories (Brewin, 2006; Craske et al., 2014).

Three interrelated maintaining processes have been consistently documented in depression: (a) unproductive processing (repetitively cycling over and analyzing negative thoughts and feelings), (b) avoidance, and (c) reward processing deficits (problems anticipating, attending to, and maintaining positive emotions). These factors lock down the system such that there is little diversity of emotions. This is an example of low variation that can stunt growth (S. C. Hayes, Monestès, & Wilson, 2017). Heightened temporal dependency or inertia of negative affect has also been reported before the onset of depression, in a depressive episode, and before relapse (Kuppens & Verduyn, 2017; Slofstra et al., 2017; Wichers et al., 2010). Depressive thoughts also cycle and recycle, with few new insights or perspectives (Watkins & Nolen-Hoeksema, 2014). The repertoire of emotion regulation strategies is similarly narrow (Aldao, Nolen-Hoeksema, & Schweizer, 2010), with a pervasive tendency to avoid and engage in stereotyped behavioral and physiological stress responses (Rottenberg, 2017).

To further perpetuate depression, there is a "positive blockade" (Disner, Beevers, Haigh, & Beck, 2011), which involves difficulty recognizing, processing, and sustaining positive emotions (Pizzagalli, 2014). Treatment can help develop the more adaptive counterparts to these maladaptive maintaining factors, which involves constructive processing of negative and positive emotions, distress tolerance, and a more flexible repertoire of coping skills and physiological responses (A. M. Hayes et al., 2015). These more adaptive processes can serve an inhibitory function by competing with or preventing the activation of the maladaptive attractor.

Together, the depressive network and maintaining processes can be viewed as a functional unit (Nowak et al., 2017) that forms a metaphorical attractor. After careful assessment of the components of the attractor, the EBCT therapist works with the client to map out the pathological network, much as is done in conflict mapping (Vallacher et al., 2015) and Schiepek et al.'s (2015) multimodal idiographic modeling in psychotherapy. Clients learn to recognize the network and what triggers it, as well as the core processes that strengthen and maintain it. Therapists also sketch out the person's positive components (or network) to illustrate how the positive system is less elaborate and harder to sustain than the depressive network. Consistent with complex systems principles, additional information about the attractor history, strength, and degree of entrenchment can guide decisions about the type of change to induce and when to do so.

Fisher and colleagues' DATA program (Fernandez et al., 2017; Fisher, 2015) could be a useful addition to treatments like EBCT, especially if other network components and maintaining and inhibiting processes were included in addition to disorder-related symptoms. Similarly, the SNS program (Schiepek et al., 2015) can accommodate a range of variables and could model such network components and processes over treatment. The SNS can capture component synchronization and pattern destabilization in real time, and that information can be fed back to clients and used in an ongoing way across the course of treatment (Schiepek et al., 2015, 2016).

By formulating a multimodal and self-perpetuating depressive pattern, clients often experience clarity and some relief, as the many different problems they have been struggling with cohere into a more manageable problem set. Comorbid problems often have overlapping components and processes that can be identified with this approach, and the clinician can target core patterns and issues in treatment rather than a disorder or a specific component of functioning (A. M. Hayes, 2015). This approach is conceptually similar to functional analysis used in behavioral therapies, but it considers a broader range of variables. As with functional analysis, the relevant elements and patterns are person-specific and can also be used nomothetically across individuals in research (S. C. Hayes et al., 2018). Progress in treatment can be assessed by measuring how these patterns change over time and whether new, more adaptive patterns develop. From this perspective, the old and new patterns can be used as measures of outcome that add idiographic detail to other more traditional symptom and disorder-oriented measures.

What Type of Change to Induce: From Linear Snapshots to Nonlinear Dynamics

With a map of the maladaptive and positive networks and the processes that lock a person in the maladaptive attractor, the next step is to formulate a plan of action—that is, what kind of change to induce. Here too, assumptions about the nature of change in therapy have been influenced by the view that people change in a gradual, linear way. The traditional view has also held that symptom reduction by the end of treatment is maintained (or not) and can therefore be assessed by quick snapshots at three- to six-month intervals. A complex systems approach opens a broader perspective that is more in line with other systems in nature. There are multiple types of change, and systems grow and evolve. If therapy is considered part of general life development, then the type of change appropriate for the problems at a given time can vary. For instance, clients might not be ready for a transformational kind of change initially, but years after treatment, they might be in a position for more substantial self-improvement. In addition, different kinds of change can be relevant at different points in treatment, as we illustrate with EBCT. The types of therapeutic change are fluid and interacting, depending on the needs, resources, and goals of a person at a given time, consistent with a process-based approach to treatment (S. C. Hayes & Hofmann, 2018).

Before initiating an intervention plan, it is critical to assess the client's readiness and resources for change. As Scheipek et al. (2015) note in their generic principles of therapeutic change, a person must be stable enough to withstand destabilization. This includes having social support, basic resources, motivation to change, and not being in crisis or in the midst of severe or destabilizing life events (see also A. M. Hayes & Strauss, 1998; Schiepek et al., 2019).

We use the metaphorical attractor landscape to characterize the process of change in psychotherapy, using depression as an example. This conceptualization can also apply to other clinical problems, especially those that tend to be recurrent or chronic, such as substance abuse, eating disorders, and personality disorders. Figure 8.1 depicts the components of the NDT model (A. M. Hayes & Andrews, in press; A. M. Hayes et al., 2015) and different types of therapeutic change. We focus on two possible attractor states and the associated networks, maladaptive and adaptive. It is possible that more than two patterns are relevant, and it is not clear whether the pathological and more adaptive states and components are indeed separate. These are important empirical questions that can be pursued, but for illustrative purposes, we follow the two-attractor modeling approach used to describe intractable conflict (Coleman, 2018) and resilience in other systems (Scheffer et al., 2018). It is also possible, and indeed likely, that the connections between nodes in a network are both positive and negative in valence, but for simplicity, we do not indicate the valence of connections between nodes in these hypothetical networks.

The right side of the first panel in Figure 8.1 depicts a deep well, similar to the concept of a depression rut that is easy to enter and difficult to exit (Holtzheimer & Mayberg, 2011). The ball, which represents the state of the system, quickly returns to the rut if perturbed. In network language, this attractor is a depressive network of cognitions, emotions, behaviors, and physiological components that is well-established, easily activated, and difficult to disengage. Maintaining processes (unproductive processing, avoidance, and a positive blockade) strengthen the network, creating self-perpetuating downward spirals. In contrast, the more positive or adaptive components shown on the left side of panel 1 are weak and loosely connected, and some nodes are not connected at all. Thus, there is no alternative attractor, and perturbations are likely to be followed by a return to the rut (system resilience). In cases where the depression well is not as deep, and the person also has a healthier way of functioning, therapy can focus on switching the person from the maladaptive to a more adaptive pattern of functioning. For others with more well-established pathological patterns, therapy might involve building a positive attractor, reducing the processes that maintain the pathological attractor, and activating and destabilizing the depressive network (see panel 2, right side) to facilitate change—for example, as in exposure therapies and emotion-focused and schema-based approaches.

What a Complex Systems Perspective Can Contribute   183

Note: Attractor landscapes are depicted with a solid line, and the ball represents the state of the system. Maladaptive and adaptive networks are depicted with nodes of cognition (C), emotion (E), behavior (B), and physiological responses (P). Larger nodes (circles) are stronger, and thicker lines represent stronger connections (direction and valence of the connections are not depicted). Panel 1 shows a maladaptive attractor with a strongly interconnected network that is maintained by amplifying feedback loops. The system tends to return to the attractor if perturbed. The maladaptive attractor in panel 2 is less strong and the adaptive attractor is more strong than in panel 1. This provides an alternative state for the ball to enter if the maladaptive network is perturbed or destabilized. With repeated activation and amplifying feedback loops (panel 3), the adaptive attractor can become stronger than the maladaptive attractor.

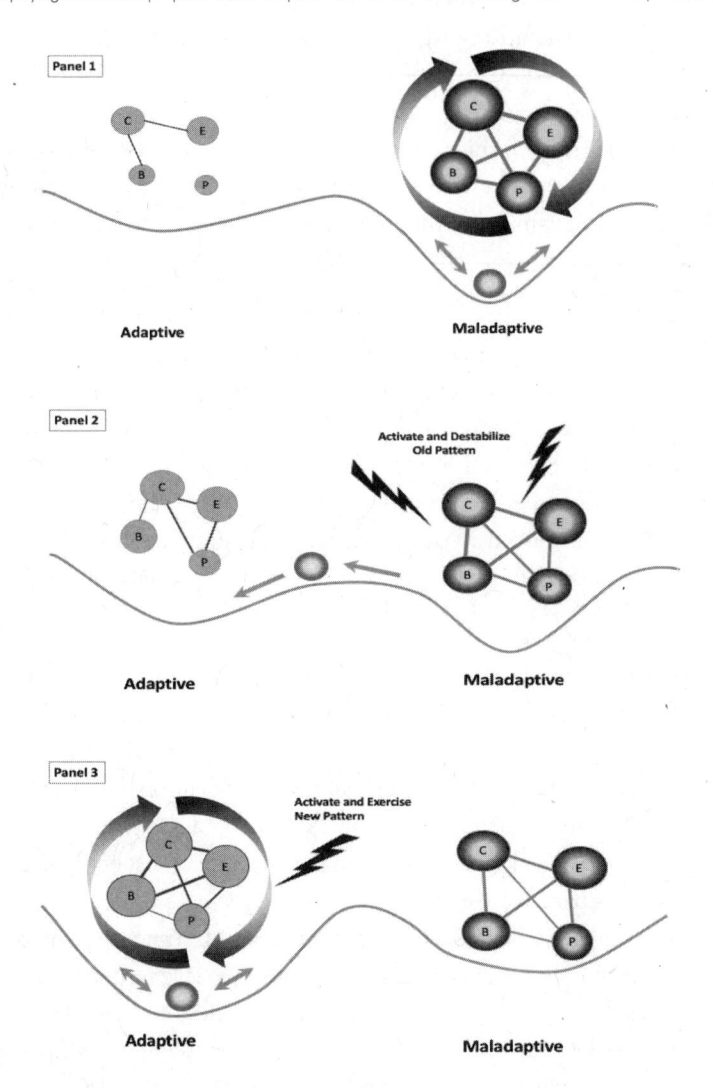

Figure 8.1. Network Destabilization and Transition (NDT) Model

Because the new attractor is initially weak, it must be repeatedly activated and exercised across different contexts, creating upward spirals of continued development (panel 3, left side), as described in variants of the "broaden and build" approach (Fredrickson & Joiner, 2018; Garland, Geschwind, Peeters, & Wichers, 2015). Repetition can strengthen the new attractor such that it becomes dominant. It can also be used to deactivate or inhibit the pathological pattern, which can still be activated, as proposed by inhibitory learning theory (Craske et al., 2014).

The attractor landscape and network metaphors can be useful for conceptualizing the different forms of therapeutic change and the kind of perturbation that can initiate movement and sustainable change. We describe in more detail below examples of different types of therapeutic change.

ADJUSTMENTS THAT DO NOT REQUIRE REORGANIZATION

Some problems require only minor adjustments to improve functioning and do not require reconfiguration of the maladaptive attractor. This type of change may be all that is needed, or it might be an adjustment that improves functioning in the short term. It is also possible that a person is not ready or does not have the resources to support more substantial modifications. With repetition, these strategies have the potential to facilitate attractor change, and some of these also come into play after recovery to prevent relapse.

Creating the Potential for More Adaptive Patterns to Develop. This can include strategies to increase readiness for change, such as motivational interviewing (Miller & Rollnick, 2012), and supportive therapies or psychoeducation. Increasing access to resources is another way to create a platform for more positive change, such as providing financial or vocational counseling, daycare, or other resources that can stabilize aspects of daily life. A stable environment, such as a safe house for domestic violence or a sober house for those struggling with substance abuse, can also help create the potential for change. Other interventions, such as the behavioral strategy of gradual shaping, are relevant, as is the concept of "nudging" people to better behavior and choices by changing the environment, policy, or contingencies (Thaler, 2018; Thaler & Sunstein, 2009). The therapeutic relationship itself can also provide these facilitative conditions (Schiepek et al., 2015).

Reducing Harm or Negative Effects of Maladaptive Patterns. Harm reduction strategies (Marlatt & Witkiewitz, 2010) are good examples of this type of modification. A heroin addict can be given clean needles to prevent infection and the spread of disease if that person is not ready to undergo full treatment for addiction. Those who self-harm can be taught other ways to handle difficult emotions that cause less damage (Lynch, Trost, Salsman, & Linehan, 2007) even if they are still mired in maladaptive patterns. Harm reduction strategies meet people where they are and can increase motivation for more change and the potential for more adaptive patterns to develop.

Changing the Threshold of Activation. This set of strategies is not designed to change attractors directly, but instead to increase or decrease attractor sensitivity. However, over time and with repetition, these strategies can change the attractor landscape by decreasing or increasing the strength of a pathological or more adaptive attractor. For instance, distress tolerance skills and mindfulness meditation can have the effect of tuning sensitivity up or down (Hölzel et al., 2011). Craske, Treanor, Conway, Zbozinek, and Vervliet's (2016) positive affect treatment is designed to repeatedly activate and increase the sensitivity of the positive emotion system and to strengthen it over time.

Deactivating or Shifting Out of the Maladaptive Attractor. Here again, the attractor is not changed directly, but clients can learn strategies that can act as a trip switch or can help them shift out of the well if they start sliding into it. In a recent paper on enhancing learning in therapy, Bruijniks, DeRubeis, Hollon, and Huibers (2019) also describe this type of change. Clients can learn when the maladaptive pattern is getting activated and unhook from it. Mindfulness and acceptance-based strategies can be used to unhook and shift out of unhelpful habits in everyday life, during therapy, and after therapy (S. C. Hayes, Strosahl, & Wilson, 2011; Segal & Teasdale, 2018). These strategies can be used to switch to more adaptive modes of functioning or to compete with or inhibit the activation of the maladaptive attractor (Brewin et al. 2006; Craske et al., 2014).

Compensating for or Overriding the Maladaptive Attractor. The old patterns can remain intact, but the person can learn or bring online skills that compensate for a deficit or problematic patterns (Bruijniks et al., 2019). For instance, in Dozier's attachment and biobehavioral catch-up program (Dozier, Bernard, & Roben, 2017), therapists teach healthy parenting styles to foster parents of maltreated infants and help these caregivers override their own maladaptive attachment patterns. Similarly, social skills training can help compensate for the flat affect and negative symptoms associated with schizophrenia (e.g., Bellack, Mueser, Gingerich, & Agresta, 2013).

TRANSITIONS THAT INDUCE REORGANIZATION AND SWITCH TO A NEW ATTRACTOR

Some problems require a more turbulent, often nonlinear, type of transition that involves destabilizing entrenched dysfunctional patterns (Gelo & Salvatore, 2016; A. M. Hayes et al., 2015; Wichers et al., 2019). For instance, in chronic and recurrent depression, patterns have been activated repeatedly across time and contexts such that they have a very strong pull and tend to dominate system dynamics. It is difficult for change to occur without a jolt to the system, which in therapy often involves creating dissonance and, as Coleman et al. (2011) describe, reaching a "threshold of inconsistency." This is a tipping point at which the challenges to the system can no longer be deflected or assimilated (see also Bruijniks et al., 2019). In transformational experiences outside of therapy, Baumeister (1994) describes a "crystallization of discontent," and in chronic substance abuse, Miller and C'de Baca (2001) describe a similar point at which dissatisfaction and distress across time and situations come together, putting the person on the verge of transition. This might be akin to the increase in synchronization (correlation between elements) and critical slowing that are early warning signs of system change in psychopathology (van de Leemput et al., 2014; Wichers et al., 2019)

The depression treatment that we have developed, EBCT (A. M. Hayes et al., 2007a, 2014), was specifically designed to induce this kind of destabilizing change. EBCT grew out of our research on the change process in cognitive behavioral therapies (CBT) for three particularly entrenched clinical problems: chronic depression, post-traumatic stress disorder, and avoidant and obsessive-compulsive personality disorders. These disorders are also characterized by three common maintaining processes: unproductive processing, avoidance, and a dysfunctional positive emotion system. EBCT is a useful way to illustrate how principles from the science of complex systems can be applied because it merges those principles in a CBT framework and induces several types of change, including the destabilizing type of transition.

After identifying the components of the person's depressive network and the maintaining processes, the first step in the change process is to prepare for it. To reduce ongoing stress generation and develop the potential for more adaptive functioning, the first phase of EBCT focuses on teaching stress management and distress tolerance skills as well as healthy lifestyle habits related to sleep, eating, exercise, and mindfulness meditation. An important task is to work directly on reducing the three processes that maintain the lockdown. This phase often brings incremental improvement in depressive symptoms and increases energy and the resources for further change.

Next, EBCT applies the second component of the NDT model (A. M. Hayes & Andrews, in press; A. M. Hayes et al., 2015) to destabilize the patterns and processes of depression and move clients toward more adaptive functioning. A combination of exposure and schema-focused techniques is used to activate the depressive network and induce dissonance by introducing new information and experiences that violate expectancies and challenge the old network (Craske et al., 2014; Foa et al., 2006). This disturbance can increase flexibility and allow for new associations and learning (cognitive-emotional processing) not possible with the previous rigidity and strong maintaining feedback loops. This type of change is preceded by a period of transient symptom exacerbation and variability that might be an early warning signal of transition (A. M. Hayes et al., 2007a; A. M. Hayes & Yasinski, 2015; Schiepek & Strunk, 2010; Wichers et al., 2019). Our research also shows that more cognitive-emotional processing during this period of destabilization predicts more improvement in symptoms in EBCT for depression (A. M. Hayes et al., 2007a) and in cognitive therapy for personality disorders (A. M. Hayes & Yasinski, 2015). Destabilizing techniques might induce the kind of variability critical for growth and continued adaptation (S. C. Hayes et al., 2017).

According to a complex systems approach and modern learning theory, the pathological network might be weaker, but it has not disappeared and can be reactivated quickly. The new learning can also serve an inhibitory function (Brewin, 2006; Craske et al., 2014) to compete with or prevent a return to the old attractor. Applying the third component of the NDT model (A. M. Hayes & Andrews, in press; A. M. Hayes et al. 2015), EBCT focuses on building and exercising the new more adaptive attractor. This involves mapping out the current positive network, living it out in therapeutic exercises and daily interactions and also elaborating it in writing exercises. Clients also apply new skills in relapse prevention drills.

In summary, the type of therapeutic change described in this section involves decreasing the processes that maintain depression, destabilizing the depressive network, and developing a more adaptive network that can serve an inhibitory function.

Conceptualizing Relapse: From Maintenance to Ongoing Change and Development

An area that has received the least attention is the process of change after the acute phase of therapy. This period is typically viewed as relatively smooth, and researchers assess the maintenance of treatment outcomes at intervals of several months. Witkiewitz and Marlatt (2007) propose that relapse has been difficult to predict because of the reliance on linear, continuous models of relapse, and they describe nonlinear methods to better capture the rocky road of recovery. Change is most fragile in the period of time after treatment, and continued and frequent monitoring of networks, maintaining and inhibitory processes, and symptoms could provide a rich source of information to better understand what happens after change is induced. If early warning signs of impending transition could be identified, then techniques such as "just-in-time" interventions could be tailored and deployed for a specific person based on that person's previous and ongoing data and patterns, as is being done after treatment for substance abuse and schizophrenia (Nahum-Shani et al., 2017). Schiepek et al. (2011) illustrate how dynamical systems methods can be used to identify early warning signs of transition and highlight points of intervention for those at high risk for suicide.

Possibilities and Challenges for the Future

Until recently, psychotherapy research has been limited by the assumption of simple linear symptom reduction and the collection of low-density data over the course of treatment. The tools of ecological momentary assessment (Ebner-Priemer, 2018) and various smartphone apps, wearable technology, and systems of passive data collection (e.g., the automatic collection of activity, location, frequency of social media usage) change that. These tools are now readily available and open many possibilities for the types of questions psychotherapy researchers can pursue and the ways in which assessment and psychotherapy can be conducted. We can now collect the density of data necessary to examine networks of pathology and health, maintaining and inhibiting processes, and system dynamics over time. We can study different types of change, whether therapy only improves pathological networks or also helps clients develop more adaptive patterns, and how therapeutic changes maintain or improve after therapy has ended. Discontinuities in patterns of symptom change can be used to reveal therapy techniques and client change processes that might be driving improvement or poor response (A. M. Hayes et al., 2007a, 2007c). A remaining challenge is to improve tools for examining changes in network connectivity dynamics when assumptions of stationarity are violated, particularly when studying destabilizing types of change.

With mobile and wireless devices, it is now possible to not only collect data in the context of one's daily life, but also to intervene in that context. Such monitoring can allow for the development and evaluation of ongoing, adaptive treatment strategies that depend on the person's response and context (Liao, Klasnja, Tewari, & Murphy, 2015). Markers of pattern stability and instability can highlight points of vulnerability and opportunity for just-in-time interventions (Nahum-Shani et al., 2017). For instance, interventions can be tailored to activate when a person's smartphone GPS detects proximity to a liquor store or another personal high-risk setting for obtaining or using the substance they had been abusing (Nahum-Shani et al., 2017).

This mobile health or "mHealth" approach takes therapy into the person's daily life, and statistical and methodological approaches are being developed to research this type of ongoing and dynamic intervention (Liao et al., 2015). Psychotherapy can advance further by adding multiple data streams that do not rely simply on frequent self-report, which can be quite burdensome. For example, Briffault, Morgiève, and Courtet (2018) describe how passively collected data can be added to an individual's health information by including monitoring of diet and fitness, activity levels, social media usage and footprint, and physical health (e.g., heart rate or glucose monitoring). Text analysis could also be added to analyze electronic communications or narrative data (Cummings, Hayes, Saint, & Park, 2014). In addition, Briffault et al. (2018) describe the possibility of using a "big data" system to gather large amounts of data across individuals that can be examined at the level of a community, city, or country. This database can reveal patterns and predictors of mental and physical health, thus making use of data from micro, macro, and meso scales to inform care.

A common framework of complex adaptive systems brings the possibility of convening teams of researchers across sciences to study a wide range of systems. The cross-disciplinary work on conflict resolution is an example of this. The recently developed Institute of Advanced Studies (IAS) in Amsterdam is an example of a team of complex systems researchers taking on mental health as one of the areas of research being conducted at micro, macro, and meso scales. This type of research not only helps the individual, but it can also have public health and policy implications.

This is an exciting time in the development of intervention science, and the theories and methods of complex system science connect our field with a range of other sciences and disciplines. The process-based approach to treatment described in this book can provide a road map forward as we move away from an overemphasis on clinical diagnoses, theoretical orientations, and single variable approaches to treatment and research.

References

Aldao, A., Nolen-Hoeksema, S., & Schweizer, S. (2010). Emotion-regulation strategies across psychopathology: A meta-analytic review. *Clinical Psychology Review, 30*(2), 217–237.

Baumeister, R. F. (1994). The crystallization of discontent in the process of major life change. In T. F. Heatherton & J. L. Weinberger (Eds.), *Can personality change?* (pp. 281–297). Washington, DC: American Psychological Association.

Beck, A. T., & Dozois, D. J. (2011). Cognitive therapy: Current status and future directions. *Annual Review of Medicine, 62*, 397–409.

Beck, A. T., Freeman, A., & Davis, D. D. (2004). *Cognitive therapy of personality disorders.* New York: Guilford Press.

Bellack, A. S., Mueser, K. T., Gingerich, S., & Agresta, J. (2013). *Social skills training for schizophrenia: A step-by-step guide.* New York: Guilford Press.

Beltz, A. M., & Gates, K. M. (2017). Network mapping with GIMME. *Multivariate Behavioral Research, 52*(6), 789–804.

Blanken, T. F., van Der Zweerde, T., van Straten, A., van Someren, E. J., Borsboom, D., & Lancee, J. (2019). Introducing network intervention analysis to investigate sequential, symptom-specific treatment effects: A demonstration in co-occurring insomnia and depression. *Psychotherapy and Psychosomatics, 88*(1), 52–54.

Borsboom, D., & Cramer, A. O. (2013). Network analysis: An integrative approach to the structure of psychopathology. *Annual Review of Clinical Psychology, 9*, 91–121.

Brewin, C. R. (2006). Understanding cognitive behaviour therapy: A retrieval competition account. *Behaviour Research and Therapy, 44*(6), 765–784.

Briffault, X., Morgiève, M., & Courtet, P. (2018). From e-health to i-health: Prospective reflections on the use of intelligent systems in mental health care. *Brain Sciences, 8*(6), 98.

Bringmann, L. F., Ferrer, E., Hamaker, E. L., Borsboom, D., & Tuerlinckx, F. (2018). Modeling nonstationary emotion dynamics in dyads using a time-varying vector-autoregressive model. *Multivariate Behavioral Research, 53*(3), 293–314.

Bringmann, L. F., Pe, M. L., Vissers, N., Ceulemans, E., Borsboom, D., Vanpaemel, W., ... Kuppens, P. (2016). Assessing temporal emotion dynamics using networks. *Assessment, 23*(4), 425–435.

Bringmann, L. F., Vissers, N., Wichers, M., Geschwind, N., Kuppens, P., Peeters, F., ... Tuerlinckx, F. (2013). A network approach to psychopathology: New insights into clinical longitudinal data. *PloS One, 8*(4), e60188.

Bruijniks, S. J., DeRubeis, R. J., Hollon, S. D., & Huibers, M. J. (2019). The potential role of learning capacity in cognitive behavior therapy for depression: A systematic review of the evidence and future directions for improving therapeutic learning. *Clinical Psychological Science, 7*(4), 668–692. doi: 10.1177/2167702619830391.

Cabrieto, J., Adolf, J., Tuerlinckx, F., Kuppens, P., & Ceulemans, E. (2018). Detecting long-lived autodependency changes in a multivariate system via change point detection and regime switching models. *Scientific Reports, 8*(1), 15637.

Carey, T. A. (2011). Exposure and reorganization: The what and how of effective psychotherapy. *Clinical Psychology Review, 31*(2), 236–248.

Castonguay, L. G., & Beutler, L. E. (2006). *Principles of therapeutic change that work.* New York: Oxford University Press.

Castonguay, L. G., & Hill, C. E. (2012). *Transformation in psychotherapy: Corrective experiences across cognitive behavioral, humanistic, and psychodynamic approaches.* Washington, DC: American Psychological Association.

Coleman, P. T. (2018). Conflict intelligence and systemic wisdom: Meta-competencies for engaging conflict in a complex, dynamic world. *Negotiation Journal, 34*(1), 7–35.

Coleman, P. T., Vallacher, R., Bartoli, A., Nowak, A., & Bui-Wrzosinska, L. (2011). Navigating the landscape of conflict: Applications of dynamical systems theory to addressing protracted conflict. In D. Körppen, N. Ropers, & H. J. Giessman (Eds.), *The non-linearity of peace processes: Theory and practice of systemic conflict transformation* (pp. 39–56). Leverkusen, Germany: Verlag Barbara Budrich.

Costantini, G., Richetin, J., Preti, E., Casini, E., Epskamp, S., & Perugini, M. (2019). Stability and variability of personality networks. A tutorial on recent developments in network psychometrics. *Personality and Individual Differences, 136,* 68–78.

Cramer, A. O., van Borkulo, C. D., Giltay, E. J., van der Maas, H. L., Kendler, K. S., Scheffer, M., & Borsboom, D. (2016). Major depression as a complex dynamic system. *PloS One, 11*(12), e0167490.

Craske, M. G., Meuret, A. E., Ritz, T., Treanor, M., & Dour, H. J. (2016). Treatment for anhedonia: A neuroscience driven approach. *Depression and Anxiety, 33*(10), 927–938.

Craske, M. G., Treanor, M., Conway, C. C., Zbozinek, T., & Vervliet, B. (2014). Maximizing exposure therapy: An inhibitory learning approach. *Behaviour Research and Therapy, 58,* 10–23.

Cuijpers, P. (2017). Psychotherapies vs. pharmacotherapies vs. combination therapies in depressive and anxiety disorders. *European Psychiatry, 41,* S6.

Cuijpers, P., Karyotaki, E., Weitz, E., Andersson, G., Hollon, S. D., & van Straten, A. (2014). The effects of psychotherapies for major depression in adults on remission, recovery and improvement: A meta-analysis. *Journal of Affective Disorders, 159,* 118–126.

Cummings, J. A., Hayes, A. M., Saint, D. S., & Park, J. (2014). Expressive writing in psychotherapy: A tool to promote and track therapeutic change. *Professional Psychology: Research and Practice, 44*(5), 1–9.

Cuthbert, B. N., & Insel, T. R. (2013). Toward the future of psychiatric diagnosis: The seven pillars of RDoC. *BMC Medicine, 11*(1), 126.

Dakos, V., van Nes, E. H., & Scheffer, M. (2013). Flickering as an early warning signal. *Theoretical Ecology, 6*(3), 309–317.

de Beurs, D. (2017). Network analysis: A novel approach to understand suicidal behaviour. *International Journal of Environmental Research and Public Health, 14*(3), 219.

Disner, S. G., Beevers, C. G., Haigh, E. A., & Beck, A. T. (2011). Neural mechanisms of the cognitive model of depression. *Nature Reviews Neuroscience, 12*(8), 467–477.

Dozier, M., Bernard, K., & Roben, C. K. (2017). Attachment and biobehavioral catch-up. In H. Steele & M. Steele (Eds.), *The handbook of attachment-based interventions* (pp. 27–49). New York: Guilford Press.

Ebner-Priemer, U. (2018). Monitoring the dynamics of real life psychopathology using ambulatory assessment. *European Neuropsychopharmacology, 28*, S86.

Epskamp, S., Borsboom, D., & Fried, E. I. (2018). Estimating psychological networks and their accuracy: A tutorial paper. *Behavior Research Methods, 50*(1), 195–212.

Epskamp, S., Rhemtulla, M., & Borsboom, D. (2017). Generalized network psychometrics: Combining network and latent variable models. *Psychometrika, 82*(4), 904–927.

Fernandez, K. C., Fisher, A. J., & Chi, C. (2017). Development and initial implementation of the Dynamic Assessment Treatment Algorithm (DATA). *PloS One, 12*(6), e0178806.

Fisher, A. J. (2015). Toward a dynamic model of psychological assessment: Implications for personalized care. *Journal of Consulting and Clinical Psychology, 83*(4), 825–836.

Fisher, A. J., Medaglia, J. D., & Jeronimus, B. F. (2018). Lack of group-to-individual generalizability is a threat to human subjects research. *Proceedings of the National Academy of Sciences, 115*(27), E6106–E6115.

Fisher, A. J., Reeves, J. W., Lawyer, G., Medaglia, J. D., & Rubel, J. A. (2017). Exploring the idiographic dynamics of mood and anxiety via network analysis. *Journal of Abnormal Psychology, 126*(8), 1044–1056.

Foa, E. B., Huppert, J. D., & Cahill, S. P. (2006). Emotional processing theory: An update. In B. O. Rothbaum (Ed.), *Pathological anxiety: Emotional processing in etiology and treatment* (pp. 3–24). New York: Guilford Press.

Fredrickson, B. L., & Joiner, T. (2018). Reflections on positive emotions and upward spirals. *Perspectives on Psychological Science, 13*(2), 194–199.

Fried, E. I., van Borkulo, C. D., Cramer, A. O. J., Boschloo, L., Schoevers, R. A., & Borsboom, D. (2017). Mental disorders as networks of problems: A review of recent insights. *Social Psychiatry and Psychiatric Epidemiology, 52*(1), 1–10.

Garland, E. L., Geschwind, N., Peeters, F., & Wichers, M. (2015). Mindfulness training promotes upward spirals of positive affect and cognition: Multilevel and autoregressive latent trajectory modeling analyses. *Frontiers in Psychology, 6*, 15.

Gelo, O. C. G., & Salvatore, S. (2016). A dynamic systems approach to psychotherapy: A meta-theoretical framework for explaining psychotherapy change processes. *Journal of Counseling Psychology, 63*(4), 379–395.

Goldfried, M. R. (1980). Toward the delineation of therapeutic change principles. *American Psychologist, 35*(11), 991–999.

Greenberg, L. S., & Watson, J. C. (2006). *Emotion-focused therapy for depression.* Washington, DC: American Psychological Association.

Greene, J. A., & Loscalzo, J. (2017). Putting the patient back together: Social medicine, network medicine, and limits of reductionism. *The New England Journal of Medicine, 377*(25), 2493–2499.

Haken, H., & Schiepek, G. (2006). *Synergetik in der Psychologie: Selbstorganisation verstehen und gestalten* (Vol. 780). Göttingen, Germany: Hogrefe.

Haken, H., & Tschacher, W. (2017). How to modify psychopathological states? Hypotheses based on complex systems theory. *Nonlinear Dynamics, Psychology, Life Sciences, 21*(1), 19–34.

Hayes, A. M. (2015). Facilitating emotional processing in depression: The application of exposure principles. *Current Opinion in Psychology, 4,* 61–66.

Hayes A. M., & Alpert, L. (2017). Biomedical bias: The importance of countervailing information and multivariate models of risk and treatment of mental illness. *Clinical Psychology: Science and Practice, 24*(1), 74–77.

Hayes, A. M., & Andrews, L. A. (in press). A complex systems approach to the study of change in psychotherapy. In E. Fried & D. Robinaugh (Eds.). Special series, Complexity in Mental Health Research: Theory, Method, and Empirical Contributions. *BMC Medicine.* Springer Nature.

Hayes, A. M., Feldman, G. C., Beevers, C. G., Laurenceau, J.-P., Cardaciotto, L., & Lewis-Smith, J. (2007a). Discontinuities and cognitive changes in an exposure-based cognitive therapy for depression. *Journal of Consulting and Clinical Psychology, 75*(3), 409–421.

Hayes, A. M., Laurenceau, J.-P., & Cardaciotto, L. (2007b). Methods for capturing the process of change. In A. M. Nezu & C. M. Nezu (Eds.), *Evidence-based outcome research: A practical guide to conducting randomized controlled trials for psychosocial interventions* (pp. 335–358). New York: Oxford University Press.

Hayes, A. M., Laurenceau, J.-P., Feldman, G., Strauss, J. L., & Cardaciotto, L. (2007c). Change is not always linear: The study of nonlinear and discontinuous patterns of change in psychotherapy. *Clinical Psychology Review, 27*(6), 715–723.

Hayes, A. M., Ready, C. B., & Yasinski, C. (2014). Exposure to emotion in depression: Exposure-based cognitive therapy. In N. Thoma & D. McKay (Eds.), *Working with emotion in cognitive behavioral therapy: Techniques for clinical practice* (pp. 121–145). New York: Guilford Press.

Hayes, A. M., & Strauss, J. L. (1998). Dynamic systems theory as a paradigm for the study of change in psychotherapy: An application to cognitive therapy for depression. *Journal of Consulting and Clinical Psychology, 66*(6), 939–947.

Hayes, A. M., & Yasinski, C. (2015). Pattern destabilization and emotional processing in cognitive therapy for personality disorders. *Frontiers in Psychology, 6,* 107.

Hayes, A. M., Yasinski, C., Barnes, J. B., & Bockting, C. L. (2015). Network destabilization and transition in depression: New methods for studying the dynamics of therapeutic change. *Clinical Psychology Review, 41,* 27–39.

Hayes, S. C., & Hofmann, S. G. (Eds.). (2018). *Process-based CBT: The science and core clinical competencies of cognitive behavioral therapy.* Oakland, CA: Context Press/New Harbinger Publications.

Hayes, S. C., Hofmann, S. G., Stanton, C. E., Carpenter, J. K., Sanford, B. T., Curtiss, J. E., & Ciarrochi, J. (2018). The role of the individual in the coming era of process-based therapy. *Behaviour Research and Therapy, 117,* 40–53. doi: 10.1016/j.brat.2018.10.005

Hayes, S. C., Monestès, J-L, & Wilson, D. S. (2017). Evolutionary principles for applied psychology. In S. C. Hayes & S. G. Hofmann (Eds.), *Process-based CBT: The science and core clinical competencies of cognitive behavioral therapy* (pp. 155–171). Oakland, CA: Context Press/New Harbinger Publications.

Hayes, S. C., Strosahl, K. D., & Wilson, K. G. (2011). *Acceptance and commitment therapy: The process and practice of mindful change.* New York: Guilford Press.

Heeren, A., & McNally, R. J. (2016). An integrative network approach to social anxiety disorder: The complex dynamic interplay among attentional bias for threat, attentional control, and symptoms. *Journal of Anxiety Disorders, 42,* 95–104.

Hofmann, S. G., Curtiss, J., & McNally, R. J. (2016). A complex network perspective on clinical science. *Perspectives on Psychological Science, 11*(5), 597–605.

Hofmann, S. G., & Hayes, S. C. (2019). The future of intervention science: Process-based therapy. *Clinical Psychological Science, 7*(1), 37–50. doi: 10.1177/2167702618772296

Hollenstein, T. (2013). *State space grids: Depicting dynamics across development.* New York: Springer Science+ Business Media.

Hollenstein, T., Lichtwarck-Aschoff, A., & Potworowski, G. (2013). A model of socioemotional flexibility at three time scales. *Emotion Review, 5*(4), 397–405.

Holmes, E. A., Ghaderi, A., Harmer, C. J., Ramchandani, P. G., Cuijpers, P., Morrison, A. P., ... Craske, M. G. (2018). The Lancet Psychiatry Commission on psychological treatments research in tomorrow's science. *The Lancet Psychiatry, 5*(3), 237–286. doi: 10.1016/S2215-0366(17)30513-8

Holtzheimer, P. E., & Mayberg, H. S. (2011). Stuck in a rut: Rethinking depression and its treatment. *Trends in Neurosciences, 34*(1), 1–9.

Hölzel, B. K., Lazar, S. W., Gard, T., Schuman-Olivier, Z., Vago, D. R., & Ott, U. (2011). How does mindfulness meditation work? Proposing mechanisms of action from a conceptual and neural perspective. *Perspectives on Psychological Science, 6*(6), 537–559.

Hoorelbeke, K., Marchetti, I., De Schryver, M., & Koster, E. H. (2016). The interplay between cognitive risk and resilience factors in remitted depression: A network analysis. *Journal of Affective Disorders, 195,* 96–104.

Insel, T. R. (2015). The NIMH experimental medicine initiative. *World Psychiatry, 14*(2), 151–153.

Joormann, J., & Tanovic, E. (2015). Cognitive vulnerability to depression: Examining cognitive control and emotion regulation. *Current Opinion in Psychology, 4,* 86–92.

Kazdin, A. E. (2009). Understanding how and why psychotherapy leads to change. *Psychotherapy Research, 19*(4–5), 418–428.

Keilholz, S., Woolrich, M. W., Chang, C., & Miller, R. (2018). Brain connectivity dynamics. Special issue, *Neuroimage, 180*(Pt B), 335–656.

Kelso, J. A. S. (1995). *Dynamic patterns: The self-organization of brain and behavior.* Cambridge, MA: MIT Press.

Kelso, J. A. S. (2012). Multistability and metastability: Understanding dynamic coordination in the brain. *Philosophical Transactions of the Royal Society, 367,* 906–918.

Kelso, J. A. S., Ding, M., & Schöner, G. (1993). Dynamic pattern formation: A primer. In L. B. Smith & E. Thelen (Eds.), *MIT Press/Bradford Books series in cognitive psychology. A dynamic systems approach to development: Applications* (pp. 13–50). Cambridge, MA: MIT Press.

Kelso, J. A. S., Dumas, G., & Tognoli, E. (2013). Outline of a general theory of behavior and brain coordination. *Neural Networks, 37,* 120–131.

Koster, E. H., De Lissnyder, E., Derakshan, N., & De Raedt, R. (2011). Understanding depressive rumination from a cognitive science perspective: The impaired disengagement hypothesis. *Clinical Psychology Review, 31*(1), 138–145.

Kozak, M. J., & Cuthbert, B. N. (2016). The NIMH research domain criteria initiative: Background, issues, and pragmatics. *Psychophysiology, 53*(3), 286–297.

Kuppens, P., & Verduyn, P. (2017). Emotion dynamics. *Current Opinion in Psychology, 17,* 22–26.

Lamey, A., Hollenstein, T., Lewis, M. D., & Granic, I. (2004). GridWare (Version 1.1) [Computer software]. Retrieved from http://statespacegrids.org.

Laska, K. M., Gurman, A. S., & Wampold, B. E. (2014). Expanding the lens of evidence-based practice in psychotherapy: A common factors perspective. *Psychotherapy, 51*(4), 467–481.

Lemmens, L. H., Galindo-Garre, F., Arntz, A., Peeters, F., Hollon, S., DeRubeis, R. J., & Huibers, M. J. (2017). Exploring mechanisms of change in cognitive therapy and interpersonal psychotherapy for adult depression. *Behaviour Research and Therapy, 94,* 81–92.

Liao, P., Klasnja, P., Tewari, A., & Murphy, S. A. (2015). Micro-randomized trials in mhealth. *ArXiv Preprint ArXiv:1504.00238.*

Lynch, T. R., Trost, W. T., Salsman, N., & Linehan, M. M. (2007). Dialectical behavior therapy for borderline personality disorder. *Annual Review of Clinical Psychology, 3,* 181–205.

Mahoney, M. J. (1991). *Human change processes.* New York: Springer.

Marlatt, G. A., & Witkiewitz, K. (2010). Update on harm-reduction policy and intervention research. *Annual Review of Clinical Psychology, 6,* 591–606.

McHugh, R. K., & Barlow, D. H. (2012). *Dissemination and implementation of evidence-based psychological interventions.* New York: Oxford University Press.

Miller, W. R., & C'de Baca, J. (2001). *Quantum change: When epiphanies and sudden insights transform ordinary lives.* New York: Guilford Press.

Miller, W. R., & Rollnick, S. (2012). *Motivational interviewing: Helping people change.* New York: Guilford Press.

Nahum-Shani, I., Smith, S. N., Spring, B. J., Collins, L. M., Witkiewitz, K., Tewari, A., & Murphy, S. A. (2017). Just-in-time adaptive interventions (JITAIs) in mobile health: Key components and design principles for ongoing health behavior support. *Annals of Behavioral Medicine, 52*(6), 446–462.

Nelson, B., McGorry, P. D., Wichers, M., Wigman, J. T., & Hartmann, J. A. (2017). Moving from static to dynamic models of the onset of mental disorder: A review. *JAMA Psychiatry, 74*(5), 528–534.

Norcross, J. C., & Wampold, B. E. (2018). A new therapy for each patient: Evidence-based relationships and responsiveness. *Journal of Clinical Psychology, 74*(11), 1889–1906.

Nowak, A., Bui-Wrzosinska, L., Coleman, P. T., Vallacher, R., Jochemczyk, L., & Bartkowski, W. (2010). Seeking sustainable solutions: Using an attractor simulation platform for teaching multi-stakeholder negotiation in complex cases. *Negotiation Journal, 26*(1), 49–68.

Nowak, A., Vallacher, R. R., Zochowski, M., & Rychwalska, A. (2017). Functional synchronization: The emergence of coordinated activity in human systems. *Frontiers in Psychology, 8*, 945.

Piccirillo, M. L., Beck, E. D., & Rodebaugh, T. L. (2019). A clinician's primer for idiographic research: Considerations and recommendations. *Behavior Therapy, 50*(5), 938–951. doi: 10.1016/j.beth.2019.02.002

Pizzagalli, D. A. (2014). Depression, stress, and anhedonia: Toward a synthesis and integrated model. *Annual Review of Clinical Psychology, 10*, 393–423.

R Core Team. (2013). *R: A language and environment for statistical computing*. Vienna, Austria: R Foundation for Statistical Computing. Retrieved from http://www.R-project.org/

Robinaugh, D. J., Hoekstra, R. H. A., Toner, E. R., & Borsboom, D. (2020). The network approach to psychopathology: a review of the literature 2008–2018 and an agenda for future research. *Psychological Medicine 50*(3) 1–14.

Rottenberg, J. (2017). Emotions in depression: What do we really know? *Annual Review of Clinical Psychology, 13*, 241–263.

Sanislow, C. A. (2016). Updating the research domain criteria. *World Psychiatry, 15*(3), 222–223.

Scheffer, M., Bolhuis, J. E., Borsboom, D., Buchman, T. G., Gijzel, S. M., Goulson, D., ... Levin, S. (2018). Quantifying resilience of humans and other animals. *Proceedings of the National Academy of Sciences, 115*(47), 11883–11890.

Scheffer, M., Carpenter, S. R., Dakos, V., & van Nes, E. H. (2015). Generic indicators of ecological resilience: Inferring the chance of a critical transition. *Annual Review of Ecology, Evolution, and Systematics, 46*, 145–167.

Scheffer, M., Carpenter, S. R., Lenton, T. M., Bascompte, J., Brock, W., Dakos, V., ... van Nes, E. H. (2012). Anticipating critical transitions. *Science, 338*(6105), 344–348.

Scheffer, M., & Westley, F. (2007). The evolutionary basis of rigidity: Locks in cells, minds, and society. *Ecology and Society, 12*(2), 36.

Schiepek, G., Aichhorn, W., Gruber, M., Strunk, G., Bachler, E., & Aas, B. (2016). Real-time monitoring of psychotherapeutic processes: Concept and compliance. *Frontiers in Psychology, 7*, 604.

Schiepek, G., Aichhorn, W., & Schöller, H. (2017). Monitoring change dynamics: A nonlinear approach to psychotherapy feedback. *Chaos and Complexity Letters, 11*(3), 355–375.

Schiepek, G., Eckert, H., Aas, B., Wallot, S., & Wallot, A. (2015). *Integrative psychotherapy: A feedback-driven dynamic systems approach*. Gottingen, Germany: Hogrefe.

Schiepek, G., Fartacek, C., Sturm, J., Kralovec, K., Fartacek, R., & Plöderl, M. (2011). Nonlinear dynamics: Theoretical perspectives and application to suicidology. *Suicide and Life-Threatening Behavior, 41*(6), 661–675.

Schiepek, G., Schöller, H., Carl, R., Aichhorn, W., & Lichtwarck-Aschoff, A. (2019). A nonlinear dynamic systems approach to psychological interventions. In E. S. Kunnen, N. M. P. de Ruiter, B. F. Jeronimus, & M. A. E. van der Gaag (Eds.), *Psychosocial development in adolescence: Insights from the dynamic systems approach* (pp. 51–68). New York: Routledge.

Schiepek, G., & Strunk, G. (2010). The identification of critical fluctuations and phase transitions in short term and coarse-grained time series—A method for the real-time monitoring of human change processes. *Biological Cybernetics, 102*(3), 197–207.

Segal, Z. V., & Teasdale, J. (2018). *Mindfulness-based cognitive therapy for depression*. New York: Guilford Press.

Slofstra, C., Klein, N. S., Nauta, M. H., Wichers, M., Batalas, N., & Bockting, C. L. H. (2017). Imagine your mood: Study design and protocol of a randomized controlled micro-trial using app-based experience sampling methodology to explore processes of change during relapse prevention interventions for recurrent depression. *Contemporary Clinical Trials Communications, 7*, 172–178.

Snippe, E., Viechtbauer, W., Geschwind, N., Klippel, A., de Jonge, P., & Wichers, M. (2017). The impact of treatments for depression on the dynamic network structure of mental states: Two randomized controlled trials. *Scientific Reports, 7*, 46523.

Teasdale, J. D. (1999). Emotional processing, three modes of mind and the prevention of relapse in depression. *Behaviour Research and Therapy, 37*(Suppl 1), S53–S77.

Thaler, R. H. (2018). Nudge, not sludge. *Science, 361*(6401), 431. doi: 10.1126/science.aau9241

Thaler, R. H., & Sunstein, C. R. (2009). *Nudge: Improving decisions about health, wealth, and happiness*. New York: Penguin.

Thelen, E., & Smith, L. B. (1996). *A dynamic systems approach to the development of cognition and action*. Cambridge, MA: MIT Press.

Tschacher, W., & Haken, H. (2019). *The Process of Psychotherapy: Causation and Chance*. New York: Springer.

Vallacher, R. R., van Geert, P., & Nowak, A. (2015). The intrinsic dynamics of psychological process. *Current Directions in Psychological Science, 24*(1), 58–64.

van de Leemput, I. A., Wichers, M., Cramer, A. O., Borsboom, D., Tuerlinckx, F., Kuppens, P., ... Aggen, S. H. (2014). Critical slowing down as early warning for the onset and termination of depression. *Proceedings of the National Academy of Sciences, 111*(1), 87–92.

van Dijk, R., Deković, M., Bunte, T. L., Schoemaker, K., Zondervan-Zwijnenburg, M., Espy, K. A., & Matthys, W. (2017). Mother-child interactions and externalizing behavior problems in preschoolers over time: Inhibitory control as a mediator. *Journal of Abnormal Child Psychology, 45*(8), 1503–1517.

Wang, R., Dearing, J. A., Langdon, P. G., Zhang, E., Yang, X., Dakos, V., & Scheffer, M. (2012). Flickering gives early warning signals of a critical transition to a eutrophic lake state. *Nature, 492*(7429), 419–422.

Watkins, E. R., & Nolen-Hoeksema, S. (2014). A habit-goal framework of depressive rumination. *Journal of Abnormal Psychology, 123*(1), 24–34.

Wichers, M. (2014). The dynamic nature of depression: A new micro-level perspective of mental disorder that meets current challenges. *Psychological Medicine, 44*(7), 1349–1360.

Wichers, M., Peeters, F., Geschwind, N., Jacobs, N., Simons, C. J. P., Derom, C., ... van Os, J. (2010). Unveiling patterns of affective responses in daily life may improve outcome prediction in depression: A momentary assessment study. *Journal of Affective Disorders, 124*(1), 191–195.

Wichers, M., Schreuder, M. J., Goekoop, R., & Groen, R. N. (2019). Can we predict the direction of sudden shifts in symptoms? Transdiagnostic implications from a complex systems perspective on psychopathology. *Psychological Medicine, 49*(3), 380–387.

Witkiewitz, K., & Marlatt, G. A. (2007). Modeling the complexity of post-treatment drinking: It's a rocky road to relapse. *Clinical Psychology Review, 27*(6), 724–738.

Young, J. E., Klosko, J. S., & Weishaar, M. E. (2003). *Schema therapy: A practitioner's guide*. New York: Guilford Press.

Zilcha-Mano, S. (2018). Major developments in methods addressing for whom psychotherapy may work and why. *Psychotherapy Research*, 1–16.

CHAPTER 9

Psychological Flexibility in Chronic Pain
Exploring the Relevance of a Process-Based Model for Treatment Development

Lance M. McCracken, PhD
Uppsala University

It is now well-known that cognitive behavioral therapy (CBT) can help people, particularly when their problems center around depression and anxiety (Butler, Chapman, Forman, & Beck, 2006; Tolin, 2010), but it can also be effective in the context of physical health conditions such as chronic pain (Williams, Eccleston, & Morley, 2012) and others. Those benefits have been demonstrated with conventional cognitive therapy methods, as well as specific approaches within CBT (such as behavioral activation; Cuijpers, van Straten, & Warmerdam, 2007) and related treatments (such as mindfulness-based treatments; Khoury et al., 2013). There is also a convincing case that the effects of CBT can be long-lasting (Hollon, Stewart, & Strunk, 2006). Nonetheless, work on developing CBT is not yet complete. Clinicians, treatment recipients, and systems of care want better, more efficient, and more accessible treatments that produce meaningful, longer-lasting effects that are reflected broadly across multiple outcome domains. In other words, the stakeholders want progress.

There are many treatment approaches to ameliorating the problems that can occur in human health and well-being. Most of these treatments are defined by specific methods that characterize each approach, in addition to broad traditions and philosophies. Some of these approaches, such as CBT, are known empirically to be helpful, but generally what this means is only that there is a positive relationship between the delivery of methods and the outcomes measured after these methods are delivered. Implicitly, the guiding research question for producing better treatments in this approach is how to identify which method is best. This is a natural question to ask, but at the same time, this is a rather blunt tool for creating progress. It suggests we need to keep comparing methods or clusters of methods to find the clearly superior one and, once we do, to invent a new one to take the next step forward. However, it can be difficult to detect small, incremental improvements between alternative treatments, and this approach does not guide us in inventing new treatments—it only tells us how to evaluate them when they appear.

The present volume, and the turn toward process-based CBT more generally (Hayes & Hofmann, 2018b), underlines how much the field is now focusing its attention on processes of change as a way to further progress. In order to create progress more quickly, there is broad agreement in CBT that we need to show *how* results are obtained (e.g., Lemmens, Muller, Arntz, & Hibers, 2016; Lemmens et al., 2017; Longmore & Worrell, 2007), for whom, and under what circumstances. These functional questions are important because they provide the basis for achieving better outcomes in the future.

Process-Based Treatment Development

Using a process-based approach as a guide to treatment development itself requires guidance. Process-based treatment development needs to meet certain success criteria that demonstrate potential utility so progress can be shown as development proceeds. A good process-based model for treatment development should include a clear and progressive theoretical model that is based on explicit philosophical assumptions and known basic psychological principles (Hayes, Levin, Plumb-Vilardaga, Villatte, & Pistorello, 2013a; Hayes, Long, Levin, & Follette, 2013b; Kazdin, 2007). Without this foundation, the development work may not join up very well, and separate streams within the research and development tradition may drift toward contradictory assumptions or goals. With a model and assumptions in hand, an empirically based approach of testing and refining the model can begin. Any useful model at this stage will contain specific component processes or facets. From a practical or applied point of view, these need to:

- be specific, validly measurable, and relate with each other in ways that are coherent with the underlying model.

- relate with outcomes of interest as a basis from which to predict and influence these outcomes.
- relate with, or sensitively reflect, changes in outcomes produced from treatment methods in order to ensure these methods are practically modifiable and coherent with the underlying theory.
- statistically mediate the effects of treatment on outcomes and eventually meet criteria as causally necessary and sufficient mechanisms of change.
- compare favorably to alternate potentially mediating processes and relate to treatment outcomes even when taking into account potentially competing models of change.
- inform the identification of moderators of treatment effects or themselves serve as moderators of treatment effects.

A model with component parts that can demonstrate these features builds a case for demonstrated utility as a process-based tool for improving treatment.

Using evidence mostly from studies of chronic pain, the current chapter will examine each of these features in relation to a particular process-based model, the psychological flexibility (PF) model. This model is a suitable process-based model to examine because it is theoretically based on a coherent set of basic psychological principles and a set of clear philosophical assumptions (Hayes, Villatte, Levin, & Hildebrandt, 2011; Hayes et al., 2013a; Vilardaga, Hayes, Levin, & Muto, 2009). Chronic pain is an appropriate condition to consider because it represents an important health problem that shares features with many other health problems—particularly chronic, disabling physical conditions—and it represents one of the earliest comprehensive applications of the PF model. Its status as a relatively early implementation of this model indicates that it provides an adequate time frame by which to provide a fair yet rigorous test of progress.

The Psychological Flexibility Model

The PF model is a model of human well-being and performance based within a contextual behavioral science approach (Hayes, Barnes-Homes, & Wilson,

2012; Hayes, Luoma, Bond, Masuda, & Lillis, 2006; Zettle, Hayes, Barnes-Holmes, & Biglan, 2016). This approach has a specific unit of analysis (the "act in context"), has specific truth criteria ("pragmatism," which is demonstrated through achievement of goals), is consistent with evolutionary science, and applies an evolutionary framework to the activity of scientists themselves (Hayes et al., 2012). It is a model in which behavior and behavior change are outcomes, not symptoms or syndromes. It emphasizes the role of the function and context of psychological events more so than their form or frequency. It includes six facets: acceptance, cognitive defusion, present-focused attention, self-as-context, values, and committed action (Hayes et al., 2006). These are also sometimes summarized as entailing behavior that is open, aware, and active (Hayes et al., 2011).

Can We Assess Facets of Psychological Flexibility?

The first question to ask in the evaluation of the PF model as a treatment development tool is to see whether facets of PF, as the model specifies them, can be assessed in a valid fashion. Evidence suggests that they can be. For example, the first published measure of acceptance in chronic pain appeared twenty years ago (McCracken, 1998). Since then, acceptance of pain has become one of the most frequently assessed variables in clinical research with chronic pain populations. The current key reference to a common measure of acceptance of chronic pain—the Chronic Pain Acceptance Questionnaire (McCracken, Vowles, & Eccleston, 2004)—has been cited more than one thousand times, and results show that the measure is well-validated.

Measures of other aspects of the PF model have gradually appeared, and in each case, they have successfully added information to the understanding of chronic pain. There are published data from measures of cognitive (de)fusion in people with chronic pain that constitute evidence for validity of the measures used, including the Cognitive Fusion Questionnaire (Gillanders et al., 2014; McCracken, Gutiérrez-Martínez, & Smyth 2013a; McCracken et al., 2014) and the Experiences Question (Fresco et al., 2007), which is a measure of decentering (McCracken, Barker, & Chilcot 2014a), a process consistent with cognitive defusion.

Likewise, there are validated methods for measuring present-moment awareness that have been used in studies of people with chronic pain, such as the Mindful Attention Awareness Scale (Brown & Ryan, 2003), which appears specific and psychometrically adequate for this purpose (e.g., McCracken, Gauntlett-Gilbert, & Vowles, 2007a; McCracken & Thompson, 2009). There is also a recently validated measure of self-as-context developed in a sample of people with chronic pain, the Self Experiences Questionnaire (Yu, McCracken, & Norton, 2016), which helps explain clinical outcomes. Validated measures of values include the Chronic Pain Values Inventory (McCracken & Yang, 2006) and the Engaged Living Scale (Trompetter et al., 2013). Finally, there is at least one validated measure of committed action, once again developed in a sample of people with chronic pain, called the Committed Action Questionnaire (Bailey, Vowles, Witkiewitz, Sowden, & Ashworth, 2016; McCracken, 2013; McCracken, Chilcot, & Norton, 2015a).

Other measures that have either been demonstrated as validated, or that were developed and validated in chronic pain samples, include the Acceptance and Action Questionnaire (Bond et al. 2011; see McCracken & Zhao-O'Brien, 2010) and the Psychological Inflexibility in Pain Scale (Wicksell, Renofalt, Olsson, Bond, & Melin, 2008b). Both measures are intended to more generally reflect PF or psychological inflexibility.

Every current measure that assesses these facets of PF has been validated through analyses that test for expected significant correlations with other facets. These analyses have generally included acceptance and often have included multiple facets as well. There is a question about whether self-report data are able to reflect the six-part PF model. Analyses of such data show that the six processes are interrelated, as specified in the model, but they cannot be detected as six statistically separate factors. For example, in one study on chronic pain, three factors emerged from a set of measures intended to comprehensively reflect PF (Vowles, Sowden, & Ashworth, 2014b). The factors identified included Defusion and Acceptance, Values and Committed Action, and Awareness (Vowles et al., 2014b). In a similar study, a higher-order "bifactor" model emerged in confirmatory factor analysis from four different measures of facets of PF (Scott, Hann, & McCracken, 2016a). The bifactor model consisted of a general Acceptance or Openness factor, as well as related and partially distinct Decentering and Committed Action factors. Interestingly, in both of these studies, the data seem to cohere more closely around the three-part "open, aware, and active" conceptualization of PF (Hayes et al., 2011) than around the six-part version.

Can Psychological Flexibility Help Us Predict and Influence Behavior?

Given that it is possible to assess the facets of PF, the next question is how good a job these measures do in explaining outcomes and suggesting treatment options. There has not yet been a comprehensive review of evidence for associations between the facets of PF and key clinical outcome variables in chronic pain. Such a review would be very desirable and informative. However, one published review—which includes twenty-three studies of acceptance measures for chronic pain—shows that acceptance is often moderately to highly associated with measures of anxiety, depression, physical and psychosocial disability, work status, medication use, and health care visits for pain (Reneman, Dijkstra, Geertzen, & Dijkstra, 2010).

Similarly, data from studies on cognitive defusion show moderate to high correlations with measures of depression, psychosocial disability, mental health, social functioning, and general health (McCracken, Gutiérrez-Martínez, & Smyth, 2013a; McCracken, Barker, & Chilcot 2014a; McCracken, DaSilva, Skillicorn, & Doherty, 2014b). These studies do not show correlations between cognitive defusion and physical functioning or disability, but they both show that cognitive defusion is able to account for significant variance in clinical outcomes independent of the contribution of pain and acceptance, particularly for depression, psychosocial disability, and mental health.

Both present-focused attention and self-as-context have also demonstrated significant associations with key outcomes of interest. Present-focused attention, as measured via mindfulness, has demonstrated moderate to high correlations with depression, anxiety, psychosocial disability, physical disability, medication use, and alertness (McCracken et al., 2007a; McCracken & Velleman, 2010). Once again, for depression, anxiety, psychosocial disability, and physical disability, the contribution to the variance in outcomes remained after controlling for the contribution of pain and acceptance. So far, measures of self-as-context have shown small to moderate correlations with depression, work and social adjustment, and pain interference in large samples of people with heterogeneous chronic pain conditions and fibromyalgia (Yu et al., 2016; Yu, Norton, Almarzooqi, & McCracken, 2017a).

Values-based action has also demonstrated moderate correlations with measures of depression, anxiety, psychosocial disability, and physical disability in a sample of people with chronic pain, with the contribution of values-based action remaining for depression and psychosocial disability after controlling for acceptance (McCracken & Yang, 2006). Finally, committed action has been shown to correlate, again moderately to highly, with depression, social functioning, mental health, and general health, and weakly with physical functioning (Åkerblom, Perrin, Rivano Fischer, & McCracken, 2016; McCracken, 2013). As demonstrated for the other facets, the role of committed action remained significant in multivariate analyses independent of the contribution of pain and acceptance as well as fear of movement.

In addition to these relatively straightforward studies regarding the relationship between facets of PF and outcome measures, there are also analyses of slightly more complex models of the facets, particularly acceptance, as interacting or contextual factors. For example, in an early study of this type, we tested a model examining the impact of fear of anxiety on chronic pain (McCracken & Keogh, 2009). We showed that fear of anxiety is generally moderately associated with pain-related anxiety, depression, and disability, but when acceptance, present-focused attention, and values-based action are taken into account in a multivariate model, these associations are reduced to non-significance. In another large study employing structural equation modeling, Fish, McGuire, Hogan, Morrison, and Stewart (2010) showed that pain-related acceptance partially mediated the relationship between pain severity and pain-related interference on emotional distress. A more recent study using similar statistical methods (Lykkegaard, Vang, Vaegter, & Andersen, 2017) found that pain acceptance mediated components of the well-known fear-avoidance model of chronic pain, helping to clarify the relations between pain and catastrophizing as well as between catastrophizing and fear-avoidance beliefs.

The results of these more complex, interactive models suggest that the effects of pain or distressing thoughts on functioning may depend on facets of PF. These results suggest that context matters: psychological events are settings that determine the influence of other psychological events. However, it is worth noting that most of the studies presented here are cross-sectional in nature and thus cannot address issues of cause and effect. They provide a basis for prediction but not necessarily influence. There are a couple of prospective studies in this area that have focused on acceptance, and both support a relationship between that aspect of PF and better functioning over time (McCracken & Eccleston, 2005; McCracken, Vowles, & Gauntlett-Gilbert, 2007b).

Are Measures of Psychological Flexibility Sensitive to Changes During Treatment?

If a set of treatment processes cannot demonstrate change in a treatment context, particularly one that is designed to produce change, then they cannot be regarded as a part of a useful process-based model. However, a failure to show change does not necessarily indicate model failure—it could indicate a failure of treatment technology or a failure of assessment instrumentation. At the same time, the measures must eventually show change based on the methods that target them or the model cannot be tested and thus is not known to be useful.

Each individual facet of PF has been found to change following methods intended to target them. Acceptance is the most studied (Daly-Eichenhardt, Scott, Howard-Jones, Nicolaou, & McCracken, 2016; McCracken, Sato, & Taylor, 2013b; McCracken, Vowles, & Eccleston, 2005; McCracken et al., 2015b; Vowles & McCracken, 2008; Vowles, McCracken, & Eccleston, 2007; Vowles, Witkiewitz, Sowden, & Ashworth, 2014c; Yu, Norton, & McCracken, 2017b), and it generally yields large, uncontrolled effect sizes and medium to large between-condition effect sizes in randomized clinical trials (RCTs) (Alonso-Fernandez, Lopez-Lopez, Lodata, Gonzalez, & Whetherell, 2016; Buhrman et al., 2013; Lin, Klatt, McCracken, & Baumeister, 2018; Luciano et al., 2014; McCracken et al., 2013b).

When it comes to the other facets of PF, studies have shown that both cognitive defusion (Daly-Eichenhardt et al., 2016; McCracken et al., 2015b; Scott, Daly, & McCracken, 2017a; Scott, McCracken, & Norton, 2016b) and present-focused attention (McCracken & Gutiérrez-Martinez, 2011) increase in treatment, with small to medium effect sizes observed. Self-as-context has been found to change in treatment as well, with small, uncontrolled effect sizes observed, but this finding is based on a single study (Yu et al., 2017b).

Finally, both values-based action (McCracken & Gutiérrez-Martinez, 2011; Vowles & McCracken, 2008; Vowles et al., 2014c) and committed action (Daly-Eichenhardt et al., 2016; McCracken et al., 2015b; Scott et al., 2016b, 2017a) show changes as well, with the former demonstrating large, uncontrolled effect sizes and the latter demonstrating consistently small ones. Taken as a whole, significant improvements in PF have been shown in RCTs, with effect sizes ranging from small/medium (Trompetter, Bohlmeijer, Veehof, & Schreurs, 2015b) to large (Wicksell, Ahlqvist, Bring, Melin, & Olsson, 2008a, 2013).

We also know that facets of PF can change in treatments that are associated with positive treatment effects, even if they were not designed specifically to produce effects on them. At least two studies have examined the effect of traditional CBT—a treatment not normally regarded as targeting PF—on acceptance, and both studies showed that acceptance exhibited significant changes, with mostly medium, uncontrolled effect sizes observed immediately following treatment and at later follow-up (Åkerblom, Perrin, Rivano Fisher, & McCracken, 2015; Baranoff, Hanrahan, Kapur, & Connor, 2012). In principle, this can be regarded as a demonstration of the generality and utility of the PF model as a guide for process-based treatment of chronic pain, especially if it can be understood how traditional CBT methods produce these process changes. However, if that cannot be determined, then it could suggest a weakness in the PF model because process-based models need to suggest treatment kernels based on theory. This will undoubtedly be a focus of research in the future.

Do Changes in Psychological Flexibility Relate to Observed Outcomes?

Most studies on changes in PF in relation to changes in outcomes employ correlational designs where a treatment is introduced without a control group and the facets of PF and outcomes are measured concurrently (e.g., McCracken et al., 2005; McCracken & Gutiérrez-Martínez, 2011; Scott et al., 2016b, 2017a; Vowles et al., 2014c; Yu et al., 2017b). These studies generally show significant but small correlations between acceptance, cognitive defusion, present-focused attention, values-based action, and committed action with outcomes including depression, anxiety, physical disability, and social functioning. However, one study that assessed results three years post-treatment found that those receiving treatment focused on PF exhibited large associations between changes in acceptance and values-based action and improvements in depression, anxiety, and psychosocial disability, as well as moderately sized associations with changes in physical disability (Vowles, McCracken, & Zhao-O'Brien, 2011).

Results from correlational analyses generally show that changes in facets of PF remain associated with changes in outcome variables even after changes in pain or level of post-treatment pain are taken into account. They also show that changes in facets of PF and outcomes appear to correlate both during the active treatment interval and during the interval from pre-treatment to follow-up (Scott et al., 2016a; Vowles & McCracken, 2008). It has also been shown that pre- to post-treatment changes in PF facets, particularly acceptance, correlate with changes in outcomes during the longer time frame from pre-treatment to follow-up at three months post-treatment, even when analyses control for pain as a predictor of outcome (McCracken & Gutiérrez-Martínez, 2011; Vowles et al., 2014c).

At least one study has approached this question of correlations between changes in PF and outcome using different, more innovative methods (Vowles, Fink, & Cohen, 2014a). This study used weekly diary ratings of PF during chronic pain treatment and looked at these ratings in relation to reliable changes in disability at a three-month follow-up. They showed that eighty-one percent of patients showed a pattern of increasing acceptance and values-based action significantly linked to reliable changes (i.e., a reduction) in disability.

The few studies of acceptance change in treatments not designed around PF have examined its relation to outcomes. For example, in a study by Baranoff and colleagues (2012), changes in acceptance showed moderate associations with changes in depression and disability post-treatment, a small association with changes in depression at follow-up, and moderate associations with changes in disability, walking speed, and sit-to-stand performance at this same time point (Baranoff et al., 2012). This change in acceptance remained a significant predictor of change in depression, anxiety, and disability even when controlling for change in pain and catastrophizing. A similar study by Åkerblom and colleagues (2015) found that changes in acceptance were correlated with changes in depression, pain interference, and pain intensity. These studies suggest that acceptance may be a broadly useful process to target in pain, perhaps providing a more proximal target for clinical interventions.

Does Psychological Flexibility Mediate Outcomes?

At least five studies have formally tested facets of PF as statistical mediators of treatment outcomes for chronic pain, and each of these studies has reported positive results, with some caveats. The first of these was a small trial ($N = 21$) of a treatment for people with chronic pain following whiplash injuries (Wicksell, Olsson, & Hayes, 2010). This study showed significant indirect effects of psychological inflexibility on life satisfaction and disability based on the currently recommended bias-corrected, non-parametric bootstrapping approach to calculating direct and indirect effects (MacKinnon, Lockwood, Hoffman, West, & Sheets, 2002; Preacher & Hayes, 2008). These researchers also addressed the issue of directionality by testing the reverse relationship—that is, that increased life satisfaction mediated the effect of psychological inflexibility on chronic pain—and found no indirect effect in that direction.

In a larger study with this same type of aim, PF was again tested as a mediator in a three-arm RCT where the primary treatment involved internet-based acceptance and commitment therapy (ACT) for chronic pain (Trompetter, Bohlmeijer, Fox, & Schreurs, 2015a). Here a non-parametric cross products of the coefficients and cross-lagged panel design was used, including outcomes for pain, pain interference, and psychological distress. They found that baseline to post-treatment changes in PF uniquely mediated changes from baseline to follow-up in each outcome. In further analyses to address the potential for causality, they showed that changes in PF significantly predicted subsequent changes in pain interference (Trompetter et al., 2015a).

Another similar three-arm trial compared guided versus unguided online treatment designed to increase PF versus a wait-list control condition (Lin et al., 2018). Using structural equation modeling, they found that changes in PF at post-treatment mediated changes at follow-up in each of the outcomes (pain interference, anxiety, depression, pain, and mental and physical health) in the active arms versus wait-list control group. A fourth trial compared ACT versus applied relaxation in the treatment of chronic pain and found that individuals in the ACT condition exhibited increased acceptance of pain, and this increased acceptance mediated the effects of treatment on physical functioning, but not life satisfaction, from baseline to follow-up six months later (Cederberg, Cernvall, Dahl, von Essen, & Ljungman, 2016).

Finally, a fifth trial compared three different conditions in the management of chronic pain: a group-based ACT treatment, pharmacological treatment, and a wait-list control (Luciano et al., 2014). Of the five different treatment outcomes they measured (fibromyalgia impact, catastrophizing, anxiety, pain, and quality of life), only one outcome—quality of life—was mediated by changes in pain acceptance in the group-based ACT condition.

These five studies represent the only RCTs that have included mediation analyses for such primary and secondary outcome measures. One could argue that the process-focused PF model has encouraged this increasing inclusion of mediation analyses, as such analyses were relatively rare in CBT trials for pain in the past (Morley & Keefe, 2007).

It should be noted that in outcome studies, the field has become used to meta-analyses rather than simple box score methods of integrating a body of work. This lack of an agreed-upon metric of mediation effect size has inhibited meta-analytic approaches to mediation, but the body of work on the meditational role of PF in chronic pain is growing rapidly, and finding ways to apply meta-analytic methods to this question appears to be a logical next step.

How Do Psychological Flexibility Measures Compare with Measures of Alternative Processes?

In the earliest studies regarding the facets of PF, questions were asked about the apparent relative utility of these facets relative to other commonly applied variables. These early studies, most of which were cross-sectional and correlational, showed that facets of PF, particularly acceptance, performed as well or better than common coping variables such as attention diversion, stress management, and cognitive restructuring (e.g., McCracken & Eccleston, 2006; McCracken et al., 2007b; Vowles & McCracken, 2010). Subsequent prospective analyses found that changes in both acceptance and catastrophizing were correlated with changes in outcomes even after controlling for changes in pain (Vowles et al., 2007). This is notable because catastrophizing is a kind of "gold standard" predictor of functioning in chronic pain, and it is perhaps the most studied and discussed variable in research on chronic pain.

When mediation analyses are conducted in studies that do not include RCT designs, this is often regarded as providing a preliminary or partial test of mediation. In one such study mentioned earlier, the PF facet of acceptance did appear to mediate the within-group effects of treatment on depression and pain interference, and it showed stronger effects compared to changes in other variables, including affective distress, perceived life control, and social support (Åkerblom et al., 2015).

With regard to formal RCTs that have tested the mediating effects of PF versus other potential mediators, one trial found that PF was the only significant mediator in comparison to pain, anxiety, depression, kinesiophobia, and self-efficacy, none of which showed significant indirect effects on the outcomes of interest (Wicksell et al., 2010). Similarly, another study found that PF showed larger indirect effects on pain interference and distress compared to catastrophizing, and only changes in PF demonstrated a relationship with subsequent changes in pain-related interference with functioning (Trompetter et al., 2015a). Finally, a third trial found an indirect effect of PF on physical functioning, and no significant indirect effects were found for alternative mediators in the form of anxiety and depression (Cederberg et al., 2016). Thus, overall, it appears that PF does as well or better than available conceptual alternatives, which is the hoped-for outcome from a relatively adequate process-based account.

Does Psychological Flexibility Moderate or Help Predict Outcomes?

When studies of chronic pain treatment attempt to find for whom treatments work best, or under what circumstances, the evidence is not clear (Day, Ehde, & Jensen, 2015). Generally, when particular treatments for chronic pain are examined, significant potential predictors or moderators of outcomes are absent among the numerous variables analyzed, leading to the tentative conclusion that the treatments are equally effective for all (Turner, Holtzman, & Mancl, 2007; Vowles et al., 2011).

In a recent systematic review of pre-treatment participant characteristics associated with treatment response—specifically with regard to trials examining contextual forms of CBT (typically ACT and mindfulness-based treatments) for chronic pain—twenty studies were identified as providing a basis for examining predictors or moderators of outcome (Gilpin, Keyes, Stahl, Greig, & McCracken, 2017). This review generally found that baseline demographic data, such as gender, age, education, pain duration, and even pain severity, were either inconsistently associated with outcomes or not associated at all. The only baseline variables that relatively and consistently correlated with outcomes were measures of psychological distress. The difficulty here is that in some treatments, high distress predicted better outcomes, while in other treatments, it was low distress that did so. Interestingly, although almost half of the studies in this review included treatments designed specifically around PF, none of the studies examined facets of PF as predictors or moderators of treatment responses (Gilpin et al., 2017).

There are also some recent studies of predictors or moderators of outcomes in treatments designed to enhance PF. These recent examples, like those conducted before, have also not examined facets of PF. Instead, they looked at psychological well-being (Trompetter et al., 2016) or neuropsychological functioning (Herbert et al., 2018) as moderators. These studies have produced positive results, finding that psychological well-being at baseline moderates pain interference six months later (Trompetter et al., 2016) and that some aspects of lower neuropsychological functioning are associated with greater improvements in depression and anxiety but not pain-related interference (Herbert et al., 2018). When interpreting these results, it is important to point out that these are moderators or predictors of the specific treatment designs being delivered, not moderators or predictors of the whole class of related treatments or of the model of treatment overall.

A recent study from our treatment center (Gilpin, Stahl, & McCracken, 2019) was large enough ($N = 609$) to allow us to explicitly examine facets of PF including acceptance, cognitive fusion, and committed action, in relation to clinical outcomes. Our analyses were both theoretically based and allowed us to detect interactive or nonlinear relations between predictors and outcomes (cf. Hofmann, Curtiss, & Hayes, 2020). When we adjusted for patient background variables and other general measures of psychological distress, we found that lower cognitive defusion at baseline was associated with greater improvements in physical functioning and pain, and greater acceptance at baseline was associated with larger improvements in emotional functioning. This appears to be the only available study of PF facets as moderators of treatment outcomes for chronic pain, and while these findings appear promising, they are limited because they were not conducted within an RCT design.

Can Psychological Flexibility Serve as a Tool for Continuous Treatment Development?

When examining PF as a process-based model, the key question is whether it can lead to conceptual and practical progress. This question can only be answered as a judgment of relative success over time (McCracken &

Morley, 2014), and success can only be examined relative to the goals that have been set. An argument can be made that it has been successful on the basis of the evidence accrued so far.

Studies of PF in relation to chronic pain represent one example of how treatment development can be shaped by adopting a particular process-focused approach. Using the PF model, the following has been shown thus far:

- There is evidence that we can validly assess each facet of PF and that these facets interrelate with each other as theory would suggest.

- There is evidence that all facets of PF are associated with outcomes of interest in chronic pain and thus provide a basis for predicting these outcomes.

- All facets PF are sensitive to change during treatment, although the evidence is very limited for some facets, and it is not possible to show simultaneous contributions from every facet.

- There is evidence that some, but not all, facets of PF statistically mediate outcomes in chronic pain treatment.

- Facets of PF perform somewhat better in analyses examining mediators of change compared to many well-known concepts such as coping, pain, fear, and general emotional distress.

- PF is about equally successful as other measures, such as catastrophizing, in predicting or tracking change.

- As of yet, there is only very limited evidence from studies of moderation or prediction to show that PF can be used as a tool for prediction of outcomes and assignment to treatment in chronic pain.

In the practical domain, indicators of progress also come from an unusual direction: the ability of the PF Model to inform change processes in the treatment provider. PF naturally shines a light on the behavior of treatment providers to a degree, or in a way, that perhaps other models have not. Let me explain.

It is not new that treatment provider behavior is important and can determine treatment effectiveness (e.g., Waller, 2009). We now know that facets of PF act as mediators in worksite well-being and performance training (Bond & Bunce, 2000; Flaxman & Bond, 2010). We further know that acceptance, present-focused awareness, and values-based action are associated with less stress and burnout, better well-being, and better functioning in daily roles among providers—and they are also associated with providers' ability to confront pain in the patients they see without that pain exerting an interfering effect on service delivery (McCracken & Yang, 2008). In one study, we also found that seventy-eight percent of providers surveyed felt that using the PF model led to benefits in their personal life (Barker & McCracken, 2014).

PF has clearly inspired clinical researchers in their choice of research questions and has influenced the services in which they work. As of 2011, there were only two very small RCTs published in this area, with only thirty-eight total participants between them. From our recent reviews, we know there are now at least thirty published treatment outcome studies, including at least eighteen RCTs, designed specifically around PF, which include a total of 1,621 participants in the RCTS alone.

Figure 9.1 is a graph of the studies conducted over time for ACT, which is only one type of treatment focused on PF. The first systematic review of RCTs of ACT for chronic pain did not appear until 2014, and all ten of the RCTs examined in this review measured some facet of PF (Hann & McCracken, 2014). A recent survey of professionals providing treatment for chronic pain has also found that twenty-eight percent emphasize primarily "newer generation" forms of CBT that include mindfulness and acceptance (Scott, Marin, Gaudiano, & McCracken, 2017b).

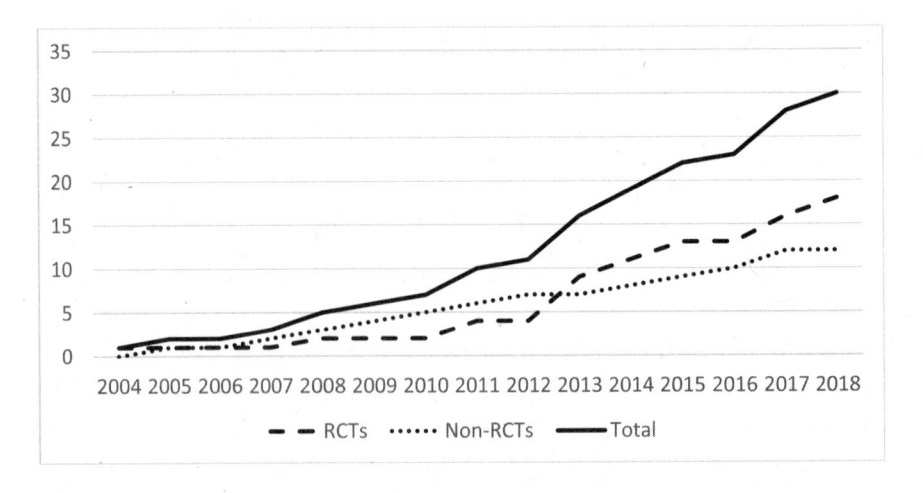

Figure 9.1. Cumulative Number of Outcome Studies of Acceptance and Commitment Therapy for Chronic Pain Published Between 2004 and 2018

From a small and relatively recent beginning, these accumulated scientific and practical results represent a significant achievement. The PF model has shown itself to be widely applicable across chronic pain populations, modes of treatment delivery, and outcomes of interest. There are now data that support the role of PF in conditions such as general or heterogeneous chronic pain, as well as in more specific conditions, such as complex regional pain syndrome (Cho, McCracken, Heiby, Moon, & Lee, 2013), headache or migraine (Almarzooqi, Chilcot, & McCracken, 2017; Dindo, Recober, Marchman, O'Hara, & Turvey, 2014), and fibromyalgia (Luciano et al., 2014; Wicksell et al., 2013; Yu et al., 2017a). PF has also demonstrated utility in specific populations or circumstances, such as older adults (Alonso-Fernandez et al., 2016; Scott et al., 2017a) and patients waiting for a surgical neuromodulation procedure for chronic pain (McCracken et al., 2015b).

When it comes to the PF model, modes of treatment delivery have included conventional individual therapy (Wicksell, Ahlqvist, Bring, Melin, & Olsson, 2008a), group therapy (McCracken et al. 2005, 2013b), Internet-based treatment (Buhrman et al., 2013; Lin et al., 2018; Trompetter et al., 2015b), and self-help manuals (Thorsell et al., 2011). Outcomes of interest have typically reflected multiple domains of emotional, physical, and social functioning, and particular cases have also been made for improved work (Dahl, Wilson, & Nilsson, 2004), sleep (Daly-Eichenhardt et al., 2016), medication reduction (Guildford, Daly-Eichenhardt, Hill, Sanderson, & McCracken, 2018), and improvement in directly assessed physical performance (Guildford, Jacobs, Daly-Eichenhardt, Scott, & McCracken, 2017).

Each of these features highlights the specific utility of the PF model, but to some degree, they also reflect the value of broadly applicable process-based approaches more generally. As clinical research has taken up the model, and clinicians learn to implement treatment based on it, the generally applicability and robustness of the model with respect to modes of application is leading to growing interest in providers and systems of care alike. Studies on the PF model have also shown benefits for both the recipient and provider, further ensuring engagement based on usefulness, personal engagement, and fit. Stated another way, the PF model is a process-based model that engages the psychological features that arguably determine use of scientific innovations (Hayes & Hofmann, 2018a).

Over the last few decades, there is evidence that the effects of CBT are not improving but falling (Johnsen & Friborg, 2015), and this trend also appears in CBT for chronic pain (Williams et al., 2012). There are a number of possible reasons for this apparent decline, including questions around fidelity and competency in delivery. Even so, a strategy for producing improvement over time is needed. The conceptual reasoning and evidence presented here suggests that taking a process-based path may represent such a strategy. Even in the hands of a very small number of research groups and people, PF as a process-based approach has changed the focus, shaped the research methods, and altered the treatment methods chosen by clinical researchers, clinicians, and systems of care around the world. As diagnostic systems, training, and provision of care move more strongly in a process-based direction, it will be interesting to see if this relative success can be replicated in other problem areas.

References

Åkerblom, S., Perrin, S., Rivano Fisher, M., & McCracken, L. M. (2015). The mediating role of acceptance in multidisciplinary cognitive-behavioral therapy for chronic pain. *The Journal of Pain, 16*, 606–615.

Åkerblom S., Perrin, S., Rivano Fischer, M., & McCracken, L. (2016). A validation and generality study of the Committed Action Questionnaire in a Swedish sample with chronic pain. *International Journal of Behavioral Medicine, 23*, 260–270.

Almarzooqi, S., Chilcot, J., & McCracken, L. M. (2017). The role of psychological flexibility in migraine headache impact and depression. *Journal of Contextual Behavioral Science, 6*, 239–243.

Alonso-Fernandez, M., Lopez-Lopez, A., Lodata, A., Gonzalez, J. L., & Whetherell, J. L. (2016). Acceptance and commitment therapy and selective optimization with compensation for institutionalized older people with chronic pain. *Pain Medicine, 17*, 264–277.

Bailey, R. W., Vowles, K. E., Witkiewitz, K., Sowden, G., & Ashworth, J. (2016). Examining committed action in chronic pain: Further validation and clinical utility of a Committed Action Questionnaire. *The Journal of Pain, 17*, 1095–1104.

Barker, E., & McCracken, L. M. (2014). From traditional cognitive behavioral therapy to acceptance and commitment therapy for chronic pain: A mixed method study of staff experiences of change. *British Journal of Pain, 8*, 98–106.

Baranoff, J., Hanrahan, S. J., Kapur, D., & Connor, J. P. (2012). Acceptance as a process variable in relation to catastrophizing in multidisciplinary pain treatment. *European Journal of Pain, 17*, 101–110.

Bond, F. W., & Bunce, D. (2000). Mediators of change in emotional-focused and problem focused worksite stress management interventions. *Journal of Occupational and Health Psychology, 5*, 156–163.

Bond, F. W., Hayes, S. C., Baer, R. A., Carpenter, K. M., Guenole, N., Orcutt, H. K., … Zettle, R. D. (2011). Preliminary psychometric properties of the Acceptance and

Action Questionnaire-II: A revised measure of psychological inflexibility and experiential avoidance. *Behavior Therapy, 42*, 676–688.

Brown, K. W., & Ryan, R. M. (2003). The benefits of being present: Mindfulness and its role in psychological well-being. *Journal of Personality and Social Psychology, 84*, 822–848.

Buhrman, M., Skoglund, A., Husell, J., Berstrom, K., Gordh, T., Hursti, T., … Andersson, G. (2013). Guided Internet-delivered acceptance and commitment therapy for chronic pain patients: A randomized controlled trial. *Behaviour Research and Therapy, 51*, 307–315.

Butler, A. C., Chapman, J. E., Forman, E. M., & Beck, A. T. (2006). The empirical status of cognitive-behavioral therapy: A review of meta-analyses. *Clinical Psychology Review, 26*, 17–31.

Cederberg, J. T., Cernvall, M., Dahl, J., von Essen, L., & Ljungman, G. (2016). Acceptance as mediator for change in acceptance and commitment therapy for persons with chronic pain? *International Journal of Behavioral Medicine, 23*, 21–29.

Cho, S., McCracken, L. M., Heiby, E. M., Moon, D., & Lee, J. (2013). Pain acceptance-based coping in complex regional pain syndrome type I: Daily relations with pain intensity, activity and mood. *Journal of Behavioral Medicine, 36*, 531–538. doi: 10.1007/s10865-012-9449-7.

Cuijpers, P., van Straten, A., & Warmerdam, L. (2007). Behavioral activation treatments of depression: A meta-analysis. *Clinical Psychology Review, 27*, 318–326.

Dahl, J., Wilson, K. G., & Nilsson, A., (2004). Acceptance and commitment therapy and the treatment of persons at risk for long term disability resulting from stress and pain symptoms: A preliminary randomized trial. *Behavior Therapy, 35*, 785–801.

Daly-Eichenhardt, A., Scott, W., Howard-Jones, M., Nicolaou, T., & McCracken, L. M. (2016). Changes in sleep problems and psychological flexibility following interdisciplinary acceptance and commitment therapy for chronic pain: An observational cohort study. *Frontiers in Psychology, 7*, 1326.

Day, M. A., Ehde, D. M., & Jensen, M. P. (2015). Psychosocial pain management moderation: The limit, activate, and enhance model. *The Journal of Pain, 16*, 947–960.

Dindo, L., Recober, A., Marchman, J., O'Hara, M. W., & Turvey, C. (2014). One-day behavioral intervention in depressed migraine patients: Effects on headache. *Headache, 54*, 528–538.

Fish, R. A., McGuire, B., Hogan, M., Morrison, T. G., & Stewart, I. (2010). Validation of the Chronic Pain Acceptance Questionnaire (CPAQ) in an Internet sample and development and validation of the CPAQ-8. *Pain, 149*, 435–443.

Flaxman, P. E., & Bond, F. W. (2010). A randomized worksite comparison of acceptance and commitment therapy and stress inoculation training. *Behaviour Research and Therapy, 48*, 816–820.

Fresco, D. M., Moore, M. T., van Dulmen, M., Segal, Z. V., Teasdale, J. D., Ma, D., & Williams, J. M. G. (2007). Initial psychometric properties of the Experiences Questionnaire: A self-report survey of decentering. *Behavior Therapy, 38*, 234–246.

Gillanders, D. T., Bolderston, H., Bond, F. W., Dempster, M., Flaxman, P. E., Campbell, L., ... Remmington, B. (2014). The development and initial validation of the Cognitive Fusion Questionnaire. *Behavior Therapy, 45*, 83–101.

Gilpin, H. R., Keyes, A., Stahl, D. R., Greig, R., & McCracken, L. M. (2017). Predictors of treatment outcome in contextual cognitive behavioural therapies for chronic pain: A systematic review. *The Journal of Pain, 18*(10), 1153–1164. doi: 10.1016/j.pain.2017.04.003

Gilpin, H. R., Stahl, D. R., & McCracken, L. M. (2019). A theoretically guided approach to identifying predictors of treatment outcome in contextual cognitive behavioural therapy for chronic pain. *European Journal of Pain, 23*, 354–366.

Guildford, B. J., Daly-Eichenhardt, A., Hill, B., Sanderson, K., & McCracken, L. M. (2018). Analgesic reduction during an interdisciplinary pain management programme: Treatment effects and processes of change. *British Journal of Pain, 12*(2), 72–86. doi: 10.1177/2049463717734016 journals.sagepub.com/home/bjp

Guildford, B. J., Jacobs, C. M., Daly-Eichenhardt, A., Scott, W., & McCracken, L. M. (2017). Assessing physical functioning on pain management programmes: The unique contribution of directly assessed physical performance measures and their relationship to self-report. *British Journal of Pain, 11*, 46–57.

Hann, K. E. J., & McCracken, L. M. (2014). A systematic review of randomized controlled trials of acceptance and commitment therapy for adults with chronic pain: Outcome domains, design quality, and efficacy. *Journal of Contextual Behavioral Science, 3*, 217–227.

Hayes, S. C., Barnes-Homes, D., & Wilson, K. G. (2012). Contextual behavioral science: Creating a science more adequate to the challenge of the human condition. *Journal of Contextual Behavioral Science, 1*, 1–16.

Hayes, S. C., & Hofmann, S. G. (2018a). A psychological model of the use of psychological intervention science: Seven rules for making a difference. *Clinical Psychology: Research and Practice, 25*(3), e12259. doi: 10.1111/cpsp.12259

Hayes, S. C., & Hofmann, S. G. (Eds.). (2018b). *Process-based CBT: The science and core clinical competencies of cognitive behavioral therapy*. Oakland, CA: Context Press/New Harbinger Publications.

Hayes, S. C., Levin, M. E., Plumb-Vilardaga, J., Villatte, J. L., & Pistorello, J. (2013a). Acceptance and commitment therapy and contextual behavioral science: Examining the progress of a distinctive model of behavioral and cognitive therapy. *Behavior Therapy, 44*(2), 180–198.

Hayes, S. C., Long, D. M., Levin, M. E., & Follette, W. C. (2013b). Treatment development: Can we find a better way? *Clinical Psychology Review, 33*, 870–882.

Hayes, S. C., Luoma, J. B., Bond, F. W., Masuda, A., & Lillis, J. (2006). Acceptance and commitment therapy: Model, processes and outcomes. *Behaviour Research and Therapy, 44*, 1–25.

Hayes, S. C., Villatte, M., Levin, M., & Hildebrandt, M. (2011). Open, aware, and active: Contextual approaches as an emerging trend in the behavioral and cognitive therapies. *Annual Review of Clinical Psychology, 7*, 141–168.

Herbert, M. S., Afari, N., Robinson, J. B., Listvinsky, A., Bondi, M. W., & Whetherell, J. L. (2018). Neuropsychological functioning and treatment outcomes in acceptance and commitment therapy for chronic pain. *The Journal of Pain, 19*(8), 852–861. doi: 10.16/j.pain.2018.02.008

Hofmann, S. G., Curtiss, J. E., & Hayes, S. C. (2020). Beyond linear mediation: Toward a dynamic network approach to study treatment processes. *Clinical Psychology Review, 76*, doi: 10.1016/j.cpr.2020.101824

Hollon, S. D., Stewart, M. O., & Strunk, D. (2006). Enduring effects for cognitive behavior therapy in the treatment of depression and anxiety. *Annual Review of Psychology, 57*, 285–315.

Johnsen, T. J., & Friborg, O. (2015). The effects of cognitive behavioral therapy as an anti-depressive treatment are falling: A meta-analysis. *Psychological Bulletin, 141*, 747–768.

Kazdin, A. E. (2007). Mediators and mechanisms of change in psychotherapy research. *Annual Review of Clinical Psychology, 3*, 1–27.

Khoury, B., Lecomte, T., Fortin, G., Masse, M., Therien, P., Bouchard, V., ... Hofmann, S. G. (2013). Mindfulness-based therapy: A comprehensive meta-analysis. *Clinical Psychology Review, 33*, 763–771.

Lemmens, L. H. J. M., Galindo-Garre, F., Arntz, A., Peeters, F., Hollon, S. D., DeRubies, R. J., & Huibers, M. J. H. (2017). Exploring mechanisms of change in cognitive therapy and interpersonal psychotherapy for adult depression. *Behaviour Research and Therapy, 94*, 81–92.

Lemmens, L. H. J. M., Muller, V. N. L. S., Arntz, A., & Hibers, M. J. H. (2016). Mechanisms of change in psychotherapy for depression: An empirical update and evaluation of research aimed at identifying psychological mediators. *Clinical Psychology Review, 50*, 95–107.

Lin, J., Klatt, L., McCracken, L. M., & Baumeister, H. (2018). Psychological flexibility mediates the effect of an online-based acceptance and commitment therapy for chronic pain: An investigation of change processes. *Pain, 159*(4), 663–672. doi: 10.1097/j.pain.00000000000001134

Longmore, R. J., & Worrell, M. (2007). Do we need to challenge thoughts in cognitive behavior therapy? *Clinical Psychology Review, 27*, 173–187.

Luciano, J. V., Gualler, J. A., Aguado, J., Lopez-del-Hoyo, Y., Olivan, B., Magallon, R., ... Garcia-Campayo, J. (2014). Effectiveness of group acceptance and commitment therapy for fibromyalgia: A 6-month randomized controlled trial (EFFIGACT study). *Pain, 155*, 693–702.

Lykkegaard, S., Vang, M. L., Vaegter, H. B., & Andersen, T. E. (2017). Pain-related acceptance as a mediator in the fear avoidance model of chronic pain: A preliminary study. *Pain Medicine, 19*(9), 1764–1771. doi: 10.1093/pm/pnx223

MacKinnon, D. P., Lockwood, C. M, Hoffman, J. M., West, S. G., & Sheets, V. (2002). A comparison of methods to test mediation and other intervening variable effects. *Psychological Methods, 7*, 83–104.

McCracken, L. M. (1998). Learning to live with the pain: Acceptance of pain predicts adjustment in persons with chronic pain. *Pain, 74*, 21–27.

McCracken, L. M. (2013). Committed action: An application of the psychological flexibility model to activity patterns in chronic pain. *The Journal of Pain, 14*, 828–835.

McCracken, L. M. & Thompson M. (2009). Components of mindfulness in patients with chronic pain. *Journal of Psychopathology and Behavioral Assessment, 31*, 75-82.

McCracken, L. M., Barker, E., & Chilcot, J. (2014a). Decentering, rumination, cognitive defusion, and psychological flexibility in people with chronic pain. *Journal of Behavioral Medicine, 37*, 1215–1225.

McCracken, L. M., Chilcot, J., & Norton, S. (2015a). Further development in the assessment of psychological flexibility: A shortened Committed Action Questionnaire (CAQ-8). *European Journal of Pain, 19*, 677–685.

McCracken, L. M., DaSilva, P., Skillicorn, B., & Doherty, R. (2014b). The Cognitive Fusion Questionnaire: A preliminary study of psychometric properties and prediction of functioning in chronic pain. *The Clinical Journal of Pain, 30*, 894–901.

McCracken, L. M., Davies, M., Scott, W., Paroli, M., Harris, S., & Sanderson, K. (2015b). Can a psychologically based treatment help people live with chronic pain when they are seeking a procedure to reduce it? *Pain Medicine, 16*, 451–459.

McCracken, L. M., & Eccleston, C. (2005). A prospective study of acceptance of pain and patient functioning with chronic pain. *Pain, 118*, 164–169.

McCracken, L. M., & Eccleston, C. (2006). A comparison of the relative utility of coping and acceptance-based measures in a sample of chronic pain sufferers. *European Journal of Pain, 10*, 23–29.

McCracken, L. M., Gauntlett-Gilbert, J., & Vowles, K. (2007a). The role of mindfulness in a contextual cognitive-behavioral analysis of chronic pain-related suffering and disability. *Pain, 131*, 63–69.

McCracken, L. M., & Gutiérrez-Martínez, O. (2011). Processes of change in psychological flexibility in an interdisciplinary group-based treatment for chronic pain based on acceptance and commitment therapy. *Behaviour Research and Therapy, 49*(4), 267–274.

McCracken, L. M., Gutiérrez-Martínez, O., & Smyth, C. (2013a). "Decentering" reflects psychological flexibility in people with chronic pain and correlates with their quality of functioning. *Health Psychology, 32*, 820–823.

McCracken, L. M., & Keogh, E. (2009). Acceptance, mindfulness, and values-based action may counteract fear and avoidance of emotions in chronic pain: An analysis of anxiety sensitivity. *The Journal of Pain, 10*, 408–415.

McCracken, L. M., & Morley, S. (2014). The psychological flexibility model: A basis for integration and progress in psychological approaches to chronic pain management. *The Journal of Pain, 15*, 221–234.

McCracken, L. M., Sato, A., & Taylor, G. J. (2013b). A trial of a brief group-based form of acceptance and commitment therapy (ACT) for chronic pain in general practice: Pilot outcome and process results. *The Journal of Pain, 14*, 1398–1406.

McCracken, L. M., & Velleman, S. (2010). Psychological flexibility in adults with chronic pain: A study of acceptance, mindfulness, and values-based action in primary care. *Pain, 148*, 141–147.

McCracken, L. M., Vowles, K. E., & Eccleston, C. (2004). Acceptance of chronic pain: Component analysis and a revised assessment method. *Pain, 107*, 159–166.

McCracken, L. M., Vowles, K. E., & Eccleston, C. (2005). Acceptance-based treatment for persons with complex longstanding chronic pain: A preliminary analysis of treatment outcome in comparison to a waiting phase. *Behaviour Research and Therapy, 43*, 1335–1346.

McCracken, L. M., Vowles, K. E., & Gauntlett-Gilbert, J. (2007b). A prospective investigation of acceptance and control-oriented coping with chronic pain. *Journal of Behavioral Medicine, 30*, 339–349.

McCracken, L. M., & Yang, S-Y. (2006). The role of values in a contextual cognitive-behavioral approach to chronic pain. *Pain, 123*, 137–145.

McCracken, L. M., & Yang S-Y. (2008). A contextual cognitive-behavioral analysis of rehabilitation workers' health and well-being: Influences of acceptance, mindfulness, and values-based action. *Rehabilitation Psychology, 53*, 479–485.

McCracken, L. M., & Zhao-O'Brien, J. (2010). General psychological acceptance and chronic pain: There is more to accept than the pain itself. *European Journal of Pain, 14*, 170–175.

Morley, S., & Keefe, F. J. (2007). Getting a handle on process and change in CBT for chronic pain. *Pain, 127*, 197–198.

Preacher, K. J., & Hayes, A. F. (2008). Asymptotic and resampling strategies for assessing and comparing indirect effects in multiple mediator models. *Behavior Research Methods, 40*, 879–891.

Reneman, M. F., Dijkstra, A., Geertzen, J. H., & Dijkstra, P. U. (2010). Psychometric properties of Chronic Pain Acceptance Questionnaires: A systematic review. *European Journal of Pain, 14*, 457–465.

Scott, W., Daly, A., & McCracken, L. M. (2017a). Treatment of chronic pain for adults 65 and over: Analyses of outcomes and changes in psychological flexibility following interdisciplinary acceptance and commitment therapy (ACT). *Pain Medicine, 18*, 252–264.

Scott, W., Hann, K. E. J., & McCracken, L. M. (2016a). A comprehensive examination of changes in psychological flexibility following acceptance and commitment therapy for chronic pain. *Journal of Contemporary Psychotherapy, 46*, 139–148.

Scott, W., Marin, F. M., Gaudiano, B., & McCracken, L. M. (2017b, June). *Practices and attitudes of professionals who provide psychological treatments for people with chronic pain: A comparison across approaches within CBT.* Paper presented to the meeting of the Association for Contextual Behavioral Science, Sevilla, Spain.

Scott, W., McCracken, L. M., & Norton, S. (2016b). A confirmatory factor analysis of facets of psychological flexibility in a sample of people seeking treatment for chronic pain. *Annals of Behavioral Medicine, 50*, 285–296.

Thorsell, J., Finnes, A., Dahl, J., Lundgren, T., Gybrant, M., Gordh, T., & Buhrman, M. (2011). A comparative study of 2 manual-based self-help interventions, acceptance and commitment therapy and applied relaxation, for persons with chronic pain. *Clinical Journal of Pain, 27*, 716–723.

Tolin, D. F. (2010). Is cognitive-behavioral therapy more effective than other therapies? A meta-analytic review. *Clinical Psychology Review, 30*, 710–720.

Trompetter, H. R., Bohlmeijer, E. T., Fox, J-P., & Schreurs, K. M. G. (2015a). Psychological flexibility and catastrophizing as associated change mechanisms during online acceptance & commitment therapy for chronic pain. *Behaviour Research and Therapy, 74*, 50–59.

Trompetter, H. R., Bohlmeijer, E. T., Veehof, M. M., & Schreurs, K. M. G. (2015b). Internet-based guided self-help intervention for chronic pain based on acceptance and commitment therapy: A randomized controlled trial. *Journal of Behavioral Medicine, 38*, 66–80.

Trompetter, H. R., ten Klooster, P. M., Schreurs, K. M. G., Fledderus, M., Westerhof, G. J., & Bohlmeijer, E. T. (2013). Measuring values and committed action with the Engaged Living Scale (ELS): Psychometric evaluation in a nonclinical and chronic pain samples. *Psychological Assessment, 25*, 1235–46.

Turner, J. A., Holtzman, S., & Mancl, L. (2007). Mediators, moderators, and predictors of therapeutic change in cognitive-behavioral therapy for chronic pain. *Pain, 127*, 276–286.

Vilardaga, R., Hayes, S. C., Levin, M. E., & Muto, T. (2009). Creating a strategy for progress: A contextual behavioral science approach. *The Behavior Analyst, 32*, 105–133.

Vowles, K. E., Fink, B. C., & Cohen, L. L. (2014a). Acceptance and commitment therapy for chronic pain: A diary study of treatment process in relation to reliable change in disability. *Journal of Contextual Behavioral Science, 3*, 74–80.

Vowles, K. E., & McCracken, L. M. (2008). Acceptance and values-based action in chronic pain: A study of treatment effectiveness and process. *Journal of Consulting and Clinical Psychology, 76*, 397–407.

Vowles, K. E., & McCracken, L. M. (2010). Comparing the role of psychological flexibility and traditional pain management coping strategies in chronic pain treatment outcomes. *Behaviour Research and Therapy, 48*, 141–146.

Vowles, K. E., McCracken, L. M., & Eccleston, C. (2007). Processes of change in chronic pain: The contributions of pain, acceptance, and catastrophizing. *European Journal of Pain, 11*, 779–787.

Vowles, K. E., McCracken, L. M., & Zhao-O'Brien, J. (2011). Acceptance and values-based action in chronic pain: A three-year follow-up analysis of treatment effectiveness and process. *Behaviour Research and Therapy, 49*, 748–755.

Vowles, K. E., Sowden, G., & Ashworth, J. (2014b). A comprehensive examination of the model underlying acceptance and commitment therapy for chronic pain. *Behavior Therapy, 45*, 390–401.

Vowles, K. E., Witkiewitz, K., Sowden, G., & Ashworth, J. (2014c). Acceptance and commitment therapy for chronic pain: Evidence of mediation and clinically significant change following an abbreviated interdisciplinary program of rehabilitation. *The Journal of Pain, 15*, 101–113.

Waller, G. (2009). Evidence-based treatment and therapist drift. *Behaviour Research and Therapy, 47*, 119–127.

Wicksell, R. K., Ahlqvist, J., Bring, A., Melin, L., & Olsson, G. L. (2008a). Can exposure and acceptance strategies improve functioning and life satisfaction in people with chronic pain and whiplash-associated disorders (WAD)? A randomized controlled trial. *Cognitive Behavior Therapy, 37,* 169–182.

Wicksell, R. K., Kemani, M., Jensen, K., Kosek, E., Kadetoff, D., Sorjonen, K., ... Olsson, G. L. (2013). Acceptance and commitment therapy for fibromyalgia: A randomized controlled trial. *European Journal of Pain, 17,* 599–611.

Wicksell, R. K., Olsson, G. L., & Hayes, S. C. (2010). Psychological flexibility as a mediator of improvement in acceptance and commitment therapy for patients with chronic pain following whiplash. *European Journal of Pain, 14*(10), 1059.e1–1059.e11.

Wicksell, R. K., Renofalt, J., Olsson, G. L., Bond, F., & Melin, L. (2008b). Avoidance and cognitive fusion—Central components in pain related disability? Development and preliminary validation of the Psychological Inflexibility in Pain Scale (PIPS). *European Journal of Pain, 12,* 491–500.

Williams, A., Eccleston, C., & Morley, S. (2012). Psychological therapies for the management of chronic pain (excluding headache) in adults. *Cochrane Database of Systematic Reviews, 11,* CD007407.

Yu, L., McCracken, L. M., & Norton, S. (2016). The Self Experiences Questionnaire (SEQ): Preliminary analyses for a measure of self in people with chronic pain. *Journal of Contextual Behavioral Science, 5,* 127–133.

Yu, L., Norton, S., Almarzooqi, S., & McCracken, L. M. (2017a). Preliminary investigation of pain acceptance and self-as-context in people with fibromyalgia. *British Journal of Pain, 11,* 134–143.

Yu, L., Norton, S., & McCracken, L. M. (2017b). Changes in "self-as-context" ("perspective-taking") occurs in acceptance and commitment therapy for people with chronic pain and is associated with improved functioning. *The Journal of Pain, 18,* 664–672.

Zettle, R. D., Hayes, S. C., Barnes-Holmes, D., & Biglan, T. (Eds.). (2016). *The Wiley handbook of contextual behavioral science.* Chichester, UK: Wiley/Blackwell.

CHAPTER 10

A Multilevel, Multimethod Approach to Testing and Refining Intervention Targets[3]

Andrew T. Gloster, PhD
University of Basel

Maria Karekla, PhD
University of Cyprus

Diagnostic systems of mental disorders have developed significantly since Kraepelin initially proposed his classification schemata (Kraepelin, 1896). This development has been received with both praise of progress (American Psychiatric Association, 2013) and criticism that it has impeded progress (Kupfer, First, & Regier, 2002).

Irrespective of how one views the current diagnostic systems of mental disorders—namely, the *Diagnostic and Statistical Manual of Mental Disorders* (DSM; American Psychiatric Association, 2013) and the *International Classification of Diseases and Related Health Problems* (ICD; World Health Organization, 2004)—it is generally agreed that these systems and diagnoses are uncoupled from treatment. For example, the introduction to the DSM-5 states that whereas diagnosis may help inform treatment, "recommendations for the selection and use of the most appropriate evidence-based treatment options for each disorder are beyond the scope of this manual" (American Psychiatric Association, 2013, p. 19). Therefore, the explicit empirical link between diagnostics and treatment is left to future research and theory.

---

[3] Author Note: This work was supported in part by a grant from the Swiss National Science Foundation (PP00P1_163716/1).

This uncoupling has generally been met with indifference. For example, an international survey found that mental health professionals perceive the DSM and ICD as useful for administrative purposes or for communicating, but they view these diagnostic systems as less useful for treatment-related activities (i.e., treatment selection or prognosis; First et al., 2018). The reasons for this indifference may include the belief that our current knowledge about treatment or etiology does not allow for direct linking to diagnoses. Further, case conceptualizations and interventions are often based on constructs or information other than the current diagnostic system (e.g., behavior analysis, psychodynamic therapy) where hypotheses about the etiology and maintenance of a client's presenting problem are generated largely within their respective theoretical framework. Thus, whereas some of the same symptoms listed within a diagnostic categorization may play a role in the conceptual framework, an explicit link to the diagnosis is seen as less important. Although some critical voices have questioned the uncoupling between diagnosis and treatment (Mullins-Sweatt & Widiger, 2009), no viable alternative has been presented to date.

Recent changes in the field of intervention science have made this issue more central, as this very book suggests. Conceptual developments, such as process-based therapy as a model of evidence-based treatment (e.g., Hayes & Hofmann, 2018; Hofmann & Hayes, 2019), are raising a different claim: that assessment procedures and therapy can and should be linked via mechanisms of action implicated in the maintenance and treatment of suffering and the promotion of well-being. Mechanisms of action refer to the change processes by which psychotherapeutic change occurs. This approach aims to directly link mechanisms of action with intervention choices and outcomes in an iterative, bottom-up process.

The goal of a process-based approach is to identify salient intervention processes that aid practitioners in promoting desirable outcomes in those they serve. By harnessing extant research findings that have already demonstrated an explicit link between mechanisms of action and outcome, there is a higher probability that when targeted again in a new context (e.g., new patient, new situation), the previous findings will generalize.

In this approach, the success of linking assessment and treatment will depend upon the degree to which basic core mechanisms of action are identified and measured. Candidate mechanisms need to be basic in the sense that they apply widely so that altering particular candidate mechanisms will be helpful in many contexts and will hold up when examined using a multi-method, multilevel approach. They also need to be basic in the sense that successfully manipulating the targeted process through intervention will generate outcomes in a predictable (though not certain) fashion. Thus, core mechanisms of action need to be malleable.

In this chapter, we examine how candidate mechanisms of action can be refined over time, and we present research recommendations that can be used in this iterative process. We will exemplify a multi-method, multilevel approach to developing interventions using the construct of psychological flexibility (PF) as an extended example. PF presents a worthwhile scaffolding for our more general points because it has been widely examined in assessment and intervention research and appears to present a reasonable beginning set of change processes around which a set of treatment module choices can be gathered.

PF refers to a range of interpersonal and intrapersonal skills that reflect the ability to "recognize and adapt to various situational demands; shift mindsets or behavioral repertoires when these strategies compromise personal or social functioning; maintain balance among important life domains; and be aware, open, and committed to behaviors that are congruent with deeply held values" (Kashdan & Rottenberg, 2010). Therefore, PF is a broad concept that helps researchers and clinicians orient toward a small set of underlying functional classes of behavior (e.g., acceptance versus avoidance; Vilardaga, Hayes, Levin, & Muto, 2009). Six interrelated classes of behavior have been most commonly proposed to contribute to PF (Hayes, Strosahl, & Wilson, 2012). These flexibility skills (and their inflexible alternatives) are:

1. acceptance (versus avoidance or suppression);

2. cognitive defusion (versus cognitive fusion and entanglement);

3. flexible attention to the here and now (versus loss of contact with the present moment or being in an "autopilot" mode of functioning);

4. having a stable and transcendental sense of self (versus attachment to a conceptualized self);

5. clarification of and living based on deeply meaningful chosen values (versus values confusion or engaging in behavior that is discrepant from one's values); and

6. committed purposeful action (versus inaction, impulsivity, or nonfunctional or persistent avoidance behavior).

We do not propose that PF is the only construct of interest that could be used as a structure for a beginning examination of a process-based diagnostic system, nor in an empirical sense do we currently know if PF will meet all of the necessary criteria for such a system. Instead, we wish to show how the behavioral classes that comprise PF appear broadly relevant for situations in and outside of the therapy room that could comprise intervention targets, and in that context, we make more general recommendations that should apply to any process-based diagnostic model.

In what follows, we will begin each section with a concrete recommendation and then show how the existing data on PF support that recommendation and why it seems relevant to any process-based alternative to the current psychiatric nosology.

Recommendation One: Target Mechanisms in Research

Treatment outcome studies aim to provide understanding about how to intervene on a specific target by comparing two or more interventions. This strategy renders evidence as to whether one intervention variant is "better" than another on chosen outcomes. Randomized controlled trials (RCTs) are typically considered the gold standard of this approach, both for psychotherapy and pharmacological interventions. Decades of RCTs have led to lists of "validated" psychotherapies (APA Presidential Task Force on Evidence-Based Practice, 2006) that, in turn, inform best practice guidelines (e.g., American Psychological Association, 2017; Bandelow et al., 2008).

The amount of evidence amassed using this strategy is staggering. It has most frequently been used to argue that a particular intervention is feasible and ethical for general categories of psychological difficulty. It is humbling to realize, however, that a mountain of evidence from RCTs tells a practitioner only that an intervention is feasible for a client with a particular condition. Whether a particular intervention is actually *applicable* to a given client depends on the degree to which a client and practitioner match the conditions examined in the study. Variations between the settings of the study and the real-world application can be many in terms of both the client (e.g., age, ethnicity, set of diagnoses, comorbidities, social network, effect of being enrolled in a study) and the method of treatment implementation (e.g., reimbursement system, therapist experience, frequency of sessions, degree of supervision, dedication to the treatment, effect of providing therapy within a study). In actuality, the sum total of these factors can *never* fully apply to an individual client and their therapist—even if the practitioner strives to implement the intervention exactly as it was in the study.

At first, the problem of generalizing or transferring research to real-world implementation may seem less of a problem for pharmacological interventions because the prescribed medication is fully standardized in the form of a pill. Once again, however, there are differences on the side of the client (e.g., entering a study, being monitored, payment, metabolism, concurrent medications) and practitioner (e.g., following a study protocol, time with the patient, explanations given). It becomes a bigger problem when there is the expectation that "idealized" studies (which maximize internal validity without adequate consideration of external validity) will transfer to real-world examples of human psychopathology.

The problem of generalization is precisely why focusing on the most salient mechanisms of change is so important. Practitioners who implement any type of intervention need to know not only that the intervention has worked for similar clients in the past, but also *why* it worked and *how* to apply that knowledge to intervene with the current client in their multifaceted context. In other words, a practitioner needs to know certain details, like which components of an intervention are crucial for a particular client, which components are necessary but not sufficient, whether a particular component can be titrated, when and in what order various components need to be presented to fit specific presentations, and so on. These questions fall within the domain of studies that examine therapy process and mechanisms of action. Relative to RCTs, there is much less scientific understanding about mechanisms of action derived from tightly controlled studies.

In attempting to understand how mechanisms exert their effects during interventions, mediation has been predominantly utilized as a statistical methodology. Statistical mediation refers to a process or pathway between an independent and a dependent variable, whereby a third intervening variable (mediator) may help account for the relationship between the independent and dependent variables (MacKinnon, Fairchild, & Fritz, 2007). In an effort to examine how and why an intervention (independent variable) exerts its influence on an outcome (dependent variable), mediation is often used to examine possible mechanisms contributing to change, but it may or may not always accomplish that task. Various mediators have been examined ranging from individual difference factors (e.g., anxiety sensitivity, distress tolerance) to theoretically driven procedures proposed to affect the outcome (e.g., exposure, relaxation). These mediators are then considered mechanisms by which a specific treatment affects the outcome. Although this constitutes an important step in exploring mechanisms of change in treatments, and it gets clinicians and researchers excited because it awakens the idea that causality is close at hand, three caveats need to be considered when examining mediational evidence.

First, it is rarely the case that only one mediator is sufficient to influence an outcome. A number of change processes may be relevant, and these may be engaged by a wide range of intervention kernels. Indeed, clinicians usually have an armament of therapeutic tools and approaches they utilize, and their proximal targets may be multiple. Thus, more complex and interactive mediation models may be needed (e.g., Kraemer, Stice, Kazdin, Offord, & Kupfer, 2001).

Second, in order for mediation to suggest evidence of a functionally important change mechanism, mediators should not be assessed at the same time as treatment outcomes. Rather, they should be assessed during the intervention and before treatment change occurs (Arch & Craske, 2008; Kazdin, 2007). It is often difficult to know how to time these assessments to accomplish that goal.

Third, statistical mediation is not synonymous with experimental control. Only after a variable is actively manipulated and experimentally influenced (e.g., in experiments or single-subject designs) can its status as a mechanism of action be verified. There are always unexamined "third variables" that could be responsible for meditational results. Thus, while mediation analyses are pragmatically useful and help iteratively refine interventions (Vilardaga et al., 2009), true causality is only possible through experimental analysis.

In addition to studies that examine mechanisms of action via statistical mediation, statistical moderation also provides important information about clients and factors that may affect treatment outcomes. Moderation specifies for whom or under what conditions a treatment works, thus delineating the context for therapeutic effects. Although this is immensely important, moderator variables (e.g., gender, socioeconomic status) tend to not be amenable to direct changes by clinicians, whereas mediator variables are more likely to present possibilities for intervention. Thus, emphasis in this chapter is placed on examining statistical mediation studies suggesting possible mechanisms via which treatment change occurs.

PF has been examined as a mediator of cognitive behavioral therapy (CBT) interventions, particularly as produced by acceptance and commitment therapy (ACT; Hayes et al., 2012). In one of the first well-crafted studies to examine statistical mediation in ACT compared to CBT, cognitive defusion was found to mediate treatment outcomes—specifically worry, quality of life, behavioral avoidance, and depression—in individuals with mixed anxiety problems (Arch, Wolitzky-Taylor, Eifert, & Craske, 2012). Similarly, experiential avoidance was found to mediate social anxiety symptoms and anhedonic depression in ACT but not CBT (Niles et al., 2014).

Present-moment awareness, or mindfulness, is another facet of PF that has been found to significantly relate to post-intervention improvements in worry and quality of life among individuals with generalized anxiety disorder (GAD; Morgan, Graham, Hayes-Skelton, Orsillo, & Roemer, 2014). This same research team also examined decentering, which is a process involved in cognitive defusion, as a mechanism of change in ACT versus applied relaxation treatment for GAD. They found that increases in decentering were associated with decreases in anxiety across both interventions and that these changes in decentering preceded changes in GAD symptoms (Hayes-Skelton, Calloway, Roemer, & Orsillo, 2015). Similarly, decentering was found to mediate the results of mindfulness-based cognitive therapy (MBCT; Segal, Williams, Teasdale, & Gemar, 2002) on relapse in patients with depression (for a review see Eisenlohr-Moul, Peters, & Baer, 2015). Additional studies have found positive evidence of statistical mediation for other aspects of PF (Hayes, Luoma, Bond, Masuda, & Lillis, 2006), though some of these studies have been criticized for not fulfilling longitudinal criteria for mediation or have not utilized formal statistical tests of mediation.

Recent work from our laboratories has attempted to address some of the problems related to timing when examining PF as a proposed mediator and assessing treatment outcomes. For example, analysis of session-by-session change using latent difference score analysis showed that increased engagement in value-based actions preceded reductions in suffering among patients with treatment-resistant panic disorder (Gloster et al., 2017). Importantly, and contrary to common conceptualizations of psychotherapy, changes in symptoms did not precede reductions in suffering, unlike changes in value-based action. In a trial comparing an ACT-based smoking cessation intervention to a wait-list control for young smokers, cognitive defusion and acceptance of smoking triggers mediated the relationship between cessation self-efficacy and intention to quit (FlexiQuit trial; Savvides & Karekla, 2014). A recent RCT for headaches found that pain acceptance, psychological inflexibility in pain, avoidance of pain, and values-based action all mediated the effects of treatment on headache disability and quality of life at three- and six-month follow-ups (Vasiliou, Karademas, Christou, Papacostas, & Karekla, under review). Finally, in an exposure-based treatment of panic disorder, PF mediated changes in clinical functioning across all stages of treatment (psychoeducation, exposure, and follow-up), even though the treatment did not directly target the skills that comprise PF (Gloster et al., 2014).

These studies are a sample of a large and growing literature showing that positive changes in PF mediate a variety of psychotherapeutic outcomes. However, not all facets of PF have been examined yet. No study has yet examined self-as-context as a mediator, although a recent, large effectiveness study suggests that it plays a role in treatment outcomes (Yu, Norton, & McCracken, 2017). Measures of self-as-context—and to a lesser degree, other aspects of PF—have only recently started to be developed and examined in terms of their psychometric properties. Additionally, most studies to date have examined only a single facet of PF, or if they examine several, then they are entered into mediation models as a single item. It is important to start examining more complex models of combinations of proposed mechanisms, which may require certain methodological changes, such as the use of complex network models (Christodoulou, Michaelides, & Karekla, 2018).

Early behavior therapists prided themselves in having one foot in the basic experimental laboratory and the other in the clinic and moving gracefully between both (Forsyth & Sabsevitz, 2002). This approach contributed greatly to our understanding of psychopathology and the discovery of successful therapeutic approaches that were grounded in science and that resulted from basic experimental manipulations. Given that one of the best ways to examine mechanisms of action is in well-controlled experimental settings, we advocate for close bidirectional ties between experimental laboratory-based research and clinical practice. Several dozen laboratory component studies have targeted elements of PF and have generally shown positive outcomes (Gloster, Hummel, Lyudmirskaya, Hauke, & Sonntag, 2012; Levin, Hildebrandt, Lillis, & Hayes, 2012). In addition, in deciphering proposed mechanisms of action, it is important that clinical studies regularly examine statistical mediation and utilize statistically rigorous methods.

We have shown that progress has been made in targeting different facets of PF as mechanisms of change. In our view, any proposed process-based alterative to the DSM will need to show similar or greater success.

Recommendation Two: Examine Events in Context

Behavior does not occur in a vacuum. Indeed, behavioral science has clearly established that responses elicited by stimuli are contingent on numerous "contextual" variables. These contextual variables have been described as "uncontrolled sights, sounds, smells, and so on" that operate in the background when pairing a conditioned stimulus with an unconditioned stimulus (Pierce & Epling, 1999, p. 86). If we define behavior as "the coherent, continuous activity of an integral organism" (Skinner, 1953, p. 15), then context may be defined as anything that exerts influence over the continuous activity of that organism. This applies to all forms of learning and transmission, including classical conditioning, operant conditioning, and relational learning (D. Barnes-Holmes, Barnes-Holmes, Luciano, & McEnteggart, 2017; Y. Barnes-Holmes, Hayes, Barnes-Holmes, & Roche, 2002), as well as genetic and epigenetic factors (Jablonka, Lamb, & Zeligowski, 2005, p. 114). Further, the term is not limited to the physical environment, but can be understood both historically and situationally.

To illustrate the importance of context, imagine the effect of yelling "stop" at a child under the following three conditions: (a) the child is a typically developing five-year-old, (b) the child is a three-month-old infant, and (c) the child is a fifteen-year-old adolescent who cannot hear. The desired impact of yelling "stop" is likely to work only in the first example because this use of language is contingent on being received by a hearing-able and verbally able person.

The importance of contextual factors can be found in various disciplines. An example from epigenetics is illustrated by examining the well-known negative impact of poor maternal care. Experiments with rodents show that biological pups of inattentive mothers have greater methylation of target genes than biological pups of attentive mothers (Meaney, 2001; Weaver et al., 2004). This can be interpreted as biological evidence of stress resulting from maternal inattention. When pups of inattentive and attentive mothers are switched after birth, however, the foster pups show methylation patterns of their adoptive mothers. In other words, any inherited "advantages" and "disadvantages" with respect to stress are now reversed. Further experiments demonstrate how these patterns extend across generations and can be reversed by "treating" the pups with substances that affect epigenetic processes such as methylation.

A clinically relevant example dramatically demonstrates the importance of context. It has been shown that the effect of "shooting up" heroin depends, in part, on the physical environment in which it occurs (Siegel, Hinson, Krank, & Mccully, 1982). When someone "shoots up" in a novel environment, they are more likely to overdose despite consuming the same amount as in their typical environment. This has been attributed to the fact that stimuli in the typical environment are part of the conditioned response to "shooting up" that dampens the response. In a novel environment, the same chemical dose is more potent for the individual, and an overdose is more likely to occur.

Research on language and cognition demonstrates another area in which context is important. Studies based on relational frame theory (D. Barnes-Holmes et al., 2017; Y. Barnes-Holmes et al., 2002) have shown how verbal cues can occasion a host of arbitrary relational responses. For example, stimuli that a person has never directly experienced can take on aversive or appetitive properties via relation framing. In the absence of relational framing, the stimulus might not elicit any response at all. Thus, relational framing is a type of contextual process involved in ongoing verbal and cognitive behavior (see also D. Barnes-Holmes & Barnes-Holmes, chapter 6 in this volume).

Despite the importance of contextual factors in explaining and influencing behavior, the study of psychopathology and psychotherapy has disproportionally focused on the individual. That is, most theories of psychopathology and therapy-related change are intrapersonal and even intrapsychic in nature. However, humans are social beings, and several studies document the bidirectional impact of patients and their social relations (Whisman & Baucom, 2012). That is, partners and families of patients are not only affected by the disorder of the patient, but they themselves can also affect the outcome of the patient's treatment (Denton et al., 2010). Even when this contextual variable is limited to the immediate family, it is not difficult to imagine that a patient who goes home to a supportive family has a greater chance of therapeutic change than someone who goes home to a criticizing and undermining family. Unfortunately, only a small minority of clinical outcome studies consider the impact of one's social environment on treatment outcomes.

With respect to PF, the impact of context on an individual and their development can be seen in a large study of adolescents ($N = 749$). Adolescents who reported increases in authoritarian parenting (low warmth, high control) over time were less psychologically flexible than peers who reported authoritative parenting (high warmth and control; Williams, Ciarrochi, & Heaven, 2012). These differences in PF, in turn, have been found to predict a wide variety of mental and behavioral health difficulties in adolescents and young adults (Levin et al., 2014). This suggests that the family context and parenting styles in particular longitudinally impact the psychological health of adolescents because these contextual factors alter PF.

Taken together, these studies point to the necessity of collecting and analyzing information about the historical and situational variables of interest. This requires conceptual work in consort with the collection of data in multiple ways, across multiple contexts, and across time—including across generations, depending on the research question. It is to the issue of time that we turn next.

Recommendation Three: Examine Events Unfolding Over Time with Intensive Analyses

Just as behavior does not occur in a vacuum, behavior is also variable across time. Stimuli change nearly constantly, and responses are not identical over time. Traditional diagnoses that appear stable when examined across weeks or years are, in fact, quite variable when assessed across days or hours (Watson, 2004) or when examined intensively within person (Molenaar, 2004). It cannot be assumed that variation that occurs between cases is generalizable to variation that occurs intraindividually (Fisher, Medaglia, & Jeronimus, 2017; Hayes et al., 2019). Instead, intraindividual variation needs to be explicitly tested (Molenaar, 2004). Thus, stability versus variability are not exclusively inherent properties of the phenomenon or diagnostic system, but they also depend on the time frame examined in a given study, as well as whether consistencies are examined within person or only at the level of collectives. In our opinion, these observations require that the science of human behavior includes within-person longitudinal analyses in at least equal measure to cross-sectional analyses across persons.

Examining variability over time in a context-sensitive manner is crucial in therapy studies that attempt to understand the effect of a given intervention. However, the vast majority of therapy studies rely on pre-treatment to post-treatment comparisons with data generated from retrospective questionnaires or interviews. If, for the sake of argument, we assume a twelve-week treatment duration, then pre-post change is "collapsed" across ninety days (2,160 hours) of a client's experience. In such a measurement approach, crucial information is lost not only about change (e.g., frequency, duration, rate of change, variability), but also about how a client begins to apply newly learned techniques, how they struggle, how their environment reacts to their attempts to change, and how these factors, in turn, accelerate or inhibit further change.

Experience sampling methodology (ESM), which is a procedure that frequently assesses behavior in one's natural environment often via an ambulatory monitoring device, is ideal to capture a rich variability of behavior as it unfolds over time within person (Stone & Shiffman, 1994; Trull & Ebner-Priemer, 2009). The time frame examined in ESM studies varies from seconds to days, depending on the focus of the study. State-of-the-art ESM studies signal participants to record data, are time stamped, and are sometimes even linked with automatic data recordings such as audio records, heart rate, or GPS location. ESM is high in ecological validity and limits biases associated with retrospective recall (Gloster et al., 2008; Miron-Shatz, Stone, & Kahneman, 2009; Rinner et al., 2019).

A few studies have examined the skills that comprise PF using ESM. For example, in one study, students reported on their social anxiety, emotion regulation, and positive events once per day for twenty-one consecutive days (Kashdan & Steger, 2006). The central research question was whether daily levels of social anxiety influenced the number of positive events experienced. Students who endorsed high levels of dispositional social anxiety at the start of the study, as assessed via a questionnaire, reported more positive events on days when they had social anxiety *and* responded with acceptance (a component of PF) than on days when they had social anxiety and responded by trying to suppress their feelings. Thus, the dispositional level alone was not enough to predict positive events. Instead, this context-sensitive, dense assessment was able to show a more nuanced pattern of behavior over time.

Recent work from our laboratories also illustrates the importance of examining events unfolding over time. Using ESM, we assessed participants with depression, those with social phobia, and those in a control group six times per day for one week. We tested whether PF (versus rigidity) would moderate the relationship between stress and interpersonal contact. Using multilevel modeling, we found that PF moderated the moment-to-moment relationship between stress and interpersonal contact (Gloster et al., under review). In particular, when individuals experienced higher levels of stress, they still engaged in interpersonal interactions if they also exhibited PF. If not, they tended to avoid interpersonal contact. This pattern was strongest for individuals with depression and social phobia but was also significant for the control group.

Although traditional psychometric approaches are useful in the examination of a hypothesized model's general structure, these approaches are unable to explore connections among a model's components. This inability has limited the exploration of proposed models of psychopathology and may have contributed to the categorical view embraced by the DSM. Innovative approaches, such as network analysis, might offer a solution for the examination of psychological constructs as a system of interconnected variables (Borsboom, 2017). Network analysis has begun to be applied to mental health problems—such as anxiety disorders (Beard et al., 2016; Heeren & McNally, 2016), post-traumatic stress disorder (McNally et al., 2015), depression (Boschloo, van Borkulo, Borsboom, & Schoevers, 2016; Fried, Epskamp, Nesse, Tuerlinckx, & Borsboom, 2016), obsessive-compulsive disorder (Ruzzano, Borsboom, & Geurts, 2015), autism (Deserno, Borsboom, Begeer, & Geurts, 2017; Ruzzano et al., 2015), and psychosis (Bak, Drukker, Hasmi, & van Jim, 2016; Isvoranu, Borsboom, van Os, & Guloksuz, 2016; Isvoranu et al., 2017)—as well as normal personality traits (Costantini et al., 2015; Cramer et al., 2012). Findings from these applications suggest that network approaches have an advantage in that they allow for the direct examination of potential underlying mechanisms of psychopathology.

We have recently reported the results of a network analysis to examine the PF model in a sample of chronic pain patients (Christodoulou et al., 2018). In that study, patients completed measures assessing all the components of the PF model. The network analysis showed strong connections among certain aspects of PF and weaker connections among others. The strongest connections were found between mindfulness and values-based action as well as between acceptance and fusion. These findings suggest that certain components of PF may be more central in the model and in their contributions toward the development of psychopathology.

These studies demonstrate that intense sampling of people's behavior over time provides insight into how behaviors, skills, and so forth function differently depending on how two or more variables interact. Such studies generate nuanced hypotheses and tests of putative mechanisms of action and further suggest crucial points during which to intervene (e.g., when X *and* Y occur). Examining mechanisms of action intensely over time is clearly related to our previous section on context, as new contexts emerge over time. The difference is one of focus chosen by the researcher or therapist. Further, the use of innovative approaches to examine networks of variables provides an opportunity to examine data within their context and in relation to other variables, thus providing further opportunities for the investigation of mechanisms of action.

Recommendation Four: Test Across Multiple Analytical Levels

Levels of research loosely refer to the degree of abstraction chosen by the researcher or practitioner to explain data. Levels range from very broad constructs (e.g., behavior, cognition, relational consistence, love, global warming) to terms that are nearly synonymous with the data itself (e.g., single nucleotide polymorphisms or SNPs, the number of lever presses per minute, reaction time, action potential, concentration of CO_2 levels). In general, lower levels tend to be generated in tight laboratory conditions. Biological and genetic variables also tend to be considered lower levels, though here, too, variation exists.

There are numerous reasons to clarify and coordinate our thinking about levels of analysis. First, explicating one's chosen level increases our understanding of what we are examining. Second, it opens the possibility that any given analysis may make sense at one level but loses explanatory value or validity at a different level. The implications of this possibility depend on the goals of the analysis. For a practitioner, this may not have immediate implications. However, for a scientific account of behavior (including a diagnostic system), contradictory findings across analytic levels suggest that theoretical work is needed. A full scientific account of a behavior needs to explain why a phenomenon responds differently at different levels of analysis. This could result in a refinement or rejection of the theory. We posit that (a) the more consistently a theory or variable can account for behavior across levels, the more broadly useful it will be, and (b) theories that are more coordinated across levels will be more "useful" than other theories that aren't. These are empirical propositions in need of experimental verification. Attention to the issue of levels has the added advantage of harnessing consorted research efforts.

To illustrate how multilevel research can be coordinated, we once again draw upon our research on the facets that comprise PF, in combination with a genetic analysis of the serotonin transporter gene (5HTT; Gloster et al., 2015). 5HTT is a regulator of serotoninergic neurotransmission that has been implicated in reward sensitivity (Wickrama, O'Neal, & Holmes, 2017). Short alleles of this polymorphism have repeatedly been associated with an increased risk of depression, suicidality, and anxiety, which has led some researchers to view the short allele as a "risk" variant. Some researchers, however, have recently argued that this interpretation is too one-sided (Belsky et al., 2009; Homberg & Lesch, 2011) and cite evidence, for example, that individuals with the short allele outperform individuals with the long allele on cognitive tasks and social conformity. This has led to the proposition that those with the short allele have higher levels of vigilance, and this serves as a common denominator that can account for both "positive" and "negative" outcomes. In other words, people with the short allele are generally more vigilant, faster, and more sensitive to their context such that the outcome of this vigilance depends on the task at hand (Enge, Fleischhauer, Lesch, Reif, & Strobel, 2011, 2014; Enge, Fleischhauer, Lesch, & Strobel, 2011).

This more contextual interpretation of the effects of the 5HTT polymorphism opened the door to exploring its relation to PF. We accomplished this within the course of an exposure-based CBT trial for patients with panic disorder and agoraphobia (Gloster et al., 2015) in which patients were asked to face their worst fears. In this trial, we found that patients with a short allele of the 5HTT polymorphism showed twice as much improvement in a measure of PF during treatment than those with the long allele. Importantly, this observed difference between the short and long allele groups was specific to PF, as allele group did not differentiate who improved with respect to panic symptoms or anxiety sensitivity. This suggests that patients in the short allele group (who were more contextually sensitive) were able to more flexibly adapt to the anxiety elicited by the exposure-based treatment.

Although replication of this finding is needed, we contend that this cohesion across levels of analysis adds a (tentative) validity to the importance of PF in various research domains.

Having found evidence for a link with a genetic polymorphism, we began to think of other ways to test the relevance of PF at another level of analysis. Because we collected data regarding the 5HTT polymorphism in a clinic setting, our sample consisted only of treatment-seeking individuals, which limited the generalizability of our findings. Thus, in order to determine whether PF is more broadly applicable to the general population, we collected data from a representative sample of over one thousand individuals in Switzerland. Participants answered questions about their physical heath, mental health, and well-being, as well as questions about risk factors (e.g., stress and lack of social support). Results showed that PF consistently moderated the relationship between stress and physical health, mental health, and well-being such that those with higher levels of PF had more desirable outcomes even if they reported higher levels of stress (Gloster, Meyer, & Lieb, 2017).

In another study involving multilevel analysis, we used physiological and self-report measures to examine emotional reactivity in women with eating disorders. Although physiological measures are often seen as more objective than self-report measures (Serfaty, Gale, Beadman, Froeliger, & Kamboj, 2018), comparing these two levels may provide important information and act as an index of PF. In our study, we found that females at high risk for developing an eating disorder presented with higher body image inflexibility and overall physiological hypersensitivity (as measured via higher heart rate and skin conductance levels) to negative affective stimuli compared to their low-risk counterparts. Lack of correspondence between self-reported affect ratings and physiological responses was considered an expression of body image inflexibility. This lack of correspondence was only found in the group at high risk for developing an eating disorder (Koushiou, 2016), suggesting that examining physiological responses in accordance with self-report may provide additional evidence regarding how PF may manifest at a physiological level.

Physiological measures have also been proposed to index individual differences in emotion regulation and coping (Donkin et al., 2011). Heart rate variability (HRV) is one particular index of physiological activity that reflects the continuous interplay between the sympathetic and parasympathetic systems and yields information about autonomic flexibility, which reflects an individual's ability to adjust to changes in the environment (Appelhans & Luecken, 2006; Denson, Grisham, & Moulds, 2011). Higher HRV is associated with the use of more adaptive emotion regulation strategies (Geisler, Vennewald, Kubiak, & Weber, 2010), which in turn, predicts positive mood, calmness, and life satisfaction.

Another potential level of analysis involves the use of imaging, such as functional magnetic resonance imaging (fMRI), to examine how behavioral variables and individual differences may relate to differences in brain anatomy and functioning among patients with specific difficulties (e.g., chronic pain, depression, obsessive-compulsive disorder). In one recent study, we attempted to investigate differences in gray matter density and resting-state functional connectivity and their interaction with PF in patients diagnosed with chronic migraines versus a control group (Karekla et al., 2019). Preliminary results suggest that PF helps explain some of the neurological differences between the two groups. This is the first study to demonstrate actual brain imaging differences in patients versus controls in relation to behavioral measures such as PF. Though more research is needed in this area before we can draw firm conclusions, imaging studies present another level of analysis that can be used to provide valuable information about anatomical and functional changes in the brain as a result of PF.

Individually, the studies we have described contribute to the literature on genetic polymorphisms, psychophysiological markers, imaging studies, and public health. Taken together, these studies begin to provide multilevel evidence that PF may represent a key mechanism of change relevant to numerous aspects of human behavior. If this proves robust in further analysis—both in and out of clinic settings and across levels—it can serve as an example of how to knit together processes of change relevant to diagnosis across levels of analysis ranging from biology to social context. We argue that any proposed process-based alterative to the DSM will need to show such properties in order to adequately facilitate interventions and to better promote mental and behavioral health.

Advantages of a Multilevel, Multi-method Approach

In this chapter, we have reviewed conditions that need to be addressed to facilitate the identification of sets of salient, functionally based mechanisms of action that promote treatment change. We posit that a multilevel, multi-method iterative approach increases the probability that identified mechanisms are relevant beyond the therapy room. The very process of exposing candidate mechanisms to the conditions described in this chapter increases their precision, and those that pass these tests have greater scope across a range of conditions and greater depth across levels of analysis.

In moving toward functional process-based alternatives to the DSM, we recommend that the following conditions be applied and tested for candidate mechanisms and models of sets of such mechanisms:

1. Target and isolate mechanisms of action. (If the target cannot be experimentally manipulated, then it will be of questionable use in interventions.)

2. Test the robustness across contexts (e.g., across various historical and situational conditions).

3. Test across different time frames to better understand how the behavior unfolds (e.g., examine behavior cross-sectionally and as it unfolds across time idiographically and utilize methodologies such as ESM).

4. Test across different levels of analysis (e.g., biological, genetic, psychophysiological, behavioral).

Using the example of PF, we have shown that implementing these recommendations raises a number of challenges. Rigorous debate will sometimes be needed in order to gain consensus about what constitutes the best unit of analysis. Different modalities of assessment will be necessary, and attention should be paid to the development of valid measures that can be used in different contexts. New methodologies may need to be explored, such as the use of complex network approaches. In all cases, assessment and treatment should constitute a continuous process of examination, evaluation, and application in an ongoing feedback loop.

These recommendations are not mutually exclusive categories. Indeed, individual studies may address multiple issues simultaneously. For example, one study can simultaneously address context via time-sensitive collection of variables that allows us to isolate antecedents and consequences of behavior across multiple levels of analysis. Our intention in making these recommendations is to help researchers and clinicians attend to the issues needed to move a process-based focus in intervention science toward a functional and contextual diagnostic nosology. It is our hope that when combined with coherent theory, the iterative approach laid out in this chapter will aid in the enormous effort needed to make meaningful progress toward our ultimate goal: to better serve those who seek our services by better coupling assessment methods and models with evidence-based interventions.

References

APA Presidential Task Force on Evidence-Based Practice. (2006). Evidence-based practice in psychology. *American Psychologist, 61*(4), 271–285. doi: 10.1037/0003-066X.61.4.271

American Psychiatric Association. (2013). *Diagnostic and statistical manual of mental disorders.* (5th ed.). Arlington, VA: Author.

American Psychological Association. (2017, February 24). Clinical practice guideline for the treatment of posttraumatic stress disorder (PTSD) in adults. Retrieved from http://www.apa.org/ptsd-guideline/ptsd.pdf

Appelhans, B. M., & Luecken, L. J. (2006). Heart rate variability as an index of regulated emotional responding. *Review of General Psychology, 10*(3), 229–240. doi: 10.1037/1089-2680.10.3.229

Arch, J. J., & Craske, M. G. (2008). Acceptance and commitment therapy and cognitive behavioral therapy for anxiety disorders: Different treatments, similar mechanisms? *Clinical Psychology: Science and Practice, 15*(4), 263–279. doi: 10.1111/j.1468-2850.2008.00137.x

Arch, J. J., Wolitzky-Taylor, K. B., Eifert, G. H., & Craske, M. G. (2012). Longitudinal treatment mediation of traditional cognitive behavioral therapy and acceptance and commitment therapy for anxiety disorders. *Behaviour Research and Therapy, 50*(7–8), 469–478. doi: 10.1016/j.brat.2012.04.007

Bak, M., Drukker, M., Hasmi, L., & van Jim, O. S. (2016). An n=1 clinical network analysis of symptoms and treatment in psychosis. *PLoS ONE, 11*(9), e0162811. doi: 10.1371/journal.pone.0162811

Bandelow, B., Zohar, J., Hollander, E., Kasper, S., Möller, H. J., Allgulander, C., ... Vega, J. (2008). World Federation of Societies of Biological Psychiatry (WFSBP) guidelines for the pharmacological treatment of anxiety, obsessive-compulsive and posttraumatic stress disorders–First revision. *World Journal of Biological Psychiatry, 9*(4), 248–312. doi: 10.1080/15622970802465807

Barnes-Holmes, D., Barnes-Holmes, Y., Luciano, C., & McEnteggart, C. (2017). From the IRAP and REC model to a multi-dimensional multi-level framework for analyzing the dynamics of arbitrarily applicable relational responding. *Journal of Contextual Behavioral Science, 6*, 434–445.

Barnes-Holmes, Y., Hayes, S. C., Barnes-Holmes, D., & Roche, B. (2002). Relational frame theory: A post-Skinnerian account of human language and cognition. In H. W. Reese & R. Kail (Eds.), *Advances in child development and behavior* (Vol. 28, pp. 101–138). New York: Academic Press.

Beard, C., Millner, A. J., Forgeard, M. J. C., Fried, E. I., Hsu, K. J., Treadway, M. T., ... Björgvinsson, T. (2016). Network analysis of depression and anxiety symptom relationships in a psychiatric sample. *Psychological Medicine, 46,* 3359–3369. doi: 10.1017/S0033291716002300

Belsky, J., Jonassaint, C., Pluess, M., Stanton, M., Brummett, B., & Williams, R. (2009). Vulnerability genes or plasticity genes? *Molecular Psychiatry, 14*(8), 746–754. doi: 10.1038/mp.2009.44

Borsboom, D. (2017). A network theory of mental disorders. *World Psychiatry, 16*(1), 5–13. doi: 10.1002/wps.20375

Boschloo, L., van Borkulo, C. D., Borsboom, D., & Schoevers, R. A. (2016). A prospective study on how symptoms in a network predict the onset of depression. *Psychotherapy and Psychosomatics, 85*(3), 183–184. doi: 10.1159/000442001

Christodoulou, A., Michaelides, M., & Karekla, M. (2018). Network analysis: A new psychometric approach to examine the underlying ACT model components. *Journal of Contextual Behavioral Science, 12,* 285–289. doi: 10.1016/J.JCBS.2018.10.002

Costantini, G., Epskamp, S., Borsboom, D., Perugini, M., Mõttus, R., Waldorp, L. J., & Cramer, A. O. J. (2015). State of the aRt personality research: A tutorial on network analysis of personality data in R. *Journal of Research in Personality, 54,* 13–29. doi: 10.1016/j.jrp.2014.07.003

Cramer, A. O. J., van der Sluis, S., Noordhof, A., Wichers, M., Geschwind, N., Aggen, S. H., ... Borsboom, D. (2012). Dimensions of normal personality as networks in search of equilibrium: You can't like parties if you don't like people. *European Journal of Personality, 26*(4), 414–431. doi: 10.1002/per.1866

Denson, T. F., Grisham, J. R., & Moulds, M. L. (2011). Cognitive reappraisal increases heart rate variability in response to an anger provocation. *Motivation and Emotion, 35*(1), 14–22. doi: 10.1007/s11031-011-9201-5

Denton, W. H., Carmody, T. J., Rush, A. J., Thase, M. E., Trivedi, M. H., Arnow, B. A., ... Keller, M. B. (2010). Dyadic discord at baseline is associated with lack of remission in the acute treatment of chronic depression. *Psychological Medicine, 40*(3), 415–424. doi: 10.1017/S0033291709990535

Deserno, M. K., Borsboom, D., Begeer, S., & Geurts, H. M. (2017). Multicausal systems ask for multicausal approaches: A network perspective on subjective well-being in individuals with autism spectrum disorder. *Autism, 21*(8), 960–971. doi: 10.1177/1362361316660309

Donkin, L., Christensen, H., Naismith, S. L., Neal, B., Hickie, I. B., & Glozier, N. (2011). A systematic review of the impact of adherence on the effectiveness of e-therapies. *Journal of Medical Internet Research, 13*(3), e52. doi: 10.2196/jmir.1772

Eisenlohr-Moul, T., Peters, J., & Baer, R. A. (2015). How do mindfulness-based interventions work? Strategies for studying mechanisms of change in clinical research. In B. D. Ostafin, M. D. Robinson, & B. P. Meier (Eds.), *Handbook of mindfulness and self-regulation* (pp. 155–170). New York: Springer.

Enge, S., Fleischhauer, M., Lesch, K-P., Reif, A., & Strobel, A. (2011). Serotonergic modulation in executive functioning: Linking genetic variations to working memory performance. *Neuropsychologia, 49,* 3776–3785. doi: 10.1016/j.neuropsychologia.2011.09.038

Enge, S., Fleischhauer, M., Lesch, K. P., Reif, A., & Strobel, A. (2014). Variation in key genes of serotonin and norepinephrine function predicts gamma-band activity during goal-directed attention. *Cerebral Cortex, 24*(5), 1195–1205. doi: 10.1093/cercor/bhs398

Enge, S., Fleischhauer, M., Lesch, K. P., & Strobel, A. (2011). On the role of serotonin and effort in voluntary attention: Evidence of genetic variation in N1 modulation. *Behavioural Brain Research, 216*(1), 122–128. doi: 10.1016/j.bbr.2010.07.021

Fisher, Medaglia, & Jeronimus, 2017, PNAS. Retrieved from: https://www.pnas.org/content/pnas/115/27/E6106.full.pdf

First, M. B., Rebello, T. J., Keeley, J. W., Bhargava, R., Dai, Y., Kulygina, M., ... Reed, G. M. (2018). Do mental health professionals use diagnostic classifications the way we think they do? A global survey. *World Psychiatry, 17*(2), 187–195. doi: 10.1002/wps.20525

Forsyth, J. P., & Sabsevitz, J. (2002). Behavior therapy: Historical perspective and overview. In M. Hersen & W. Sledge (Eds.), *Encyclopedia of psychotherapy* (2nd ed., pp. 259–275). New York: Academic Press.

Fried, E. I., Epskamp, S., Nesse, R. M., Tuerlinckx, F., & Borsboom, D. (2016). What are "good" depression symptoms? Comparing the centrality of DSM and non-DSM symptoms of depression in a network analysis. *Journal of Affective Disorders, 189*, 314–320. doi: 10.1016/J.JAD.2015.09.005

Geisler, F. C. M., Vennewald, N., Kubiak, T., & Weber, H. (2010). The impact of heart rate variability on subjective well-being is mediated by emotion regulation. *Personality and Individual Differences, 49*(7), 723–728. doi: 10.1016/j.paid.2010.06.015

Gloster, A. T., Gerlach, A. L., Hamm, A., Höfler, M., Alpers, G. W., Kircher, T., ... Reif, A. (2015). 5HTT is associated with the phenotype psychological flexibility: Results from a randomized clinical trial. *European Archives of Psychiatry and Clinical Neuroscience, 265*(5), 399–406. doi: 10.1007/s00406-015-0575-3

Gloster, A. T., Hummel, K. V., Lyudmirskaya, I., Hauke, C., & Sonntag, R. (2012). Aspects of exposure therapy in acceptance and commitment therapy. In P. Neudeck & H-U. Wittchen (Eds.), *Exposure therapy: Rethinking the model–Refining the method* (pp. --------------). New York: Springer.

Gloster, A. T., Klotsche, J., Ciarrochi, J., Eifert, G., Sonntag, R., Wittchen, H-U., & Hoyer, J. (2017). Increasing valued behaviors precedes reduction in suffering: Findings from a randomized controlled trial using ACT. *Behaviour Research and Therapy, 91*, 64–71. doi: 10.1016/j.brat.2017.01.013

Gloster, A. T., Klotsche, J., Gerlach, A. L., Hamm, A., Ströhle, A., Gauggel, S., ... Wittchen, H-U. (2014). Timing matters: Change depends on the stage of treatment in cognitive behavioral therapy for panic disorder with agoraphobia. *Journal of Consulting and Clinical Psychology, 82*(1), 141–153. doi: 10.1037/a0034555

Gloster, A. T., Meyer, A., Karekla, M., Hoyer, J., Mikoteit, T., Hatzinger, M., & Lieb, R. (under review). Having my stress & seeing you too: Daily stress, social interaction, & flexible vs. rigid response style.

Gloster, A. T., Meyer, A., & Lieb, R. (2017). Psychological flexibility as a malleable public health target: Evidence from a representative sample. *Journal of Contextual Behavioral Science, 6*, 166–171. doi: 10.1016/j.jcbs.2017.02.003

Gloster, A. T., Richard, D. C. S., Himle, J., Koch, E., Anson, H., Lokers, L., & Thornton, J. (2008). Accuracy of retrospective memory and covariation estimation in patients with obsessive-compulsive disorder. *Behaviour Research and Therapy, 46*(5), 642–655. doi: 10.1016/j.brat.2008.02.010

Hayes-Skelton, S. A., Calloway, A., Roemer, L., & Orsillo, S. M. (2015). Decentering as a potential common mechanism across two therapies for generalized anxiety disorder. *Journal of Consulting and Clinical Psychology, 83*(2), 395–404. doi: 10.1037/a0038305

Hayes, S. C., & Hofmann, S. G. (Eds.). (2018). *Process-based CBT: The science and core clinical competencies of cognitive behavioral therapy.* Oakland, CA: Context Press/New Harbinger Publications.

Hayes, S. C., Hofmann, S. G., Stanton, C. E., Carpenter, J. K., Sanford, B. T., Curtiss, J. E., & Ciarrochi, J. (2019). The role of the individual in the coming era of process-based therapy. *Behaviour Research and Therapy, 117,* 40–53. doi: 10.1016/j.brat.2018.10.005

Hayes, S. C., Luoma, J. B., Bond, F. W., Masuda, A., & Lillis, J. (2006). Acceptance and commitment therapy: Model, processes and outcomes. *Behaviour Research and Therapy, 44,* 1–25. doi: 10.1016/j.brat.2005.06.006

Hayes, S. C., Strosahl, K., & Wilson, K. G. (2012). *Acceptance and commitment therapy: The process and practice of mindful change* (2nd ed.). New York: Guilford Press.

Heeren, A., & McNally, R. J. (2016). An integrative network approach to social anxiety disorder: The complex dynamic interplay among attentional bias for threat, attentional control, and symptoms. *Journal of Anxiety Disorders, 42,* 95–104. doi: 10.1016/j.janxdis.2016.06.009

Hofmann, S. G., & Hayes, S. C. (2019). The future of intervention science: Process-based therapy. *Clinical Psychological Science, 7*(1), 37–50. doi: 10.1177/2167702618772296

Homberg, J. R., & Lesch, K. P. (2011). Looking on the bright side of serotonin transporter gene variation. *Biological Psychiatry, 69*(6), 513–519. doi: 10.1016/j.biopsych.2010.09.024

Isvoranu, A. M., Borsboom, D., van Os, J., & Guloksuz, S. (2016). A network approach to environmental impact in psychotic disorder: Brief theoretical framework. *Schizophrenia Bulletin, 42*(4), 870–873. doi: 10.1093/schbul/sbw049

Isvoranu, A. M., van Borkulo, C. D., Boyette, L-L., Wigman, J. T. W., Vinkers, C. H., & Borsboom, D. (2017). A network approach to psychosis: Pathways between childhood trauma and psychotic symptoms. *Schizophrenia Bulletin, 43*(1), 187–196. doi: 10.1093/schbul/sbw055

Jablonka, E., Lamb, M. J., & Zeligowski, A. (2005). *Evolution in four dimensions: Genetic, epigenetic, behavioral, and symbolic variation in the history of life.* Cambridge, MA: MIT Press.

Karekla, M., Vasileiou, V., Papacostas, S., Christou, G., Constantinidou, F., Eracleous, E., ... Constantinou, N. (2019, March). Altered grey matter density and resting-state functional connectivity among headache sufferers vs. matched controls. Poster presented at the Society for Behavioral Medicine Conference, Washington DC, USA.

Kashdan, T. B., & Rottenberg, J. (2010). Psychological flexibility as a fundamental aspect of health. *Clinical Psychology Review, 30*(7), 865–878. doi: 10.1016/j.cpr.2010.03.001

Kashdan, T. B., & Steger, M. F. (2006). Expanding the topography of social anxiety. *Psychological Science, 17*(2), 120–128. doi: 10.1111/j.1467-9280.2006.01674.x

Kazdin, A. E. (2007). Mediators and mechanisms of change in psychotherapy research. *Annual Review of Clinical Psychology, 3,* 1–27. doi: 10.1146/annurev.clinpsy.3.022806.091432

Koushiou, M. (2016). *Eating disorder risk: The role of sensitivity to negative affect and body-image inflexibility* (Unpublished doctoral dissertation). University of Cyprus: Nicosia, Cyprus.

Kraemer, H. C., Stice, E., Kazdin, A., Offord, D., & Kupfer, D. (2001). How do risk factors work together? Mediators, moderators, and independent, overlapping, and proxy risk factors. *American Journal of Psychiatry, 158*(6), 848–856. doi: 10.1176/appi.ajp.158.6.848

Kraepelin, E. (1896). *Lehrbuch de psychiatrie.* Leipzig, Germany: Barth.

Kupfer, D. J., First, M. B., & Regier, D. A. (2002). Introduction. In D. J. Kupfer, M. B. First, & D. A. Regier (Eds.), *A research agenda for DSM-V* (pp. xv–xxiii). Washington DC: American Psychiatric Association.

Levin, M. E., Hildebrandt, M. J., Lillis, J., & Hayes, S. C. (2012). The impact of treatment components suggested by the psychological flexibility model: A meta-analysis of laboratory-based component studies. *Behavior Therapy, 43*(4), 741–756. doi: 10.1016/j.beth.2012.05.003

Levin, M. E., MacLane, C., Daflos, S., Seeley, J. R., Hayes, S. C., Biglan, A., & Pistorello, J. (2014). Examining psychological inflexibility as a transdiagnostic process across psychological disorders. *Journal of Contextual Behavioral Science, 3*(3), 155–163. doi: 10.1016/j.jcbs.2014.06.003

MacKinnon, D. P., Fairchild, A. J., & Fritz, M. S. (2007). Mediation analysis. *Annual Review of Psychology, 58*(1), 593–614. doi: 10.1146/annurev.psych.58.110405.085542

McNally, R. J., Robinaugh, D. J., Wu, G. W. Y., Wang, L., Deserno, M. K., & Borsboom, D. (2015). Mental disorders as causal systems: A network approach to posttraumatic stress disorder. *Clinical Psychological Science, 3*(6), 836–849. doi: 10.1177/2167702614553230

Meaney, M. J. (2001). Maternal care, gene expression, and the transmission of individual differences in stress reactivity across generations. *Annual Review of Neuroscience, 24*(1), 1161–1192. doi: 10.1146/annurev.neuro.24.1.1161

Miron-Shatz, T., Stone, A., & Kahneman, D. (2009). Memories of yesterday's emotions: Does the valence of experience affect the memory-experience gap? *Emotion, 9*(6), 885–891. doi: 10.1037/a0017823

Molenaar, P. C. M. (2004). A manifesto on psychology as idiographic science: Bringing the person back into scientific psychology, this time forever. *Measurement: Interdisciplinary Research & Perspective, 2*(4), 201–218. doi: 10.1207/s15366359mea0204_1

Morgan, L. P. K., Graham, J. R., Hayes-Skelton, S. A., Orsillo, S. M., & Roemer, L. (2014). Relationships between amount of post-intervention mindfulness practice and follow-up outcome variables in an acceptance-based behavior therapy for generalized anxiety disorder: The importance of informal practice. *Journal of Contextual Behavioral Science, 3*(3), 173–178. doi: 10.1016/j.jcbs.2014.05.001

Mullins-Sweatt, S. N., & Widiger, T. A. (2009). Clinical utility and DSM-V. *Psychological Assessment, 21*(3), 302–312. doi: 10.1037/a0016607

Niles, A. N., Burklund, L. J., Arch, J. J., Lieberman, M. D., Saxbe, D., & Craske, M. G. (2014). Cognitive mediators of treatment for social anxiety disorder: Comparing acceptance and commitment therapy and cognitive-behavioral therapy. *Behavior Therapy, 45*(5), 664–677. doi: 10.1016/j.beth.2014.04.006

Pierce, W. D., & Epling, W. F. (1999). *Behavior analysis and learning* (2nd ed.). Upper Saddle River, NJ: Prentice Hall.

Rinner, M. T. B., Meyer, A. H., Mikoteit, T., Hoyer, J., Imboden, C., Hatzinger, M., … Gloster, A. T. (2019). General or specific? The memory-experience gap for individuals diagnosed with a major depressive disorder or a social phobia diagnosis, and individuals without such diagnoses. *Memory, 27*(9), 1194–1203. doi: 10.1080/09658211.2019.1640252

Ruzzano, L., Borsboom, D., & Geurts, H. M. (2015). Repetitive behaviors in autism and obsessive-compulsive disorder: New perspectives from a network analysis. *Journal of Autism and Developmental Disorders, 45*(1), 192–202. doi: 10.1007/s10803-014-2204-9

Savvides, S. N., & Karekla, M. (2014). Evaluating an acceptance and commitment therapy internet-based intervention for smoking cessation in young adults. *European Health Psychologist, 17*(S), 415.

Segal, Z. V., Williams, J. M. G., Teasdale, J. D., & Gemar, M. C. (2002). Mindfulness-based cognitive therapy for depression: A new approach to preventing relapse. *Clinical Psychology & Psychotherapy, 9*(2), 123–125. doi: 10.1080/713869628

Serfaty, S., Gale, G., Beadman, M., Froeliger, B., & Kamboj, S. K. (2018). Mindfulness, acceptance and defusion strategies in smokers: A systematic review of laboratory studies. *Mindfulness, 9*(1), 44–58. doi: 10.1007/s12671-017-0767-1

Siegel, S., Hinson, R. E., Krank, M. D., & Mccully, J. (1982). Heroin "overdose" death: Contribution of drug-associated environmental cues. *Science, 216*(4544), 436–437.

Skinner, B. F. (1953). *Science and human behavior.* New York: The Free Press.

Stone, A. A., & Shiffman, S. (1994). Ecological momentary assessment (EMA) in behavorial medicine. *Annals of Behavioral Medicine, 16,* 199–202.

Trull, T. J., & Ebner-Priemer, U. W. (2009). Using experience sampling methods/ecological momentary assessment (ESM/EMA) in clinical assessment and clinical research: Introduction to the special section. *Psychological Assessment, 21*(4), 457–462. doi: 10.1037/a0017653

Vilardaga, R., Hayes, S. C., Levin, M. E., & Muto, T. (2009). Creating a strategy for progress: A contextual behavioral science approach. *The Behavior Analyst, 32*(1), 105–133.

Vasiliou, S. V., Karademas, E.V., Christou, Y., Papacostas, S., & Karekla, M. (under review). Acceptance and commitment therapy for primary headache sufferers: A randomized controlled trial of efficacy.

Watson, D. (2004). Stability versus change, dependability versus error: Issues in the assessment of personality over time. *Journal of Research in Personality, 38*(4), 319–350. doi: 10.1016/j.jrp.2004.03.001

Weaver, I. C. G., Cervoni, N., Champagne, F. A., D'Alessio, A. C., Sharma, S., Seckl, J. R., ... Meaney, M. J. (2004). Epigenetic programming by maternal behavior. *Nature Neuroscience, 7*(8), 847–854. doi: 10.1038/nn1276

Whisman, M. A., & Baucom, D. H. (2012). Intimate relationships and psychopathology. *Clinical Child and Family Psychology Review, 15*(1), 4–13. doi: 10.1007/s10567-011-0107-2

Wickrama, K., O'Neal, C. W., & Holmes, C. J. (2017). Towards a heuristic research model linking early socioeconomic adversity and youth cumulative disease risk: An integrative review. *Adolescent Research Review, 2*(3), 161–179. doi: 10.1007/s40894-017-0054-3

Williams, K. E., Ciarrochi, J., & Heaven, P. C. L. (2012). Inflexible parents, inflexible kids: A 6-year longitudinal study of parenting style and the development of psychological flexibility in adolescents. *Journal of Youth and Adolescence, 41*(8), 1053–1066. doi: 10.1007/s10964-012-9744-0

World Health Organization. (2004). ICD-10: international statistical classification of diseases and related health problems: tenth revision. (2nd ed.). World Health Organization.

Yu, L., Norton, S., & McCracken, L. M. (2017). Change in "self-as-context" ("perspective-taking") occurs in acceptance and commitment therapy for people with chronic pain and is associated with improved functioning. *The Journal of Pain, 18*(6), 664–672. doi: 10.1016/j.jpain.2017.01.005

CHAPTER 11

Building a Process-Based Diagnostic System
An Extended Evolutionary Approach

Steven C. Hayes, PhD
University of Nevada, Reno

Stefan G. Hofmann, PhD
Boston University

Joseph Ciarrochi, PhD
Australian Catholic University

In the first chapter of this book, we argued that the world of evidence-based therapy was changing. In the pages that have followed, all of the chapter authors have, in one way or another, agreed.

Few intervention scientists still believe that an adequate field of evidence-based therapy will emerge from the continued evaluation and deployment of psychosocial protocols and medications focused on psychiatric syndromes. That era created progress, but it is hard to imagine that a decade or two on the same course will create much more. Do we really need the scores of new protocols that will undoubtedly emerge? Will the reorganization, elimination, and emergence of various sub-syndromes matter? Evidence suggests that effect sizes have fallen over the last three or four decades (e.g., Friborg & Johnsen, 2017; Johnsen & Friborg, 2015; Hofmann, Curtiss, Carpenter, & Kind, 2017), and no one would argue that the effectiveness of intervention is *improving*. But isn't improvement what we should expect of a progressive field of applied science?

Researchers and practitioners are shifting away from the "protocols-for-syndromes" strategy because intervention science has stagnated. The shift is palpable to any unbiased observer. Heralded by the Research Domain Criteria approach of the National Institute of Mental Health (RDoC; Insel et al., 2010) described in Chapter 2, this shift has shaken the field of evidence-based therapy to its roots. The field needs a new way forward, and as of yet, there is not agreement on a viable alternative.

The present volume is part of a larger effort to create this new path. It marks a return to the roots of evidence-based intervention. With respect to the roots of the behavioral and cognitive therapies, at least, it did not matter much which wing one came from. The message from the founders was similar.

Consider these quotes from the 1960s and '70s.

From the cognitive wing, Aaron Beck admonished therapists to "distinguish between a system of psychotherapy and a simple cluster of techniques," noting that such a system should have "a clear blueprint of the general principles and specific procedures of treatment" and that "a well-developed system provides (a) a comprehensive theory or model of psychopathology and (b) a detailed description of and guide to therapeutic techniques related to this model" (1976, p. 278 for all quotes).

The behavior modifiers of the time agreed. In their initial defining article on behavior analysis, Don Baer, Mont Wolf, and Todd Risley said that a defining quality of evidence-based behavioral interventions is that "the published descriptions of its procedures are not only precisely technological, but also strive for relevance to principle," and they warned against the use of a mere "collection of tricks" unrelated to basic principles because these "historically have been difficult to expand systematically" (1968, p. 96 for all quotes).

Behavior therapists of the time likewise wanted to know "what treatment, by whom, is most effective for this individual with that specific problem, under which set of circumstances, and how does it come about?" (Paul, 1969, p. 44), and they defined behavior therapy as experientially tested intervention methods linked to and explained by "operationally defined learning theory" (Franks & Wilson, 1974, p. 7).

Every wing of the behavioral and cognitive therapies began its scientific and practical journey with a commitment both to evidence-based procedures and to evidence-based theories, models, principles, and processes of change. Syndromal diagnosis interrupted that journey, but we should remember that these original purposes were not canceled out or obliterated by the syndromal strategy. Intervention science still hoped to get to processes of change, functional diagnosis, and intervention kernels. The detour into "protocols for syndromes" was not homegrown by evidence-based psychotherapists—its origins were in academic psychiatry—but at the beginning, one could plausibly hope that it could have been the needed impetus to achieve the vision of the founders of evidence-based therapy.

Syndromes and the Purposes of Diagnosis

Topographically focused diagnosis and classification is a primitive scientific strategy sometimes deployed early in the development of a scientific field when functional knowledge is limited. With academic medicine, theorists cluster problems into sets of empirically related complaints ("symptoms") and formal features ("signs") with the hope of identifying etiological causes of these sets, mechanistic details of their course, and coherent responses to different types of treatment, gradually producing a *functional* understanding in place of a mere topographical description. When these features are clear, we are no longer dealing with syndromes but with functional entities called diseases.

Topographical classification had shown itself to be a useful beginning strategy in the history of science, but it faltered when few functional processes gave rise to a variety of topographies, or when a topography could be produced by a variety of functional processes. The fields of botany and oncology contain well-known example of these limits.

In botany, consider toadflax and peloric toadflax. These two plants look similar except for their completely different flowers. Carl Linnaeus argued in the 1700s that they were different species. In the mid 1800s, Darwin showed that the peloric variety bred true, supporting Linnaeus.

We now know that these plants are genetically identical. They have a dramatically different appearance and can breed true because of heritable *epigenetic* differences. Appearances could never have resolved this issue or directed researchers to its source. The epimutation responsible for peloric toadflax was apparent only when scientists identified epigenetic mechanisms in the lab and developed accurate assessments of these mechanisms. Then, it was a simple matter to test the two flowers and understand why genetically identical plants could look so different.

In a similar example, treatment success with many varieties of cancer did not soar until the underlying mechanisms of tumor growth were better understood. Mere appearances of different tumors and lesions did not lead to this understanding—it came from studying oncogenes and other processes that lead to the development of cancer. Appearances did not direct researchers toward the underlying processes because they led to far too many topographical appearances.

Our point is that syndromal classification is merely a strategy. That strategy is not hostile to the ultimate scientific and practical goals of evidence-based therapy, but it is largely orthogonal to them in fact. Mental health research has been galvanized for half a century by the assumption that human suffering reflects different latent diseases that might be functionally understood by studying categories of syndromal diagnosis. At this point in the volume, it is worth reviewing what we would hope for from diagnosis so we can assess the viability of the process-based alternative and compare it to the progressivity in a syndromal approach (for more on the broader context of a process-based approach, see Hayes & Hofmann, 2018). Syndromal diagnosis promised progress in every area that diagnosis hoped to address, but it only delivered in one or two.

A Common Language

One promise of a diagnostic nosology is having a common language that funders, providers, researchers, and the public can use to describe people and their problems. In principle, any reliable diagnostic system can provide this. The *Diagnostic and Statistical Manual of Mental Disorders* (DSM) was indeed successful in getting its terms adopted, but a more granular examination shows clear signs of difficulty in this area. For example, the most common DSM-IV diagnosis in clinical practice was "NOS" or "not otherwise specified" (e.g., Fairburn & Bohn, 2005), and a similar pattern is unfolding in the DSM-5 with a new manifestation of this term known as "not elsewhere classified" (American Psychiatric Association, 2013). Further, in many areas, the DSM still shows low reliability of diagnostic categories and high levels of unexplained comorbidity (Hyman, 2010; Jacobi et al., 2004).

Destigmatization and Empowerment

Theorists have frequently argued that the latent-disease assumptions that are built into syndromal diagnosis reduce enacted and self-stigma and thus empower people who are facing mental health issues. The actual data are less supportive. People are indeed less likely to blame the individual when they believe that mental health issues are the result of latent disease (Corrigan et al., 2002).

That benefit, however, comes at a very high long-term cost. Over time, belief in a latent disease *increases* some aspects of stigma and self-stigma, such as feeling that it is impossible to change, fearing that a person is dangerous, or reducing life horizons (Ben-Zeev, Young, & Corrigan, 2010; Corrigan & Watson, 2004). Patients can also experience "diagnostic overshadowing," in which physicians misattribute physical health problems to mental health issues (Thornicroft, Rose, & Kassam, 2007).

We can lay many of these problems at the feet of reification (Hyman, 2010). Syndromes are abstractions, but we treat them as concrete entities people *have*. The latent-diseases connotation exacerbates this tendency by giving syndromes pseudoscientific causal power for the very patterns of behavior that led to the diagnostic labels themselves. In the popular mind, if not in that of therapists, depression is a cause of depressed mood, obsessive-compulsive disorder (OCD) is a cause of obsessions, panic disorder is a cause of anxiety, and so on.

Once people are in this mindset, it is easy to think medications are a required treatment since latent diseases are a biomedical concept. In the United States, over ninety percent of those suffering with mental health issues receive medications, and two-thirds of those receive nothing else (Olfson & Marcus, 2010). Given the known and long-lasting side effects of psychoactive medications, these ratios are upside down from what an objective analysis of treatment benefits would lead us toward. Meanwhile, whereas psychosocial interventions for DSM syndromes and sub-syndromes are ever more specific, there is hardly a category of syndromes for which selective serotonin reuptake inhibitors (SSRIs) are not prescribed, undermining the supposition that syndromes are biomedical diseases in hiding.

Conceptual Utility and Causal Understanding

The hope of syndromes is that we will learn about etiological causes, mechanistic details of their course, and coherent responses to different types of treatment. A clear sign of success would be for at least a few syndromal entities to transition to diseases status. That never happens. The last condition to undergo that transition was general paresis, and untreated syphilis is not a modern issue. Because of the widespread use of a few medications, response to treatment in a statistical sense has become less and less related to diagnosis over time, not more.

The DSM-5 workgroup concluded that there were no sensitive and specific biomarkers for any of the DSM syndromal entities (Kupfer, First, & Regier, 2002), a situation that remains unchanged. A recent study with full genomic analyses of up to a quarter of a million people found that the thirteen most commonly studied "candidate genes" relevant to major depression were no more likely to relate to this condition than were thirteen randomly selected genes (Border et al., 2019).

The billions of dollars of funding that have been poured into syndromal research have yielded interesting and useful data about how mental health problems often unfold as well as data on how processes of change can lead to their exacerbation or amelioration, but these findings do not, on the whole, line up with syndromal classification per se. Furthermore, in the absence of a clearer focus on processes of change, many of these data are buried and given little attention.

Treatment Utility and Progress

Ideally, diagnosis would help providers select treatments that maximize outcomes (the "treatment utility" of assessment; Hayes, Nelson, & Jarrett, 1987) and also allow them to optimize and tailor their interventions. It would also allow for the development of new and more effective treatment methods with better outcomes ("treatment progress"). With syndromal diagnosis, that simply has not occurred. The DSM itself declares that the system does not have known treatment utility.

Building a Process-Based Alternative

In chapter 1, we laid out the bones of a process-based alternative to the DSM. The chapters that followed have supported the basic outlines of such an approach. In this section, we review the process-based proposal and how it connects to current trends before we return to the Extended Evolutionary Meta-Model (EEMM) to see if we can use it as a beginning framework for process-based diagnosis.

In chapter 1, we argued that processes of change are theory-based, dynamic, progressive, contextually bound, modifiable, and multilevel changes or mechanisms that occur in predictable, empirically established sequences oriented toward desirable outcomes. We argued that, in order to assemble known processes into a useful process-based system, we need to focus on those processes of change that are high in precision, scope, and depth; that are immediately and repeatedly measurable; that have been vetted ideographically and not just at the level of collectives; that have been shown to be functionally important in the achievement of outcomes; and that have coherent moderators. We proposed a meta-model of both adaptive and maladaptive sets of processes of change with six psychological dimensions and two additional levels of analysis crossed with the four key evolutionary issues of variation, selection, retention, and context. We can understand specific models of change processes in terms of this meta-model. At their best, process-based models assemble a variety of existing processes of change into sets that are philosophically consistent and clear, that are potent and relatively comprehensive in the range of dimensions and levels they can adequately address, and that are broadly applicable across problem and prosperity goals—that is, they are "transdiagnostic" and beyond. These models are "versatile" in that they address **V**ariation and **R**etention of what is **S**elected in **C**ontext at the right **D**imension and **L**evel (VRSCDL; Hayes, Stanton, Sanford, Law, & Ta, in press) and can be used to ask evolutionarily sensible (Tinbergen, 1963) questions regarding the *function, history, development,* and *proximal mechanisms* of processes of change and how they can combine to produce particular behavioral conditions or phenotypes.

The RDoC initiative described in chapter 2 also took a multidimensional and multilevel approach. The emphasis in that chapter was on physical and psychosocial elements that might contribute to neurodevelopmental processes that RDocC presumes to underlie psychopathology. That emphasis can be seen in Figure 2.1, in which neural development involving genes, molecules, and cells is linked to behavioral dimensions via brain circuits. This is a bet on the progressivity of an elemental realist view of human complexity driven by a "back-to-the-lab" strategy to uncover the processes that lead to latent diseases. The jury is still out on this approach, and while we applaud the focus on processes of change, we are concerned that it would be better to link these processes from the beginning to practical issues of treatment selection and impact.

Chapter 3 began this pragmatic approach by exploring a social constructionist and systems perspective on a process-based approach. While not explicitly linked to an extended evolutionary synthesis, it is worth noting the many overlaps. Chapter 3 emphasized the role of context and of the dynamical systems nature of psychopathology. From the evolutionary perspective described in chapter 1, psychopathology refers to a set of self-sustaining biopsychosocial processes that restrict healthy variation, selection, or retention, and these processes are sensitive to context and occur in a variety of dimensions or levels relevant to psychological functioning. In brief, it is an adaptive peak that prevents further positive behavioral development via normal evolutionary processes. Chapter 3 takes a very similar stance, even though it begins from a different philosophical viewpoint. In particular, chapter 3 emphasizes that psychopathology involves "solutions" that create problems in a vicious cycle. The author presents mastery by avoidance as an archetypal example. He suggests that all successful models and therapies note, interrupt, and redirect vicious cycles in order to note, create, and support virtuous cycles. This idea fits fully within the functional and contextual approach encouraged by an extended evolutionary perspective.

Chapter 4 distinguished vulnerability mechanisms (established and relatively unchangeable susceptibilities to stress) from processes of change or "response mechanisms." Vulnerability mechanisms are moderators of change processes. We agree that moderators are key, although only extensive research will allow this sorting, and some of the vulnerability mechanisms listed—such as distress tolerance or even some personality traits (see Roberts & Mroczek, 2008)—are on a continuum with change processes.

Chapters 5 and 6 explored how human cognition might impact other dimensions of psychological functioning. There is a good reason that we call mental health problems "mental": Almost always, language and cognition play some role in psychopathology. We see this in the pervasive impact of cognitive expectations, which therapists can alter to increase treatment impact in areas such as anxiety and depression (chapter 5). We also see this in how cognitive processes establish and alter one's sense of self—a dimension of known importance to psychopathology (chapter 6). These chapters make it clear that any adequate process model needs to include verbal and self-related processes.

In chapter 7, the authors explored individual variability in emotions and how this variation is influenced by temperamental, social, and cultural factors. They argue that biologically established temperamental factors interact with familial and cultural factors to shape emotion and its role across the lifespan in a specific, idiographic way. Emotional problems are themselves bound by these interactions. The chapter provides support for the idea that process models need to be vetted idiographically and not just at the level of collectives (Hayes et al., 2019).

Chapter 8 showed how a complex systems approach offers conceptual and methodological tools to create a process-based diagnostic system. Evolutionary theory is a special case of complex network analysis, and thus it is not surprising that the theoretical concepts that flow from a complex network (e.g., resilience, fluctuation, tipping points, and so on) all resonate with issues of contextually situated multidimensional, multilevel variation, selection, and retention. Chapter 8 underlined issues of self-sustaining cycles (both vicious and virtuous, as discussed in chapters 1 and 3) and the need to create system perturbation.

Chapters 9 and 10 explored one of the better-known process-based models: psychological flexibility (PF). The PF model has core sets of change processes focused on each of the six psychological dimensions in the EEMM. These chapters give rigidity and flexibility (issues of variation) clear attention, with measures and intervention kernels noted. Accordingly, we view research on PF as a "proof of concept" of a process-based approach. Chapter 9 explored its success in chronic pain, while chapter 10 showed how a contextually bound, idiographic, longitudinal, and multilevel approach is yielding applied progress.

We did not select the authors of this volume with consilience as an explicit goal, but the review we have just done shows that this is very much what emerged. A process-based approach thought of in extended evolutionary terms naturally extends across the empirical and conceptual issues that we need to face in a process-based approach to diagnosis. However, two questions remain: Can we turn it into a practical system? And, importantly, would such a system be acceptable to different wings of psychotherapy (e.g., psychodynamic, cognitive-behavioral, acceptance-based)? If we can say yes to both questions, then we have a diagnostic pathway forward that could transcend theoretical and philosophical orientations. It would allow people to communicate across islands and work together to build an intervention science more adequate to the human condition.

The Deathstar Project

Our first major step to see if this is possible has been to conduct a massive meta-analysis of mediators of treatment outcomes. We included every known major (and often minor) therapy in the search terms. This allowed us to address two important questions: First, what do different psychotherapies consider to be the key mechanisms of action? And, second, can we understand these mechanisms within the evolutionary process umbrella?

Mediation is the primary way researchers have examined processes of change in treatment outcomes. As a method, it admittedly leaves much to be desired (Hayes et al., 2019), as mediation can only handle a tiny number of variables (generally only one mediator is examined empirically), and researchers assume processes of change are related in a linear, non-recursive way to treatment and, subsequently, to outcome. We only consider change processes at the level of the collective, despite the non-ergodic nature of human processes of change, thus violating a key assumption of process-based analysis (Hofmann, Curtiss, & Hayes, in press). Despite the weaknesses of mediation analysis, though, we have committed to a complete meta-analysis of the world's scientific literature on mediation to help launch a process-based diagnostic alternative to the DSM because of the important attributes of meditational results and the strengths of a comprehensive meta-analysis in this area.

Before we describe the project in more detail, as well as the data it is yielding, it is worth thinking through how different this approach is to syndromal diagnosis. By starting at the pragmatic end of the hoped-for outcome of classification—that is, treatment utility—and then backing up into a conceptual and categorical scheme, we can design a process-based alternative from the beginning to achieve all of the key goals of diagnosis we reviewed earlier in this chapter. We can note them in reverse order.

A process can have treatment utility only if we can reliably measure it and show it to mediate the link between clinical intervention and outcome. This is a major reason we focused on mediational research. To this day, syndromal diagnosis does not have known treatment utility. Mediators, in contrast, are processes of change with proven treatment utility: by definition, they are functionally important pathways to outcomes that have been differentially moved by intervention and that have been shown to relate to outcomes when controlling for treatment.

If we can systematize these processes underneath the umbrella of an extended evolutionary synthesis, then we will have concepts of known pragmatic importance that can take advantage of the consilience that evolutionary theory provides (Wilson, 1999). Coherent concepts leading to pragmatic outcomes is a virtual operational definition of conceptual utility. If we can examine proposed mediators of change from a wide variety of clinical frameworks, and yet understand them within the EEMM, then we will have demonstrated conceptual consilience.

What about destigmatization and empowerment? Focusing on moderators combined with multilevel, multidimensional change processes found in history and circumstance is a destigmatizing way to consider a life story. Biomedicalization of human problems, by contrast, is inert or harmful to reduced stigma (Pescosolido et al., 2010). Furthermore, because processes of *change* are (by definition) not passive entities, process-based diagnosis is far less likely to be disempowering to the person than is syndromal diagnosis. Most often, processes of change are things people *do*, not things people *have*. Moderators and context alter how these processes of change apply, allowing greater cultural and individual sensitivity.

Our process-based model gives us a common language. We see no reason that it cannot quickly lead to ways of describing "disorders" based on adaptive peaks. For example, we can see the time coming when people may speak of cognitive inflexibility disorders, experiential avoidance disorders, and so on.

The What and Why of the Deathstar Project

We named the Deathstar project after the Star Wars artificial planet that was gigantic, took forever to build, loomed in outer space, and could severely disrupt ongoing activities. Deathstar is a large meta-analysis that seeks to identify the known mediators of intentional behavior change in mental and behavioral health. It addresses several questions, such as: What mediators have the strongest support? Can we organize mediators in terms of evolutionary theory? What moderates mediator effectiveness?

The review is inclusive. It includes all bona fide psychotherapeutic intervention/experimental studies, as well as all psychotherapeutic orientations and major therapeutic outcomes, including anxiety, depression, behavioral change, work effectiveness, psychosocial disability, valued living, quality of life, and recidivism/relapse. Using very broad search criteria, we identified nearly 55,000 potential mediational studies. Multiple raters conducted abstract screenings, resulting in nearly 110,000 independent ratings from which they identified approximately 1,500 articles that potentially meet criteria for mediation.

We are now reading and categorizing the studies that may contain mediators. The screening will determine the final number, but we already know that some of these studies will not be legitimate mediational studies and that the same mediator will be identified in several studies. Thus, although the number is not yet known, we will likely be dealing with many scores (if not hundreds) of mediators drawn from several hundred studies of mediation.

Categorizing Studies of Mediation

We will categorize each of these studies according to the EEMM. We also plan to consider all mediators sorted into physiological or sociocultural level to see if a dimensional system emerges for these levels.

Because our approach to the construction of a process-based alternative to the DSM has been largely empirical (other than seeking a way to do so within the potential consilience provided by an extended evolutionary account), we can only broadly characterize where this approach is taking us. Consider the following six mediators, each of which we identified in the first dozen studies to be fully screened: change in obsessive beliefs, cognitive defusion, mindful awareness, change in intrusive thoughts, anxiety sensitivity, and frequency of mindfulness practice. These six concepts apply easily to cognitive, attentional, and affective dimensions. With the exception of the last concept, each is focused on fostering healthy variation. Mindful awareness and anxiety sensitivity carry with them issues of positive and negative contextual sensitivity; frequency of mindfulness practice addresses a retention process in the form of habit formation.

When we develop a reliable scoring system based on the meta-model for all identified mediations, we suspect that most of the cells will contain several processes to consider. If we identify moderators and dynamical or interactive features, then we will link each of these change processes in a cell to other dimensions, levels, or columns. The assessment tools used for each process will provide a preliminary form of assessment for researchers and practitioners to consider. At that point, we can consider the degree to which existing models of therapeutic change can bear on a coherent summary of these processes.

Because every single process identified by the Deathstar project will have already been shown to have moved by a specific form of treatment, we will also then have a list of interventions methods that researchers have shown to move processes in each cell. Thus, it seems likely that we will be able to link most cells to measures, processes of change, and intervention methods or kernels, at least broadly. All other things being equal, models that efficiently cover more of this matrix will be more useful; those that cover less of it will be less useful.

Even before we can present a fully organized empirical account of the world's literature on mediation, however, we can still explore what such a system might yield. Even with a limited set of processes to consider, the EEMM approach suggests a way forward.

Process-Based Diagnosis and Therapy: The Basic Approach

We have defined *therapeutic processes of change* as a set of theory-based, dynamic, progressive, context-dependent, and multilevel changes that occur in predictable, empirically established sequences oriented toward the desirable outcomes (Hofmann & Hayes, 2019). As we noted in chapter 1, these processes are:

- *theory-based* because they are associated with a clear statement of relations among events and lead to testable predictions and method of influence;

- *dynamic* because processes may involve feedback loops and nonlinear changes;

- *progressive* because they may need to be arranged in an order to reach the treatment goal;

- *contextually bound and modifiable* to focus on their implications for practical changes and intervention kernels within reach of practitioners; and

- *multilevel* because some processes supersede or are nested within others.

In this process-based approach, psychological problems are not person-invariant expressions of a latent disease. Instead, we understand psychopathology as context-specific problems in variation, selection, and retention issues that can occur in a variety of dimensions and levels. This is the core idea of the Extended Evolutionary Meta-Model shown in Figure 11.1 (repeated from chapter 1) that we base on evolutionary science, adapted to psychopathology and psychotherapy.

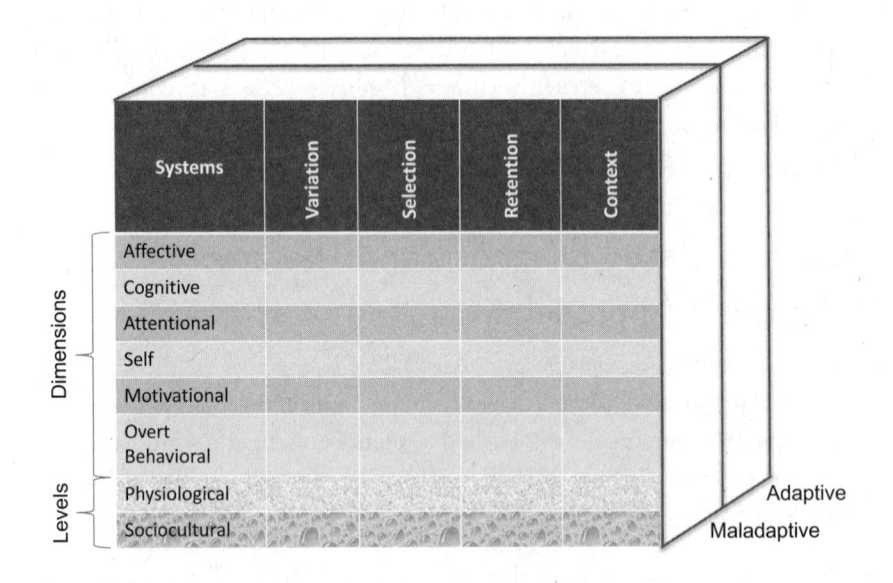

Figure 11.1. The Extended Evolutionary Meta-Model of Processes of Change
(© Steven C. Hayes and Stefan G. Hofmann. Used by permission.)

Because we need to link processes of change to the idiographic level, a good place to begin in process-based diagnosis is to link identified problems by using a complex network approach to foster a functional analysis of an individual's presenting problems. We can then apply the EEMM framework while considering all relevant past and present contributing factors such as early life history, attachment styles, traumas, medical issues, beliefs, behavioral patterns, and so on.

We can provide a practical example. In one of our process-based therapy workshops, a participant sent the network shown in Figure 11.2. She listed the features of the case and guessed about what led to what with a variety of directional arrows. The specific problems are depicted as nodes connected through arrows (what are called "edges" in complex networks) that can form unidirectional and bidirectional relationships.

When developing such client-based networks, we encourage clinicians to begin with descriptive language and even the words of the client to capture the essence of the primary concerns. Some of the edges and nodes might be emboldened to illustrate the centrality of a problem and its functional connection with other nodes. At this point in the process, linking the network to data and sequence is more important than a process-based interpretation. Before we return to process, let's consider the treatment purpose of network thinking.

We think of treatment as a dynamic change of the complex network from maladaptation to adaptation. In such dynamic networks, we encode temporal information in the edges or arrows. This conveys insight into the time-series relationships between nodes. Temporal networks can provide information about relationships between nodes across different measurement windows, which might reveal whether certain nodes predict other nodes.

We can do this conceptually but also empirically during a high temporal density baseline assessment. When done empirically, we specify directed edges to represent partial regression coefficients connecting different nodes. Both autoregressive and cross-lagged effects are possible because each node is regressed onto both itself and other time-lagged nodes.

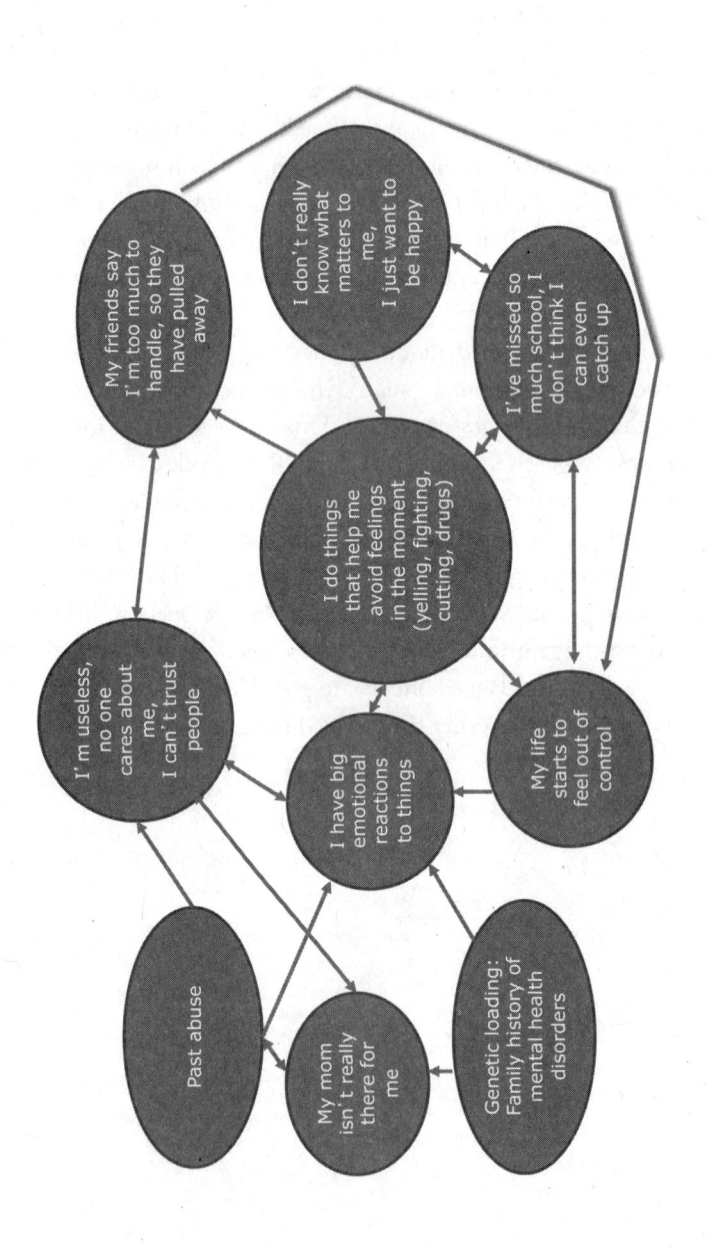

Figure 11.2. A Client Network

(© Steven C. Hayes and Stefan G. Hofmann. Used by permission.)

We thus find processes of change in the "edges" (the arrows) or in larger sub-networks. In accord with the ideas in this volume, a focus should be on parts of the network that could be self-amplifying (negatively so in problem diagnosis, but positively so in treatment planning). Any double-headed arrow can be self-amplifying. So too can any network of three or more nodes in which an output from one could be an input to another, and then to another, and then back to the first one in a kind of merry-go-round fashion. We focus on these self-amplifying parts because, in resonance with the systems approach described in chapter 3, we view psychopathology as context-specific problems in variation, selection, and retention issues. In considering maintaining factors, diagnosis thus needs to focus on self-amplifying aspects of the network.

So too does treatment planning. Network changes can happen suddenly when repeated (or single) strong perturbations cause the complex network to lose its resilience, going over a tipping point into a different attractor state. We can depict such a change in the stability of a network as a ball rolling across a valley and hill (see Figure 11.3).

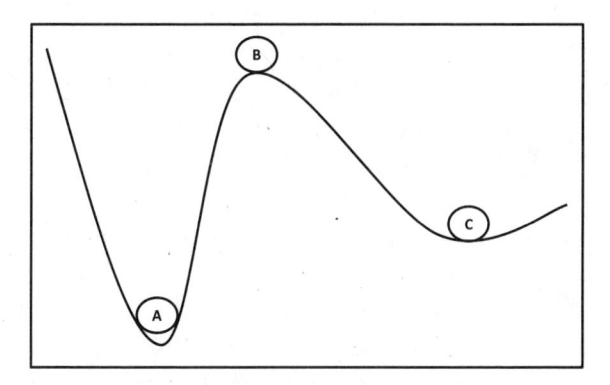

Figure 11.3. Changes in Network Stability.
From a complex network perspective, change from a non-pathological to a pathological stage may be depicted by a ball moving from one stable state (position A) over a tipping point (position B) to another stable state (position C).

A network is more resilient and stable if the valley is deep (position A) because it requires more effort to move the ball out of the valley and over the hill. Once the ball reaches the tipping point (position B), a sudden and dramatic shift can occur even after a small additional perturbation. As a result, the network undergoes a dramatic shift, leading to a new, alternative, and stable state (position C). Depending on a variety of factors, the new state may be more or less resilient to change. The example shown in Figure 11.3 suggests that the new network structure is relatively less resilient to change because the valley is shallow (position C), and we require less effort to move the ball out of the valley. If this is applied to a psychopathological network, it would be good news for our client because less effort is necessary to reinstate the non-pathological state.

Example

To illustrate how a network analysis could feed a new form of diagnosis, one might imagine a client who became depressed after a recent relationship break-up. As depicted in Figure 11.4, suppose a client is going through a divorce and as a result is worrying, feeling depressed, and lonely. Most central to his problems are his feelings of loneliness and negative self-perception. Both variables have edges (relationships with other nodes) that are stronger in magnitude than other nodes, as reflected by the thickness of the arrows depicted. In addition, these nodes are more influential than the other variables in accounting for the functioning of the network, as shown by the thickness of the node borders. These variables can also be bidirectionally related, as shown by the connections between loneliness and negative self-perception and between negative self-perception and feelings of depression. Thus, the client's break-up led to more loneliness, which then entered a recursive and self-amplifying relationship with negative self-perception and feelings of depression.

From an EEMM approach, repertoire-narrowing issues of self, affect, and social dimensions occupy critical nodes. Given this, the therapist may decide that it is important to intervene on the client's negative self-perception and loneliness, as these are the two influential nodes in the network.

Suppose the therapist believes that a key feature of this network is that loneliness is leading to a narrow, negative, and rigid view of the self as being unworthy or unlovable, fostering both a self-amplifying process with depressed mood (with depressed mood being both a result of this view of the self and a goad exacerbating it) and a further sense of social disconnection and feelings of loneliness.

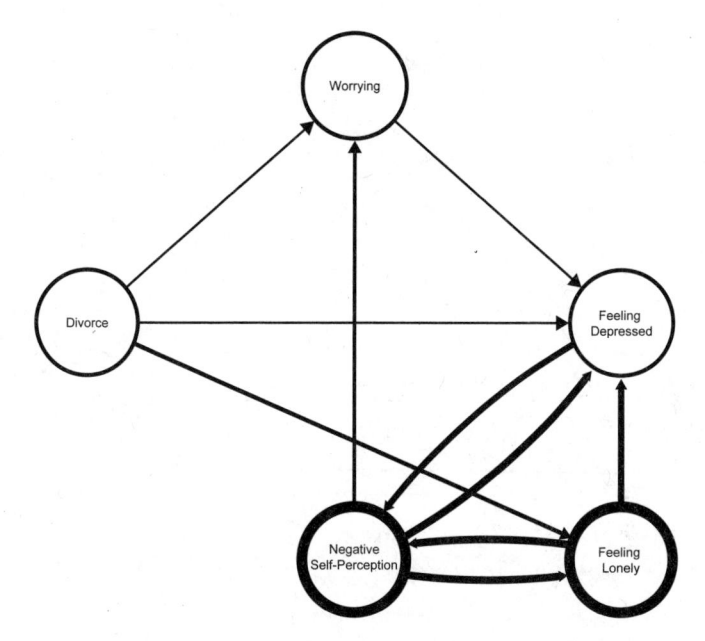

Figure 11.4. Network Structure of an Example Client

(© Steven C. Hayes, Stefan G. Hofmann & Joseph Ciarrochi. Used by permission.)

Focusing on this process account, several techniques might be conceivable to perturbate the system. Suppose the therapist introduces self-compassion meditation as a treatment strategy and teaches the client to apply this skill when he feels lonely, perhaps while remembering how he felt as a lonely child so as to be more kind to himself. The goal might be to introduce another competing view of the self in which loneliness is not proof of being unworthy or unlovable; instead, it is an indication of a time when the client needs greater self-kindness and compassion. This perturbates the system by changing the functional roles of the needed nodes in the network. Suppose that the client's network now reflects the presence of this more adaptive process. It might change the network significantly, undermining the relationship of loneliness to depression and negative views of the self and fostering its relationship to self-compassion. If self-compassion, in turn, reduces a sense of loneliness and poor self-image and moderates the relationship between worry and depressed mood, then a new and more adaptive network arrangement might emerge with self-amplifying adaptive features (see Figure 11.5).

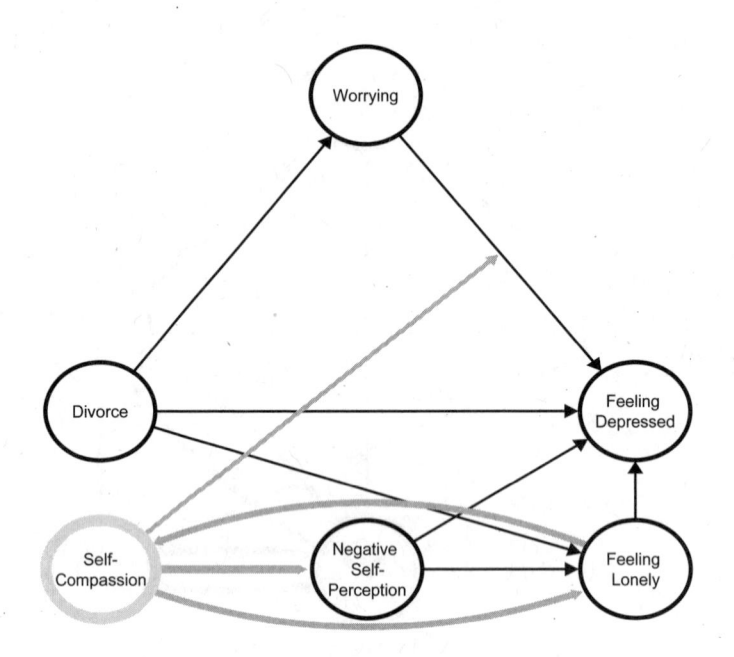

Figure 11.5. Applying Network Thinking to the Example Client

(© Steven C. Hayes, Stefan G. Hofmann & Joseph Ciarrochi. Used by permission.)

This example illustrates how a new form of functional analysis might emerge from process-based diagnosis. Maladaptive nodes, edges, and self-amplifying sub-networks become weaker, as suggested by (a) thinner borders and (b) a reduction in the existence or strength of harmful edges (i.e., negative self-perception to worrying, loneliness leading to negative self-perception, and negative self-perception to feeling depressed). The two features that were originally most influential (i.e., loneliness and negative self-perception) have lost their dominance in this network except as inputs to the now dominant node of self-compassion.

It is important to feed complex network analyses the right information, assessed with high fidelity and frequency. Thus, the practitioner needs both adequate theory and assessment technology to mount the use of dynamical systems in case conceptualization. To date, many of the network analyses have been based on assessments focused on self-reports of syndromal features (e.g., signs and symptoms) as distinct from contextual factors, biological measures, overt behavioral measures, or measures focused specifically on change processes such as cognitive flexibility or emotional openness. We need high temporal density measures for change processes to be modeled as nodes in complex networks. Traditional psychometrics is likely not adequate filter since it too is based on implausible ergodic assumptions (Molenaar, 2008). Any weakness in assessment limits a network-based case conceptualization and its treatment utility. Thus, this new form of process-based diagnosis will inexorably lead to a number of major changes in evidence-based therapy.

Applying the Extended Evolutionary Meta-Model in Clinical Situations

Even before the results of the Deathstar project become known, the EEMM combined with idiographic network analysis provides a structure for a treatment-relevant approach to process-based diagnosis. We can organize an approach to *process-based diagnosis* with the following nine steps:

1. Select a theory or model within which to conduct treatment-relevant process-based diagnosis, focusing on models that are reasonably comprehensive as considered within the EEMM and that best fit the setting, population, and background of the practitioner.

2. Using case description and the formal practical repeated measurements that best fit the case (including measures drawn directly from session transcripts and client behavior in session), and considering the client's goals, describe the longitudinal relationships among the features of the case. Wherever possible, rely on empirically established relationships at the idiographic level. Be relatively inclusive of features, provided they may be relevant to known processes of change and to client goals and fit with provider competence as specified by step 1.

3. Assess a range of strengths and weakness in the client's repertoire linked to processes of change in the relevant dimensions and levels in the meta-model, within the theory or model being applied by the practitioner.

4. Considering the client's goals, organize the network of features of the case into known change processes and moderators of these

processes, focusing in particular on self-amplifying sub-networks within the network. Add measures of process and outcomes as needed. Collect additional information if needed.

5. Organize these processes into an integrative, process-based account of the development and maintenance of the maladaptive network. This account is the functional analysis of the case. It is the process-based diagnosis.

6. Consider how to perturbate the dominant features of the network expressed in process-based terms, either directly or indirectly, but make particular consideration of changes that are available, known to respond to intervention, likely to be retained, likely to alter the idiographic functional relations within the maladaptive parts of the client network, and likely to enter idiographically, self-amplifying features of a new adaptive network.

7. Considering the therapeutic context and relationship, select a series of intervention kernels or methods that are most likely to perturbate the network in that fashion.

8. Intervene while continuing to repeatedly measure key change processes, the therapeutic context and relationship, and progress toward client goals.

9. Recycle based on both process and outcome impact.

As knowledge of processes of change increase and measures become more sophisticated, many of these steps can become more automated and empirical. For example, as automated measures of outcomes or settings (or repeated measures of processes of change) advance, step 2 may become more routine, and steps 3 through 7 may be more driven by big data. In just a few months, we hope to offer a comprehensive empirical list of processes of change within specified dimensions and levels. We expect to find some overlap in more conceptual attempts, such as that expressed in chapter 4.

Our existing clientele cannot wait for the future. Thus, in process-based training, we have found it useful to teach idiographic conceptual network analysis and to then link the self-amplifying parts of these networks to the meta-model and repeated assessments.

Consider the network shown in Figure 11.2. You will notice that the nodes of this network are simply features of the case that seem possibly important. Any well-trained practitioner could generate the bones of such a network for any of their clients. We have not changed so much as a word from the network we were sent.

Because chapters 9 and 10 were on the PF model (Hayes, Strosahl, & Wilson, 2012), it is not difficult for us to try to apply that model to this network. We show the psychopathological version of PF in preliminary form within the EEMM in Figure 11.6. Each of the six inflexibility processes restricts healthy variation in each of the six dimensions in the meta-model. They also all alter healthy selection, retention, and context-sensitivity processes, but they appear to do so most especially in the areas we have indicated. If we apply these concepts to the network in Figure 11.2, then Figure 11.7 is relatively easy to generate. Three self-amplifying edges or sub-networks stand out, each interlinked and connected to plausible moderators.

Dimensions / Levels	Systems	Variation	Selection	Retention	Context
Dimensions	Affective	Experiential Avoidance	X	X	X
	Cognitive	Fusion	X	X	X
	Attentional	Inflexible Attention			X
	Self	Conceptualized Self			X
	Motivational	Absent or Unclear Values	X		
	Overt Behavioral	Impulsivity / Inaction / Avoidant Persistence		X	
Levels	Physiological				
	Sociocultural				

Adaptive / Maladaptive

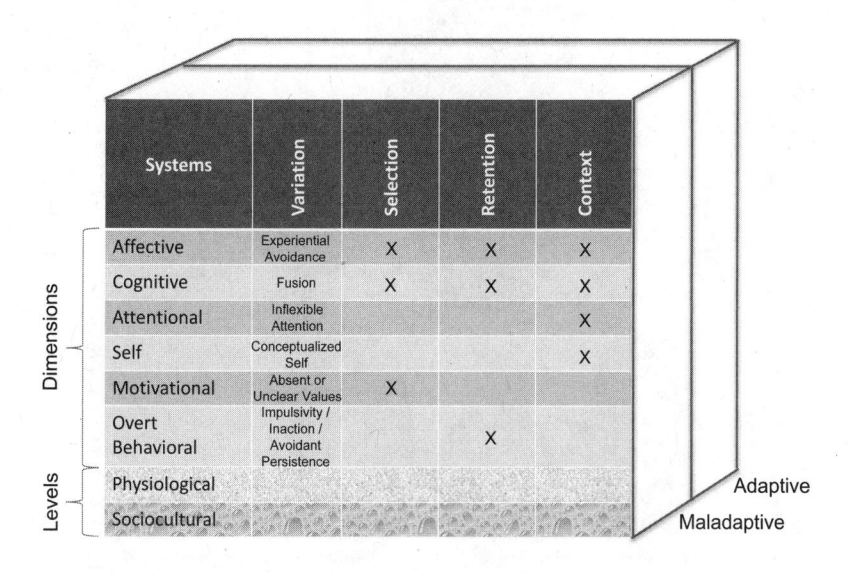

Figure 11.6. The Maladaptive Version of the Psychological Flexibility Model, Organized in Terms of the EMMM.

(© Steven C. Hayes and Stefan G. Hofmann. Used by permission.)

274 Beyond the DSM

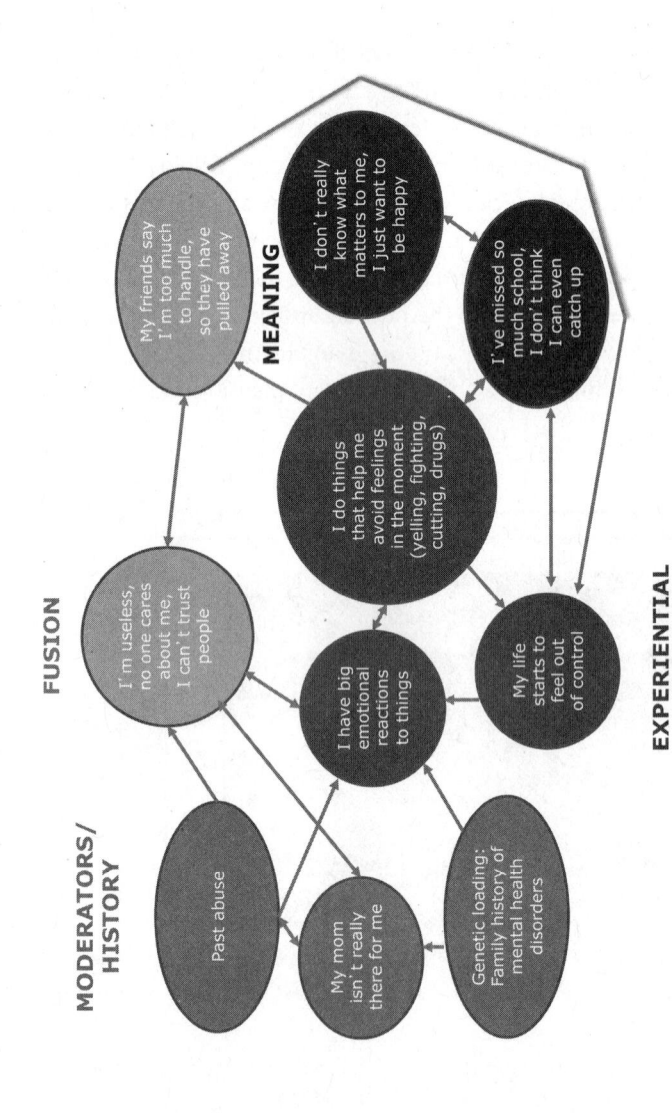

Figure 11.7. The Client Network in Figure 11.2 Considered in Terms of the Model Shown in Figure 11.6

(© Steven C. Hayes and Stefan G. Hofmann. Used by permission.)

In the context of Figure 11.6, a person-specific process-based diagnosis is now possible. This person shows affective, self, and cognitive inflexibility, likely initially fostered by abuse. Avoidance is used in the affective domain to a pathological degree and has self-amplified. Yelling, fighting, cutting, and drug use all dampen excessive emotional reactions at the cost of feeling out of control and exacerbating emotional responses themselves. Meanwhile, this core negative process is supported by a dominant core set of thoughts that craft a view of the self and others: *I'm useless, no one cares, and people are untrustworthy*. The behavioral impact of these change processes on school leads to a sense of lack of motivation and a "just be happy" stance that actually fosters drug use and other destructive forms of self-soothing. Said in a few words within the model shown in Figure 11.6, this case represents an abuse-fostered experiential avoidance and social trust disorder that is supported by a fusion with a conceptualized self and conceptualized others and an absence of chosen values.

In session, the therapist might test this analysis even before intervention. For example, the therapist might watch out for avoidance of emotional content in session by the client through the situational equivalent of "yelling and fighting," such as quarrelling with the therapist when difficult material is raised. If the therapist shows concern and caring in such situations, then it might be worth noting if this leads the client to exhibit a "you don't care about me" posture with the therapist. Thus, in-session behaviors might become de facto measures of change processes and be integrated into the evidence base for a process-based diagnosis.

In terms of treatment selection, it is worth emphasizing that, unlike traditional syndromal diagnosis, all of these processes are changeable. The therapist could directly target core features of destructive emotional avoidance—perhaps by teaching and modeling acceptance or distress tolerance skills. An alternative might be to enter into a deep values-based conversation, perhaps even linking it to the past abuse so issues of trust can be shifted from "I can trust people" to "I can trust myself to add in my deepest interests." That might increase school-based behavior, reduce the excesses of "yelling, fighting, cutting, and drug use," and maintain healthy friendships. If the therapist chooses to focus on either acceptance- or values-based work, then they could use both the therapeutic relationship and intervention kernels to change these processes, and then assess the impact on processes and outcomes.

Conclusion

We believe the field of intervention science already has the elements of a process-based alternative to the DSM in its hands. In this chapter, we have shown how we can proceed empirically and conceptually, beginning with what we know about processes of change and combining that knowledge with empirical and conceptual idiographic network analysis. Many aspects of the nine-step process-based diagnosis approach have already been tested. For example, we know that basing interventions on empirically established idiographic functional relations leads to better clinical outcomes (e.g., Fisher, 2015; Fisher, Medaglia, & Jeronimus, 2018). We know that using intervention kernels linked to client need, rather than entire named protocols, is more efficient and effective (e.g., Weisz et al., 2012).

What we want from a diagnostic system is not what we are getting from psychiatric syndromes. It is time to take the field in a bold new direction.

References

American Psychiatric Association. (2013). *Diagnostic and statistical manual of mental disorders* (5th ed). Arlington, VA: Author.

Baer, D. M., Wolf, M. M., & Risley, T. R. (1968). Some current dimensions of applied behavior analysis. *Journal of Applied Behavior Analysis, 1*, 91–97.

Beck, A. T. (1976). *Cognitive therapy and the emotional disorders.* New York: Penguin.

Ben-Zeev, D., Young, M. A., & Corrigan, P. W. (2010). DSM-V and the stigma of mental illness. *Journal of Mental Health, 19*(4), 318–327. doi: 10.3109/09638237.2010.492484

Border, R., Johnson, E. C., Evans, L. M., Smolen, A., Berley, N., Sullivan, P. F., & Keller, M. C. (2019). No support for historical candidate gene or candidate gene-by-interaction hypotheses for major depression across multiple large samples. *American Journal of Psychiatry, 176*(5), 376–387. doi: 10.1176/appi.ajp.2018.18070881

Corrigan, P. W., Rowan, D., Green, A., Lundin, R., River, P., Uphoff-Wasowski, K., ... Kubiak, M. A. (2002). Challenging two mental illness stigmas: Personal responsibility and dangerousness. *Schizophrenia Bulletin, 28*(2), 293–309.

Corrigan, P. W., & Watson, A. C. (2004). At issue: Stop the stigma: Call mental illness a brain disease. *Schizophrenia Bulletin, 30*, 477–479.

Franks, C. M., & Wilson, G. T. (1974). *Annual review of behavior therapy: Theory and practice.* New York: Brunner/Mazel.

Fairburn, C. G., & Bohn, K. (2005). Eating disorder NOS (EDNOS): An example of the troublesome "not otherwise specified" (NOS) category in DSM-IV. *Behaviour Research and Therapy, 43*(6), 691–701. doi: 10.1016/j.brat.2004.06.011

Fisher, A. J. (2015) Toward a dynamic model of psychological assessment: Implications for personalized care. *Journal of Consulting and Clinical Psychology, 83*, 825–836. doi: 10.1037/ccp0000026.

Fisher, A. J., Medaglia, J. D., & Jeronimus, B. F. (2018). Lack of group-to-individual generalizability is a threat to human subjects research. *Proceedings of the National Academy of Sciences, 115*(27), E6106–E6115.

Friborg, O., & Johnsen, T. J. (2017). The effect of cognitive-behavioral therapy as an antidepressive treatment is falling: Reply to Ljòtsson et al. (2017) and Cristea et al. (2017). *Psychological Bulletin, 143*(3), 341–345. doi: 10.1037/bul0000090

Hayes, S. C., & Hofmann, S. G. (Eds.). (2018). *Process-based CBT: The science and core clinical competencies of cognitive behavioral therapy*. Oakland: Context Press/New Harbinger Publications.

Hayes, S. C., Hofmann, S. G., Stanton, C. E., Carpenter, J. K., Sanford, B. T., Curtiss, J. E., & Ciarrochi, J. (2019). The role of the individual in the coming era of process-based therapy. *Behaviour Research and Therapy, 117*, 40–53. doi: 10.1016/j.brat.2018.10.005

Hayes, S. C., Nelson, R. O., & Jarrett, R. (1987). Treatment utility of assessment: A functional approach to evaluating the quality of assessment. *American Psychologist, 42*, 963–974. doi: 10.1037//0003-066X.42.11.963

Hayes, S. C., Stanton, C. E., Sanford, B. T., Law, S., & Ta, J. (in press). Becoming more versatile: Using evolutionary science to suggest innovations in ACT. Chapter to appear in M. E. Levin, M. P. Twohig, & J. Krafft (Eds), *Recent Innovations in ACT*. Oakland, CA: New Harbinger Publications.

Hayes, S. C., Strosahl, K., & Wilson, K. G. (2012). *Acceptance and commitment therapy: The process and practice of mindful change* (2nd ed.). New York: Guilford Press.

Hofmann, S. G., Curtiss, J., Carpenter, J. K., & Kind, S. (2017). Effect of treatments for depression on quality of life: A meta-analysis. *Cognitive Behaviour Therapy, 46*(4), 265–286. doi: 10.1080/16506073.2017.1304445

Hofmann, S. G., Curtiss, J. E., & Hayes, S. C. (in press). Beyond linear mediation: Toward a dynamic network approach to study treatment processes. *Clinical Psychological Science*. doi:10.1016/j.cpr.2020.101824

Hofmann, S. G., & Hayes, S. C. (2019). The future of intervention science: Process-based therapy. *Clinical Psychological Science, 7*(1), 37–50. doi: 10.1177/2167702618772296

Hyman, S. E. (2010). The diagnosis of mental disorders: The problem of reification. *Annual Review of Clinical Psychology, 6*, 155–79. doi: 10.1146/annurev.clinpsy.3.022806.091532

Insel, T., Cuthbert, B., Carvey, M., Heinssen, R., Pine, D. S., Quinn, K., ... Wang, P. (2010). Research Domain Criteria (RDoC): Toward a new classification framework for research on mental disorders. *American Journal of Psychiatry, 167*(7), 748–751. doi: 10.1176/appi.ajp.2010.09091379

Jacobi, F., Wittchen, H-U., Hölting, C., Höfler, M., Pfister, H., Müller, N., & Lieb, R. (2004). Prevalence, co-morbidity and correlates of mental disorders in the general population: Results from the German Health Interview and Examination Survey (GHS). *Psychological Medicine, 34*(4), 597–611. doi: 10.1017/S0033291703001399

Johnsen, T. J., & Friborg, O. (2015). The effects of cognitive behavioral therapy as an anti-depressive treatment is falling: A meta-analysis. *Psychological Bulletin, 141*(4), 747–768.

Kupfer, D. J., First, M. B., & Regier, D. A. (2002). Introduction. In D. J. Kupfer, M. B. First, & D. A. Regier (Eds.), *A research agenda for DSM-V* (pp. xv–xxiii). Washington DC: American Psychiatric Association.

Molenaar, P. (2008). Consequences of the ergodic theorems for classical test theory, factor analysis, and the analysis of developmental processes. In S. M. Hofer & D. F. Alwin (Eds.), *Handbook of cognitive aging: Interdisciplinary perspectives* (pp. 90–104). Thousand Oaks, CA: SAGE. doi: 10.4135/9781412976589.n5

Olfson, M., & Marcus, S. C. (2010). National trends in outpatient psychotherapy. *American Journal of Psychiatry, 167*(12), 1456–1463. doi: 10.1176/appi.ajp.2010.10040570

Paul, G. L. (1969). Behavior modification research: Design and tactics. In C. M. Franks (Ed.), *Behavior therapy: Appraisal and status* (pp. 29–62). New York: McGraw-Hill.

Pescosolido, B. A., Martin, J. K., Long, J. S., Medina, T. R., Phelan, J. C., & Link, B. G. (2010). "A disease like any other"? A decade of change in public reactions to schizophrenia, depression, and alcohol dependence. *American Journal of Psychiatry, 167*(11), 1321–1330. doi: 10.1176/appi.ajp.2010.09121743

Roberts, B. W., & Mroczek, D. (2008). Personality trait change in adulthood. *Current Directions in Psychological Science, 17*(1), 31–35.

Thornicroft, G., Rose, D., & Kassam, A. (2007). Discrimination in health care against people with mental illness. *International Review of Psychiatry, 19*(2), 113–122. doi: 10.1080/09540260701278937

Tinbergen, N. (1963). On aims and methods of ethology. *Zeitschrift für Tierpsychologie/Journal of Animal Psychology, 20*(4), 410–433.

Weisz, J. R., Chorpita, B. F., Palinkas, L. A., Schoenwald, S. K., Miranda, J., Bearman, S. K. ... Gibbons, R. D. (2012). Testing standard and modular designs for psychotherapy treating depression, anxiety, and conduct problems in youth: A randomized effectiveness trial. *Archives of General Psychiatry, 69*(3), 274–282.

Wilson, E. O. (1999). *Consilience: The unity of knowledge.* New York: Vintage.

Editor **Steven C. Hayes, PhD**, is Nevada Foundation Professor in the department of psychology at the University of Nevada, Reno. He has been president of numerous professional organizations, is author of forty-five books and nearly 650 scientific articles, and is among the most cited living psychologists. He has shown in his research how language and thought leads to human suffering, and is originator and codeveloper of acceptance and commitment therapy (ACT): a powerful therapy method that is useful in a wide variety of areas; relational frame theory (RFT): an empirical program in language and cognition; and process-based therapy (with Stefan G. Hofmann).

Editor **Stefan G. Hofmann, PhD**, is professor of psychology in the department of psychological and brain sciences at Boston University. He has been president of numerous professional organizations, and is currently editor in chief of *Cognitive Therapy and Research*. He has published more than 400 peer-reviewed journal articles and twenty books. He is a highly cited researcher, and has received many awards, including the Humboldt Research Award. His research focuses on the mechanism of treatment change, translating discoveries from neuroscience into clinical applications, emotion regulation, and cultural expressions of psychopathology. He is codeveloper (with Steven C. Hayes) of process-based therapy.

Index

A

about this book, 17–18, 257–259
acceptance: emotion, 145; pain-related, 205; PF studies on, 206, 207, 208, 210, 231; suppression or avoidance vs., 227
Acceptance and Action Questionnaire, 203
acceptance and commitment therapy (ACT), 51; outcome studies based on, 209, 214; relational frame theory and, 119, 126
adjunctive skills training, 93
American Psychological Association, 49, 50
analogies, therapeutic use of, 124–125
analysis: correlational, 207–208; dynamical system, 70, 173; functional, 181; mediation, 208–210, 229–232; multilevel, 238–241; network, 8, 174–176, 237, 268–271; time series, 70; transcript, 8, 69
Andrews, Leigh A., 165
anticipatory reactions, 99
anxiety disorders: chronic pain and, 205; contextual sensitivity and, 262; expectations related to, 100; exposure therapy for, 104; RDoC-themed research on, 36; TDMs linked to, 85, 86, 87, 88, 89
appraisal theory, 141
arbitrarily applicable relational responding (AARR), 119
arousal/regulatory systems, 27
assessment: ecological momentary, 69, 188; psychological flexibility, 202–203; RDoC approach to, 34

assumptions: continuity, 115–116, 117, 118, 119; philosophical, 11–12
attention deficit/hyperactivity disorder, 36
attractor, 169, 170–171, 173
attractor landscapes, 171, 182–184
authoritarian parenting, 147, 235
authoritative parenting, 147, 235

B

Baer, Don, 252
Barlow, David, 49
Barnes-Holmes, Dermot, 115
Barnes-Holmes, Yvonne, 115
Barthel, Abigail L., 137
Beck, Aaron T., 58, 97, 252
behavior: contextual factors and, 234; examining over time, 235–238; Skinner's definition of, 233
behavior therapy, 2–3, 252
behavioral activation, 51, 58
behavioral genetics, 14
behavioral observation, 8
behavioral science, 115
Bergin and Garfield's Handbook of Psychotherapy and Behavior Change (Lambert), 49
bifactor model, 203
big data methods, 39, 189
biomedicalization of problems, 261
borderline personality disorder (BPD), 85, 86, 151
botany, field of, 253
bottom-up approach, 69
brain: imaging studies of, 241; predictions generated by, 99, 102
BSNIP study, 35–36, 39
butterfly effect, 64

C

cancer treatment, 253–254
candidate mechanisms, 226–227, 242
caregiver responses, 147
case formulation model, 77
catastrophizing, 210
CBT. *See* cognitive behavioral therapy
change: cascading results of, 64; considering types of, 181–187; constancy/stability and, 63, 65; core strategies for, 92; first- vs. second-order, 55–57, 60, 71; minor adjustments as type of, 184–186; principles of system, 168–172; relapses following, 188. *See also* processes of change
Changes to the RDoC Matrix (CMAT) workgroup, 37
chronic pain: effectiveness of CBT for, 199; expectations related to, 101, 102, 105; fear-avoidance model of, 205; psychological flexibility and, 201–216
Chronic Pain Acceptance Questionnaire, 202
Chronic Pain Values Inventory, 203
Ciarrochi, Joseph, 1, 251
client-based networks, 264–267, 268–271, 274
Clinical Handbook of Psychological Disorders (Barlow), 49
cognitive behavioral therapy (CBT): changes based on TDM classification, 90–91; cognitive frame offered in, 60; decline in effectiveness of, 215–216; depression treatment with, 105; evidence supporting use of, 3–4, 51; for intolerance of uncertainty, 75–76; modern behavioral science and, 116; transdiagnostic protocols based on, 75–76
cognitive defusion, 202, 204, 206, 227, 231

Cognitive Fusion Questionnaire, 202
cognitive immunization strategies, 109, 112
cognitive systems, 27, 97
cognitive therapy, 58
coherence of relational responding, 129
coherent moderators, 10
collectivistic cultures, 142–143
combinatorial entailment, 120
committed action, 203, 205, 206, 227
Committed Action Questionnaire, 203
common factors, 50
common language, 254
common problems, 56, 57
compassion-oriented strategies, 145, 269
complex network approach, 68, 70
complex systems perspective, 168–190; change induction process, 181–187; future possibilities and challenges, 188–190; indicators of dynamic resilience, 172; measurement methods, 172–176; metaphorical descriptions, 171; networks and processes, 177–181; principles of system change, 168–172; psychotherapeutic application, 176–187; relapse prediction, 188
complexity of relational responding, 129
Comprehensive Coping Inventory-Revised (CCI-R), 83; preliminary validation study, 83–85; symptoms related to subscales of, 85–89
computational psychiatry, 38–39
conflict mapping, 171, 180
context: change processes understood in, 15, 64; definition of, 233; examining events in, 233–235; problem patterns and cultural, 66; variation and selective retention in, 15
contextual cues, 120
contextual variables, 233

contingency learning, 15
continuity assumption, 115–116, 117, 118, 119
coordination relations, 124–125
correcting experiences, 106
correlational analyses, 207–208
culture: emotion influenced by, 141–144, 151–152; problem patterns related to, 66
culture-bound syndromes, 151
Cuthbert, Bruce, 23

D

Deathstar project, 261–263
decentering process, 231
deictic stimulus relations, 126–127
depression: complex system perspective on, 178–181; decentering process for, 231; EBCT treatment for, 186–187; evidence-supported treatments for, 57–59; expectations related to, 100–101, 105; maintaining processes in, 179; process and change in, 59–61; research on genes related to, 256; rumination-focused CBT for, 76; TDMs linked to, 85, 86, 87, 89
Depression, Anxiety, and Stress Scale (DASS), 86–88
depth of change process, 5
derived responses, 128–129
destigmatization, 254–255, 261
developmental processes, 28
diagnosis: common language of, 254; process-based, 264, 270, 271–272, 275, 276; purposes of, 253–256; syndromal, 1, 2, 252, 254–256; uncoupling of treatment and, 225–226
Diagnostic and Statistical Manual of Mental Disorders (DSM), 1; common language as promise of, 254; medical model underlying, 71; problems with, 24, 74, 225
diagnostic overshadowing, 255

Doan, Stacey N., 137
Dynamic Assessment Treatment Algorithm (DATA), 174, 180
dynamical system analyses, 70, 173

E

early warning signals, 172, 173
eating disorders, 240
ecological momentary assessment (EMA), 69, 188
EEMM. *See* Extended Evolutionary Meta-Model
effortful control, 148
Ellis, Albert, 97
emotion, 137–152; cultural influences on, 141–144, 151–152; expression of, 143–144, 147; human experience of, 137–138; individual variability in, 138–139, 148–149; infant temperament and, 139, 148–149; psychopathology and, 148–152; regulation of, 144–147, 150, 151; social influences on, 139–141, 149–151
emotional flexibility, 146–147
emotional schemas, 75
emotionality/neuroticism, 148
emotion-focused therapy (EFT), 51, 60
empathic joining, 60
empowerment, 255, 261
enabling technology, 41
Engaged Living Scale, 203
environmental factors, 28, 30–31
equivalence relations, 118, 120
ergodic theorem, 7, 9
evidence-based therapy, 2–4, 251, 252
evidence-supported relationships (ESRs), 50
evidence-supported treatments (ESTs), 49, 57–59
evolutionary science, 14–17; behavioral genetics and, 14; extended meta-model based on, 16–17; six key concepts from, 15–16

expectations, 97–112; case example of modifying, 106–108; disorder descriptions and, 109; interventions to violate, 104–106, 109–110, 111; mental disorders related to, 100–102; special role of, 97–99; treatment selection and, 109–110; ViolEx-model of, 103, 105
experience sampling methodology (ESM), 69, 236–237
Experiences Questionnaire, 202
experiential avoidance, 75, 146, 231
exposure therapy, 51, 104–105
exposure-based cognitive therapy (EBCT), 178, 180, 186–187
expression of emotions, 143–144, 147
Extended Evolutionary Meta-Model (EEMM), 16–17, 256, 264, 271–273

F

fear-avoidance model, 205
feedback loops, 179
first-order change, 55–56, 60
5HTT polymorphism study, 239–240
flexibility: emotional, 146–147; relational response, 129. *See also* psychological flexibility
frames, therapeutic, 60–61
Frank, Rochelle I., 73
Fraser, J. Scott, 47
functional analysis, 181, 270
functional connectivity methods, 176
functional magnetic resonance imaging (fMRI), 241
functional pathways of change, 9–10

G

Garvey, Marjorie, 23
General Vulnerabilities Questionnaire (GVQ), 82
generalization problem, 229
generalized anxiety disorder (GAD), 231
genomic mapping, 14

Gloster, Andrew T., 225
Gottman, John, 64
GridWare program, 173
grief, complex, 101
Group Iterative Multiple Model Estimation (GIMME) method, 8
group theory, 59
Guide to Treatments That Work, A (Nathan and Gorman), 49

H

harm reduction, 184–185
Hayes, Adele M., 165
Hayes, Steven C., 1, 251
HDML framework, 131–132
Heart and Soul of Change, The (Duncan, Miller, Wampold, and Hubble), 50
heart rate variability (HRV), 240
Hegel, G. W. F., 53
Heraclitus, 53, 54, 63, 65
HERE-THERE relations, 126
Hofmann, Stefan G., 1, 137, 251

I

idiographic processes, 6–8, 131, 145, 276
individualistic cultures, 142–143
infant temperament, 139, 148–149
inhibitory learning, 116–117
in-session measures, 8
Institute of Advanced Studies (IAS), 189
instructional control, 116, 117
International Classification of Diseases and Related Health Problems (ICD), 1, 24, 225
interpersonal emotion regulation, 144, 146, 150
interpersonal therapy (IPT), 51, 58, 60
intervention science, 9, 252–253, 276
interventions: delivering based on RDoC, 32–35;

expectation-violation, 104–106, 109–110, 111; functional categorization of, 92–93
intolerance of uncertainty, 75
intractable conflict, 171, 182
intrapersonal processes, 144, 145–146
I-YOU relations, 126

J

Jobs, Steve, 41

K

Karekla, Maria, 225
Kuhn, Thomas, 47, 52, 71

L

language: continuity assumption and, 117; diagnostic use of common, 254; mental state, 140
learning: contingency, 15; inhibitory, 116–117
Leibniz, Gottfried, 53
levels of analysis, 238–241
lifespan development, 32
Linnaeus, Carl, 253

M

manualized treatments, 73
McCracken, Lance M., 199
McEnteggart, Ciara, 115
McKay, Matthew, 73
MDML framework, 127, 128–132
measurement: of change processes, 8–9; complex systems theory, 172–176; instruments for TDM, 82–83; multi-measurement designs, 29; psychological flexibility, 202–211
mechanisms of action, 226–227, 229, 232, 238, 242
mediation: categorizing studies of, 262–263; explanatory overview of, 229–230; meta-analysis of, 260, 261–262; psychological flexibility and, 208–210, 231–232; statistical, 229–230, 231
mediator variables, 74, 230
medical model, 47–48, 55, 61, 71
medications, psychoactive, 255
mental disorders: contemporary model of, 24–25; developmental processes and, 28; environmental influences on, 28, 30–31; expectations related to, 100–102. *See also* psychopathology
mental state language, 140
meta-analysis on mediation, 260, 261–262
meta-level alliance, 66–67
metaphors: complex system theory, 171, 182; therapeutic use of, 124–125
Mind and Emotions Protocol, 83
Mindful Attention Awareness Scale, 203
mindfulness, 76, 92, 185, 204, 231, 262
mindfulness-based therapy, 51, 60, 185, 231
mixed methods design, 74
mobile health (mHealth) approach, 189
models of change processes, 10–13; essential characteristics of, 12–13; Extended Evolutionary Meta-Model, 16–17, 256, 264, 271–273; philosophical assumptions in, 11–12
moderator variables, 74, 230, 261
Morris, Sarah, 23
multilevel analysis, 238–241
multilevel, multi-method approach, 227, 241–242
multilevel selection, 16
multiple exemplar training, 121
Murphy, Eric, 23
mutual entailment, 120, 128, 129–130

N

National Advisory Mental Health Council (NAMHC), 37

National Institute of Mental Health (NIMH): Data Archive, 39–40; National Advisory Mental Health Council, 37; Research Domain Criteria, 2, 23–41, 74, 166, 252
Natya Shastra (ancient Indian text), 137
negative emotions, 140, 143, 144
negative feedback loops, 64
negative valence systems, 27
network analyses, 8, 174–176, 237, 268–271
network destabilization and transition (NDT) model, 178, 182–184, 187
network intervention analysis (NIA), 175
network theory, 171, 177
networks: analysis of, 8, 174–176, 237, 268–271; examples of client-based, 264–267, 268–271, 274; pathological, 177–179, 267, 268; stability changes in, 267–268; temporal, 265
niche construction, 15–16
NIMH. *See* National Institute of Mental Health
nomothetic generalizations, 8
NOW-THEN relations, 126

O

objectivism, 48
observers, systems defined by, 62–63
obsessive-compulsive disorder (OCD), 101, 102
organicist metaphor, 11

P

pain. *See* chronic pain
panic disorder, 100, 101, 231, 232
paradigm shifts, 47–48, 51–52, 70–71
parents: authoritative vs. authoritarian, 147, 235; cultural influence of, 143; emotional development related to, 147, 149–150; teaching parenting styles to, 185; verbal self and abusive, 127

pathological networks, 177–179, 267, 268
patterns: attractor, 169; process view of, 68–69; self-similar, 63–64; shifts in, 62, 63
Paul, Gordon, 3
perfectionism, CBT for, 76
perseverative processes, 85, 87–88
Personality Assessment Inventory (PAI), 85–86
PF. *See* psychological flexibility
phase transitions, 170
phobias, 101
placebo effects, 98
positive blockade, 180
positive emotions, 140, 143, 144
positive feedback loops, 64
positive valence systems, 27
post-traumatic stress disorder (PTSD), 101, 102
precision of change process, 5
predictions, 99, 102, 109, 111
present-focused attention, 203, 204, 206, 227, 231
PRISM project, 39
Process and Reality (Whitehead), 53
process view, 53–55; principles of, 62–65; research approaches from, 67–70, 167–168; summary points about, 54; systems-oriented, 54, 59, 61, 65; treatment development based on, 200–201
process-based diagnosis, 264, 270, 271–272, 275, 276
process-based therapy, 70, 123–124, 145, 152, 226
processes of change, 3, 4–13; characteristics of, 4–5; coherent moderators and, 10; contextual and historical view of, 9; Extended Evolutionary Meta-Model of, 16–17, 256, 264, 271–273; functional pathways of, 9–10; idiographic processes and, 6–8; measurement of,

8–9, 172–176; models of, 10–13; paradigm shift to, 53–71; PF model informing, 213; process-based diagnosis and, 261; requirements for adequate, 5–6; therapeutic, 263–264
protocols-for-syndromes strategy, 2, 3, 252, 253
psychoactive medications, 255
psychological flexibility (PF), 201–216; assessing facets of, 202–203; classes of behavior related to, 227–228; contextual factors in, 235; experience sampling of, 236–237; explanation of model of, 201–202; measures of alternative processes vs., 210–211; moderation or predication of outcomes based on, 211–212; multilevel analysis of, 239–241; observed outcomes related to changes in, 207–208; predicting and influencing behavior based on, 204–205; psychopathological version of, 273; sensitivity of measures to changes in, 206–207; studies on mediation of outcomes by, 208–210, 231–232; treatment development based on, 212–216
psychological inflexibility, 75, 203, 209
Psychological Inflexibility in Pain Scale, 203
psychological suffering, 118, 123, 126, 132
psychopathology: context and, 234–235; cultural influences and, 151–152; emotion processes and, 148–152; evolutionary perspective and, 258; infant temperament and, 148–149; network theory and, 177–189; RDoC approach to, 27–28, 30, 33, 40, 166; social influences and, 149–151. *See also* mental disorders
psychotherapy: common factors in, 50; complex systems approach to, 176–188; contextual variables in, 234–235; future of research in, 188–190; medical model of, 47–48; nature of the problem in, 48–52; process-based approach to, 167–168; shifting patterns as goal of, 63; therapeutic rationales in, 50–51, 55, 67; traditional approach to research in, 165–166; unifying through process paradigm, 62
Psychotherapy Relationships That Work (Norcross), 50
psychotic disorders, 35–36

R

randomized controlled trials (RCTs), 2, 73, 206, 209–210, 214, 228
RDoC. *See* Research Domain Criteria
reactivity phenotype, 36
reappraisal of emotions, 145
reflective functioning, 141
regulation of emotion, 144–147, 150, 151
reinforcement contingencies, 116
relapse prediction, 188
relating relations, 124, 125, 128
relational frame theory (RFT), 116, 119–121; analogy/metaphor and, 124; contextual factors in, 234; MDML framework and, 128, 131; rule-governed behavior and, 123; transformation of functions and, 122; verbal self and, 126, 127
relational framing, 119, 120, 121, 128, 234
relational networking, 128
relational responding, 128
religion, benefits of, 147
Rescher, Nicholas, 53, 54
research: future possibilities in psychotherapy, 188–190; process-based approach to, 67–70, 167–168; targeting mechanisms in, 228–233;

traditional approach to psychotherapy, 165–166
Research Domain Criteria (RDoC), 2, 23–41, 252; expectations and, 109; framework for, 26–28; future evolution of, 37–40; matrix constructs, 28–31; motivation for developing, 23–26, 166; RDoC-themed research findings, 35–36; study design based on, 31–32; transdiagnostic approach and, 74–75; treatment and, 32–35
resilience, system, 172
resolutions, 56–57
response mechanisms, 79, 80–81, 83
retention processes, 15
RFT. *See* relational frame theory
Rief, Winfried, 97
Risley, Todd, 252
ROEing, concept of, 131
rule-governed behavior, 116, 117, 118–119, 123–124, 126
rumination-focused CBT, 76

S

safety behaviors, 150
scope of change process, 5
second-order change, 56–57, 60, 71
selection processes, 15, 16
Self Experiences Questionnaire, 203
self, stable sense of, 126
self-as-context, 203, 204, 206, 227, 232
self-compassion, 269
self-conscious emotions, 143
self-construal, 141–142
self-regulatory strategies, 145
self-report measures, 8–9, 203
self-similar patterns, 63
sensorimotor systems, 27
Sherrill, Joel, 23
sibling relationships, 147
Sidman, Murray, 116, 118
Skinner, B. F., 116, 117
smoking cessation, 231–232

Social Baseline Theory, 146
social constructivist view, 55, 141
social influences on emotion, 139–141, 149–151
social processes, 27
social skills training, 185
social traps, 170
Society of Clinical Psychology, 49
socioeconomic status, 147
somaticizing disorders, 85, 86
Sommers, David, 23
specific factors, 49–50
statistical mediation, 229–230, 231
statistical moderation, 230
stigma and self-stigma, 255–256
stimulus equivalence, 116, 118, 119
strange attractors, 56
stress, TDMs linked to, 87, 88
stressors, identifying, 81
Structure of Scientific Revolutions, The (Kuhn), 47
suppression of emotions, 145, 146
symbolic generalization, 121
symbolic relations, 122
syndromal diagnosis, 1, 2, 252, 254–256
Synergetic Navigation System (SNS), 173, 180
system change: principles of, 168–172. *See also* complex systems perspective
systems-oriented process view, 54, 59, 61, 65

T

TDMs. *See* transdiagnostic mechanisms
temperament, 139, 148–149
temporal networks, 265
therapeutic procedures, 68
therapeutic processes, 68, 131, 263
therapeutic rationales, 50–51, 55, 67
therapy. *See* psychotherapy
thoughts, fusion with, 126
threshold of inconsistency, 186
time, examining events over, 235–238
time series analyses, 70

Tinbergen, Niko, 15, 16
tipping points, 170
topographical classification, 253
transcript analyses, 8, 69
transdiagnostic approaches:
　classification systems, 75, 81–82;
　functional categorization of
　interventions, 92–93; process-based
　CBT changes, 90–91; TDM-targeted
　treatment planning, 89–90;
　transdiagnostic road map, 77–89;
　treatment protocols, 75–77
transdiagnostic mechanisms (TDMs),
　75–91; case formulation diagram, 78;
　changes to CBT based on, 90–91;
　classification system, 81–82;
　definition of, 77; measurement
　instruments, 82–83; overview table
　of, 79; planning treatment of, 89–90;
　research on CCI-R for measuring,
　83–89; response mechanisms, 79,
　80–81, 83; treatments focused on,
　75–77, 89–90; vulnerability
　mechanisms, 79, 80–81, 82
transference hypothesis, 106
transformation of functions, 121–122,
　131
transformation of stimulus functions,
　120, 125
transitions, system, 170, 172–173
treatment: evidence-supported, 49,
　57–59; expectations and selection of,
　109–110; process-based development
　of, 200–201, 212–216; RDoC
framework and, 32–35; selection
process for, 275; uncoupling of
diagnosis and, 225–226; utility of,
260
tripartite model, 75

U

uncertainty, intolerance of, 75
unification, process-based, 61–62
Unified Protocol, 76

V

Vaidyanathan, Uma, 23
values-based action, 204–205, 206, 207,
　227, 231
vaporware, 10
variation, 15
Venkatesh, Shruthi M., 137
Verbal Behavior (Skinner), 117
verbal operants, 117
verbal self, 126–127
vicious cycles, 56, 61, 62
ViolEx-model, 103, 105
virtuous cycles, 57, 62
VRSCDL features, 15–16, 257
vulnerability mechanisms, 79, 80–81,
　82, 258

W

Wagner, Ann, 23
Whitehead, Alfred North, 53, 62
Wolf, Mont, 252
working alliance, 60, 66

MORE BOOKS from NEW HARBINGER PUBLICATIONS

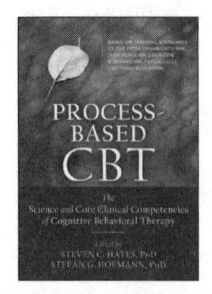

PROCESS-BASED CBT
The Science & Core Clinical Competencies of Cognitive Behavioral Therapy
978-1626255968 / US $69.95
CONTEXT PRESS
An Imprint of New Harbinger Publications

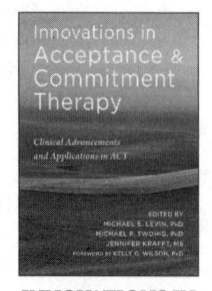

INNOVATIONS IN ACCEPTANCE & COMMITMENT THERAPY
Clinical Advancements & Applications in ACT
978-1684033102 / US $69.95
CONTEXT PRESS
An Imprint of New Harbinger Publications

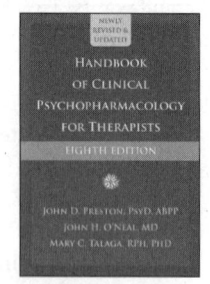

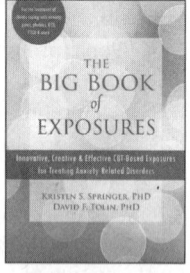

HANDBOOK OF CLINICAL PSYCHOPHARMACOLOGY FOR THERAPISTS, EIGHTH EDITION
978-1626259256 / US $59.95

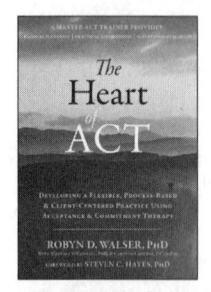

THE HEART OF ACT
Developing a Flexible, Process-Based & Client-Centered Practice Using Acceptance & Commitment Therapy
978-1684030392 / US $49.95
CONTEXT PRESS
An Imprint of New Harbinger Publications

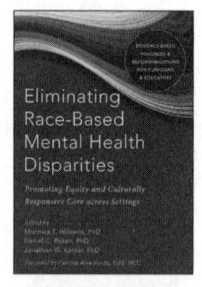

ELIMINATING RACE-BASED MENTAL HEALTH DISPARITIES
Promoting Equity & Culturally Responsive Care across Settings
978-1684031962 / US $89.95
CONTEXT PRESS
An Imprint of New Harbinger Publications

THE BIG BOOK OF EXPOSURES
Innovative, Creative & Effective CBT-Based Exposures for Treating Anxiety-Related Disorders
978-1684033737 / US $49.95

newharbingerpublications
1-800-748-6273 / newharbinger.com

(VISA, MC, AMEX / prices subject to change without notice)

Follow Us

QUICK TIPS for THERAPISTS
Fast and free solutions to common client situations mental health professionals encounter every day

Written by leading clinicians, Quick Tips for Therapists are short e-mails, sent twice a month, to help enhance your client sessions. **Visit newharbinger.com/quicktips to sign up today!**

Sign up for our Book Alerts at newharbinger.com/bookalerts